Color Atlas of
Differential Diagnosis in
Dermatopathology

Color Atlas of Differential Diagnosis in Dermatopathology

Loren E Clarke MD

Vice President of Medical Affairs
Dermatology Unit Myriad Genetics, Inc/MYGN
Salt Lake City, Utah, USA

Jennie T Clarke MD

Associate Professor of Dermatology
Milton S Hershey Medical Center
Penn State University
Hershey, Pennsylvania, USA

Klaus F Helm MD

Professor of Dermatology and Pathology
Milton S Hershey Medical Center
Penn State University
Hershey, Pennsylvania, USA

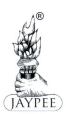

JAYPEE BROTHERS MEDICAL PUBLISHERS (P) LTD

New Delhi • London • Philadelphia • Panama

Jaypee Brothers Medical Publishers (P) Ltd

Headquarters

Jaypee Brothers Medical Publishers (P) Ltd
4838/24, Ansari Road, Daryaganj
New Delhi 110 002, India
Phone: +91-11-43574357
Fax: +91-11-43574314
Email: jaypee@jaypeebrothers.com

Overseas Offices

J.P. Medical Ltd
83, Victoria Street, London
SW1H 0HW (UK)
Phone: +44-2031708910
Fax: +02-03-0086180
Email: info@jpmedpub.com

Jaypee-Highlights.
Medical Publishers Inc
City of Knowledge, Bld. 237
Clayton, Panama City, Panama
Phone: +1 507-301-0496
Fax: +1 507-301-0499
Email: cservice@jphmedical.com

Jaypee Medical Inc.
The Bourse
111 South Independence Mall East
Suite 835, Philadelphia, PA 19106, USA
Phone: +1 267-519-9789
Email: jpmed.us@gmail.com

Jaypee Brothers
Medical Publishers (P) Ltd
17/1-B Babar Road, Block-B
Shaymali, Mohammadpur
Dhaka-1207, Bangladesh
Mobile: +08801912003485
Email: jaypeedhaka@gmail.com

Jaypee Brothers
Medical Publishers (P) Ltd
Shorakhute, Kathmandu
Nepal
Phone: +00977-9841528578
Email: jaypee.nepal@gmail.com

Website: www.jaypeebrothers.com
Website: www.jaypeedigital.com

Inquiries for bulk sales may be solicited at: jaypee@jaypeebrothers.com

Color Atlas of Differential Diagnosis in Dermatopathology

First Edition: **2014**
ISBN 978-93-5090-845-7
Printed at : Ajanta Offset & Packagings Ltd., New Delhi

Dedicated to

Katie and Kyle

Ava and Alaina

— *Loren E Clarke and Jennie T Clarke*

— *Klaus F Helm*

Preface

Color Atlas of Differential Diagnosis in Dermatopathology is based upon a simple algorithmic approach that simplifies diagnosis of dermatological diseases. This unique atlas uses pathologic findings correlated with clinical information to arrive at a precise diagnosis. The book is divided into 15 chapters based upon common histopathologic findings such as psoriasiform dermatitis, lichenoid tissue reaction, panniculitis, vasculitis, blistering skin diseases, adnexal neoplasms, and pigmented lesions. Color images illustrate the histological patterns along with clinical photographs. Criteria required to make an accurate diagnosis are listed in an easy-to-use outline form. Potential pitfalls in diagnosis are covered along with diagnostic pearls.

Loren E Clarke
Jennie T Clarke
Klaus F Helm

Acknowledgments

We would like to acknowledge the residents and faculty in Dermatology for help in supplying some of the clinical pictures, and we would like to thank the numerous editors at M/s Jaypee Brothers Medical Publishers (P) Ltd, New Delhi, India, in helping with the manuscript.

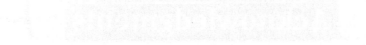

Contents

CHAPTER 1

Normal Skin Pattern

When the histology looks like normal skin

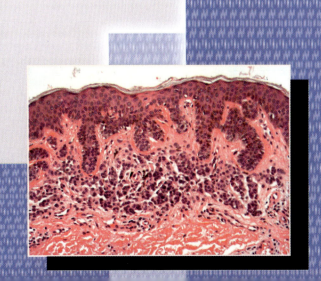

INTRODUCTION

Occasionally, a biopsy is encountered that looks unremarkable on low power and resembles "normal skin". In these cases, the possibility of a sampling error could be considered. However, a variety of diseases are associated with minimal histologic findings or requires closer scrutiny to notice abnormalities (Box 1.1). Definitive diagnosis often requires clinical pathologic correlation. A systematic approach starting with examination of the stratum corneum, epidermis, dermis and then the fat may be useful to elucidate a specific diagnosis.

Box 1.1: Differential diagnosis of normal appearing skin
• Amyloidosis
• Anetoderma
• Anhidrotic ectodermal dysplasia
• Argyria
• Atrophoderma
• Becker's nevus
• Café au lait
• Chrysiasis
• Connective tissue nevus/collagenoma
• Cutis laxa
• Erythrasma
• Injection of filler
• Focal dermal hypoplasia (Goltz's syndrome)
• Ichthyosis
• Lipodystrophy
• Morphea
• Myxedema
• Ochronosis
• Focal acral hypokeratosis
• Postinflammatory pigmentary alteration
• Pseudoxanthoma elasticum
• Scleroderma
• Scleredema
• Telangiectasia
• Telangiectasia macularis eruptiva perstans
• Urticaria
• Tattoo
• Tinea versicolor
• Trauma
• Vitiligo

FINDINGS WITHIN STRATUM CORNEUM

- Tinea versicolor (Figs 1.1A to C)
- Erythrasma (Figs 1.2A to C).

Disorders of Epidermis and Stratum Corneum

- Ichthyosis (Figs 1.3A and B)
- Focal acral hypokeratosis (Fig. 1.4)
- Keratoderma (Figs 1.5A and B).

Disorder Involving Epidermal Pigmentation

- Vitiligo (Figs 1.6A to D)
- Idiopathic guttate hypomelanosis: Small faint white macules on lower extremity (Figs 1.7A to C)
- Café au lait macule (Figs 1.8A to C)
- Becker's nevus (Figs 1.9A to C).

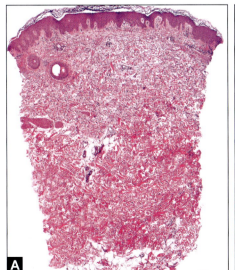
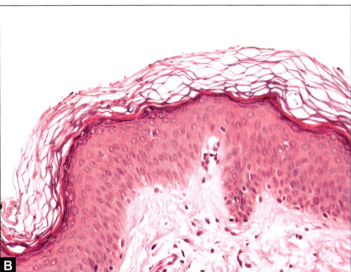

Figs 1.1A and B

Color Atlas of Differential Diagnosis of Dermatopathology

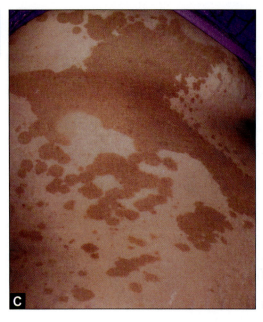

Figs 1.1A to C: Tinea versicolor. (A) Low power: normal skin appearance; (B) High power: hyphae within the stratum corneum; (C) Hyperpigmented patches on trunk giving patient multicolored appearance.

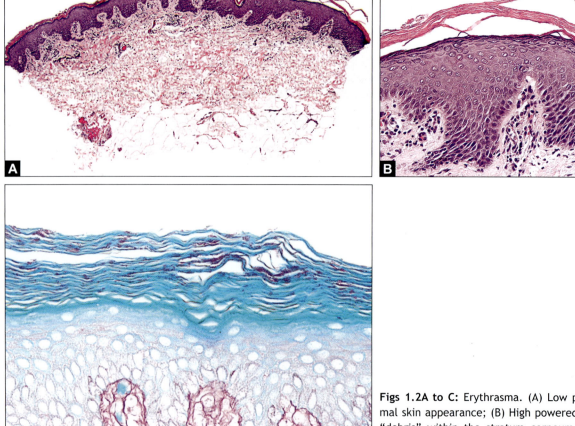

Figs 1.2A to C: Erythrasma. (A) Low power with normal skin appearance; (B) High powered H and E shows "debris" within the stratum corneum in erythrasma; (C) Periodic acid-Schiff stain demonstrates filamentous bacteria within the stratum corneum.

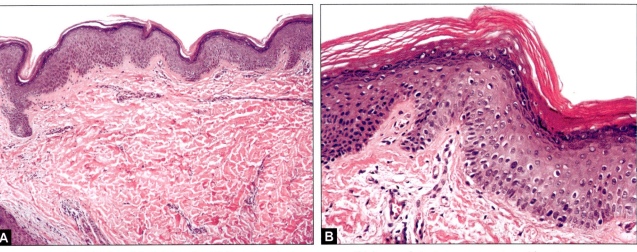

Figs 1.3A and B: Ichthyosis. (A) Hyperkeratosis: compare thickness of stratum corneum to epidermis; (B) Stratum corneum appears more compact then in "normal skin" also some areas of follicular plugging.

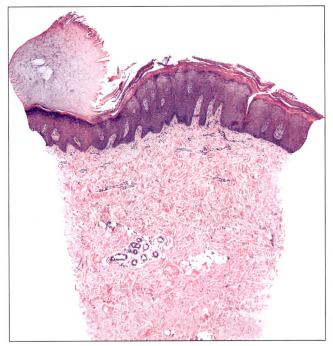

Fig. 1.4: Circumscribed focal acral hypokeratosis. Abrupt loss of stratum corneum in lesional skin tag.

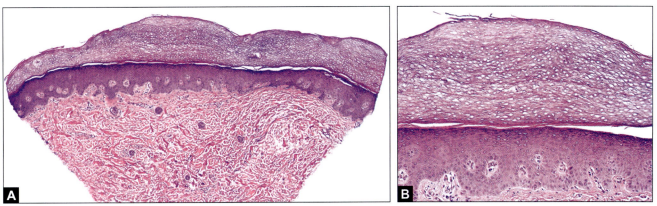

Figs 1.5A and B: Keratoderma. (A) Orthohyperkeratosis; (B) Notice thickness of stratum corneum relative to thickness of epidermis.

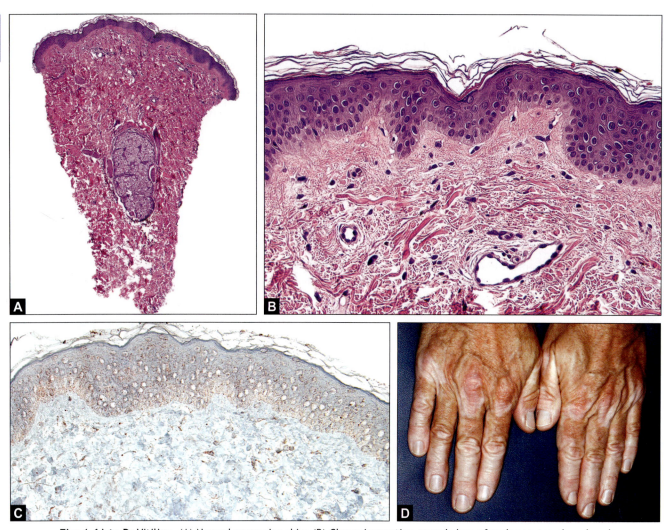

Figs 1.6A to D: Vitiligo. (A) Normal appearing skin; (B) Closer inspection reveals loss of melanocytes along basal layer of epidermis; (C) Melan-A stain confirms absence of melanocytes; (D) Porcelain white patches.

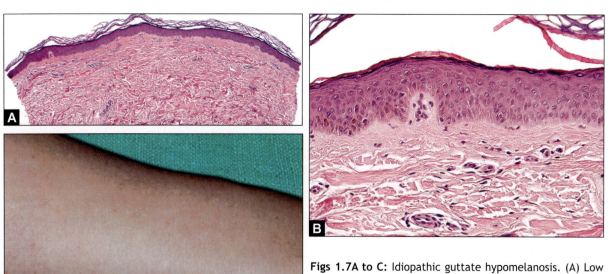

Figs 1.7A to C: Idiopathic guttate hypomelanosis. (A) Low power; (B) High power (note pigmentation along the basal layers of epidermis on left part of biopsy not right part); (C) Faint hypopigmented macules on lower extremity.

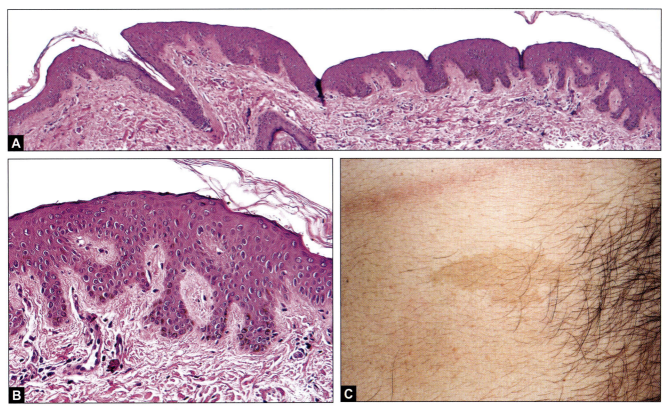

Figs 1.8A to C: Café au lait macule. (A and B) Low and high powered with increased pigmentation along the basal layers of the epidermis (C) Clinical: Brown coffee colored macule.

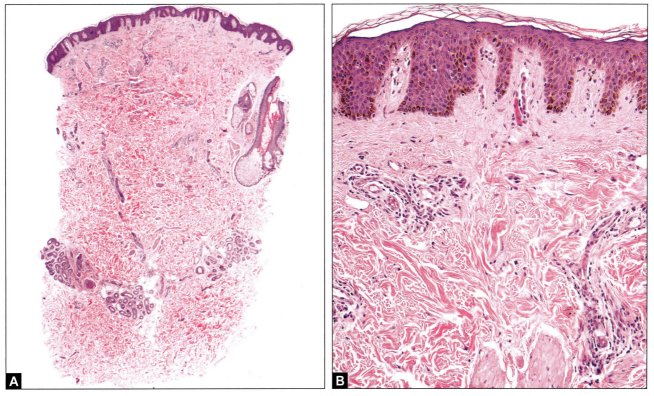

Figs 1.9A and B

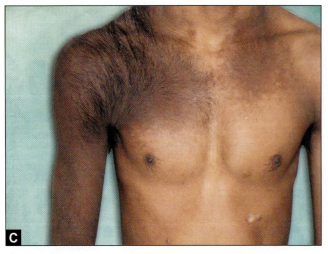

Figs 1.9A to C: Becker's nevus. (A) Increased pigmentation along the basal layers of anastomosing epidermal rete ridges; (B) Flat bottom rete ridges is clue to diagnosis; (C) Becker's nevus on shoulder picture.
Courtesy: Dr Renee Straub

FINDINGS WITHIN THE DERMIS

- Melanophages:
  - Postinflammatory pigmentary alteration (Figs 1.10A to C)
  - *Clue to deposition*: Lichen amyloidosis, macular amyloidosis (Figs 1.11A to D)
- *Siderophages*: Trauma
- Other pigment deposition:
  - Tattoo (Figs 1.12A and B)
  - Drug induced pigmentation (Figs 1.13A to C)
  - Argyria (Figs 1.14A and B)
  - Chrysiasis (Figs 1.15A and B)
  - Ochronosis
- Deposition disorders:
  - Amyloid (Figs 1.11A to D)
  - *Mucin*: Scleredema (Figs 1.16A and B)
- Mixed inflammatory infiltrate
  - Urticaria (Figs 1.17A to D)
- Altered Collagen:
  - Connective tissue nevus/collagenoma (Figs 1.18A and B)
  - Morphea/scleroderma/atrophoderma (Figs 1.19A to C)
  - Injection due to filler (Figs 1.20A and B)
- Altered Elastic Fibers:
  - *Absence*: Disorders of elastolysis
    - Cutis laxa (Figs 1.21A and B)
    - Mid dermal elastolysis
    - Anetoderma (Figs 1.22A to E)
  - *Increased*: Connective tissue nevus/Buchske-Ollendorff syndrome
  - *Calcified*: Pseudoxanthoma elasticum (Figs 1.23A to C).
- Fat cells within the dermis:
  - Focal dermal hypoplasia (Figs 1.24A and B)
  - Nevus lipomatosus superficialis (lesion usually mamillated)

- Telangiectatic blood vessels:
  - *No other finding*: Causes for telangiectasias
    - Idiopathic, essential, genetic, connective tissue disease
  - *Mast cells and rare eosinophil present*: Telangiectasia macularis eruptiva perstans (Figs 1.25A to C)
- Sweat glands absent: Anhidrotic ectodermal dysplasia.

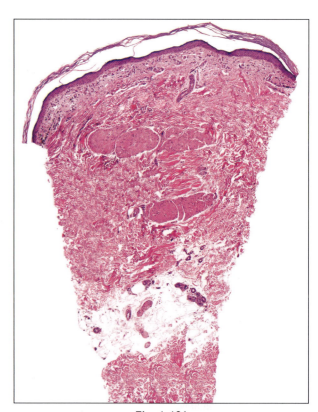

Fig. 1.10A

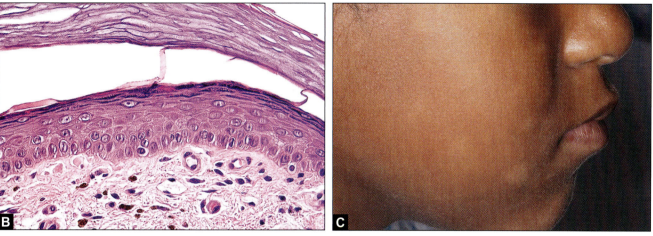

Figs 1.10A to C: Postinflammatory pigmentary alteration. (A) Melanophages within the dermis along with sparse inflammatory infiltrate. (B) High power note colloid bodies and melanophages; (C) Clinical figure.

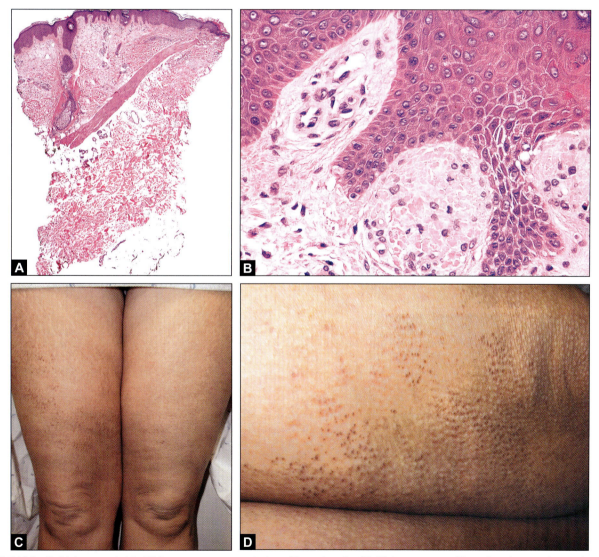

Figs 1.11A to D: Lichen amyloid. (A) Low power: expanded papillary dermis; (B) High power: papillary dermis contains eosinophilic globules separated by clefts; (C) Lichen amyloidosis; (D) Lichen amyloidosis with lichenified papules on lower legs.

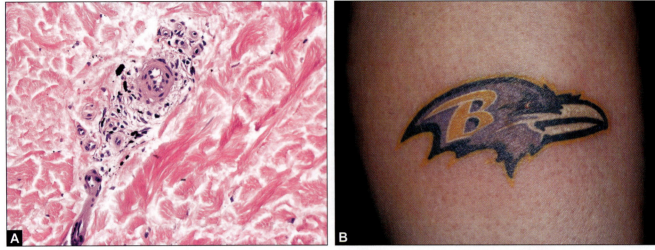

Figs 1.12A and B: Tattoo. (A) Black graining material within dermis; (B) Clinical figure.

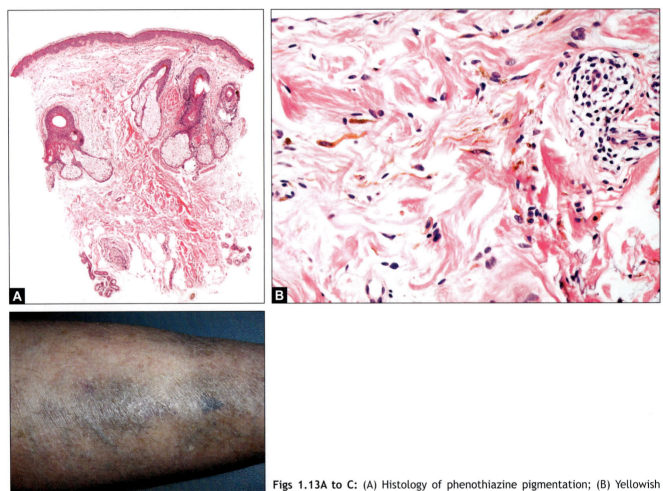

Figs 1.13A to C: (A) Histology of phenothiazine pigmentation; (B) Yellowish brown dermal pigment; (C) Blue grey hyperpigmentation due to plaquenil.

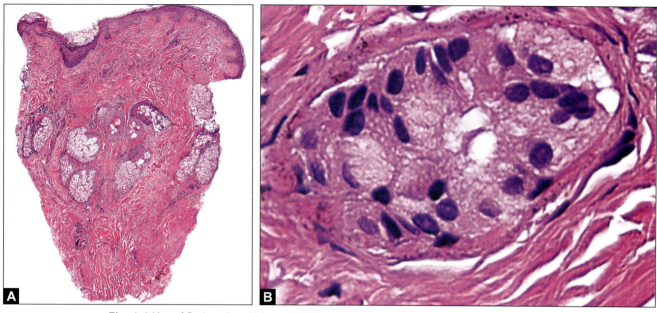

Figs 1.14A and B: Argyria. (A) Low power; (B) High power-black granules predilection for basement membrane zone around eccrine glands.

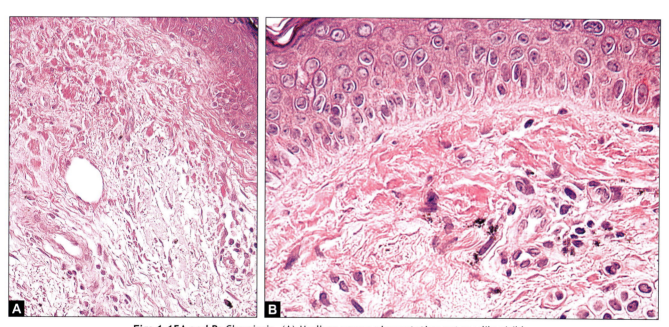

Figs 1.15A and B: Chrysiasis. (A) Medium power pigmentation not readily visible; (B) Higher power, black granules visible in dermis.

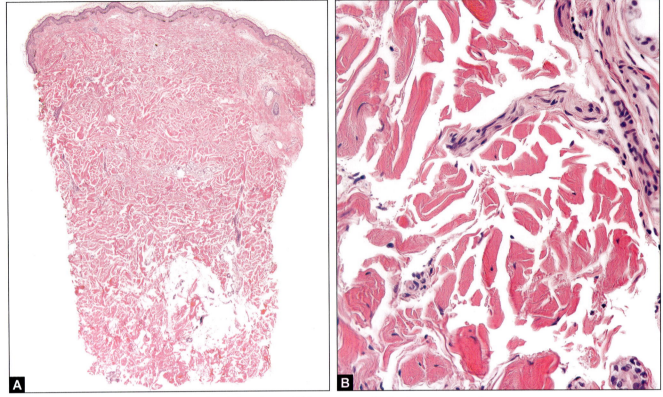

Figs 1.16A and B: Scleredema. (A) Low power; (B) Mucin appears as clear spaces with faint stringy pale blue material between collagen bundles.

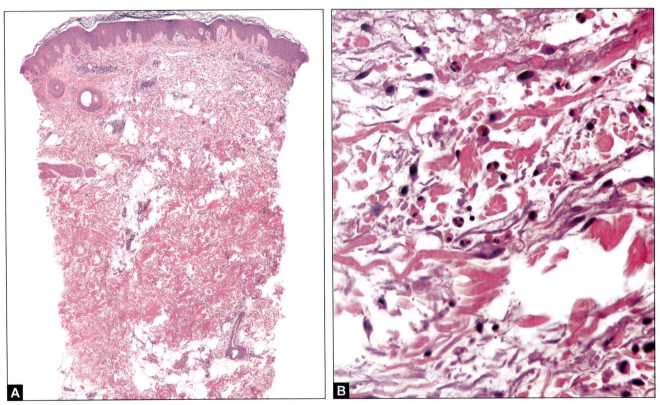

Figs 1.17A and B

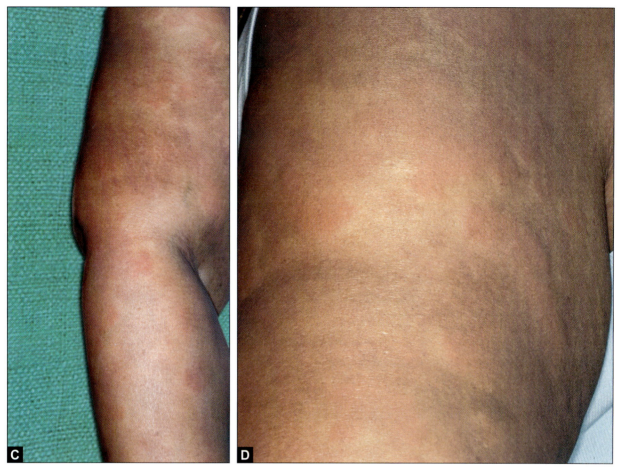

Figs 1.17A to D: Urticaria. (A) Low power; (B) High power sparse
mixed inflammatory infiltrate; (C and D) Clinical figures.

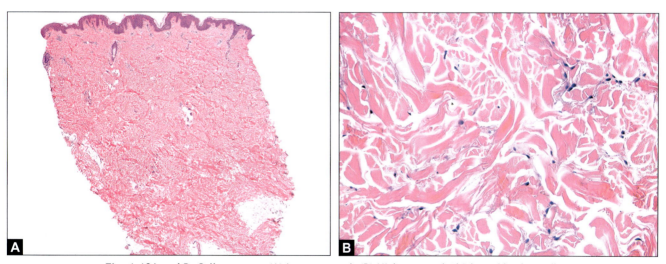

Figs 1.18A and B: Collagenoma. (A) Low powered; (B) High powered: thickened haphazardly
organized collagen bundles clue to diagnosis.

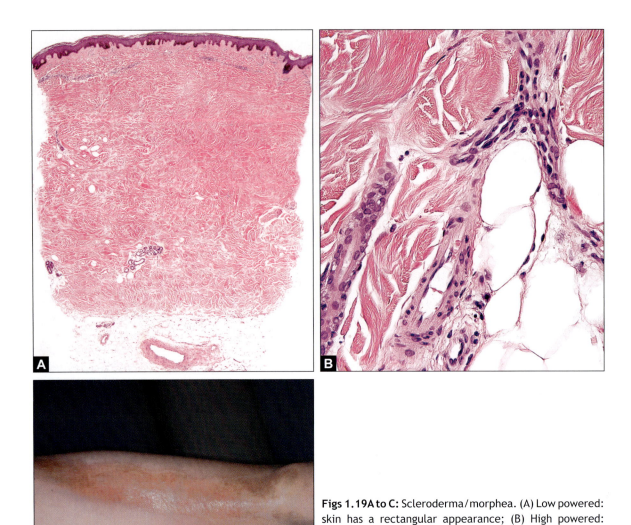

Figs 1.19A to C: Scleroderma/morphea. (A) Low powered: skin has a rectangular appearance; (B) High powered: decreased space between collagen bundles along with sclerotic collagen bundles and inflammatory infiltrate concentrated along dermal subcutaneous junction; (C) Clinical figure of linear morphea.

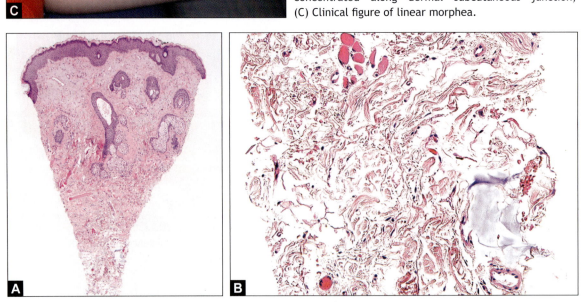

Figs 1.20A and B: Filler material restylane. (A) Low power; (B) High power: basophilic material seen at base of biopsy.

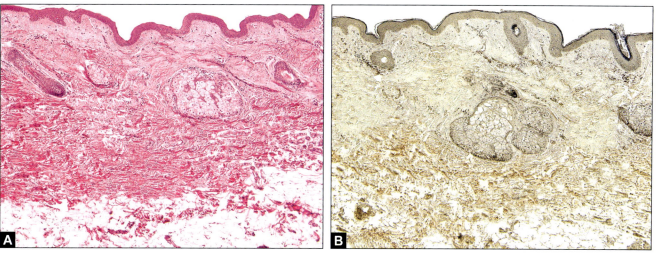

Figs 1.21A and B: Cutis laxa. (A) Low power; (B) Elastic tissue stain low power demonstrates loss of elastic fibers.

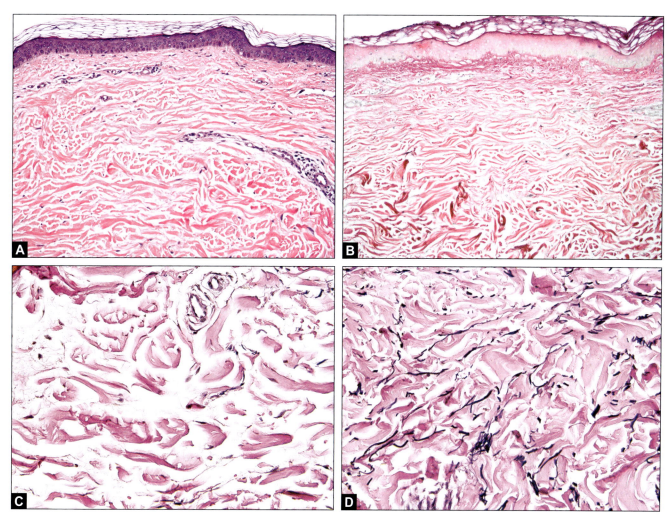

Figs 1.22A to D

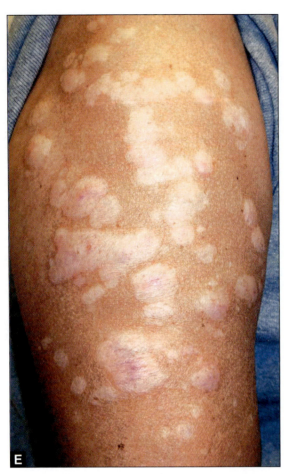

Figs 1.22A to E: Anetoderma. (A) Low power; (B) Low power elastic stain; (C) High power elastic stain of involved skin (notice decreased elastic fibers in contrast to 1.22D); (D) Uninvolved skin in patient with anetoderma: high power elastic stain; (E) Papules and nodules which are soft and compressible.

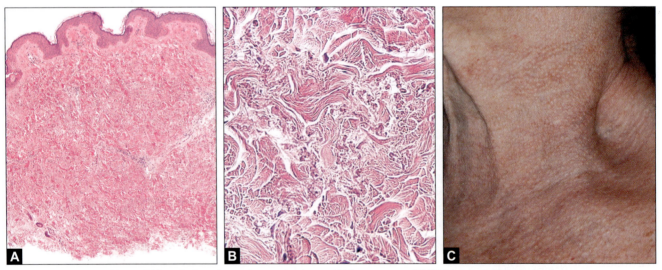

Figs 1.23A to C: Pseudoxanthoma elasticum. (A) Low power; (B) High power: Fragmented calcified elastic fibers; (C) Neck with yellow chicken wire like plaques.

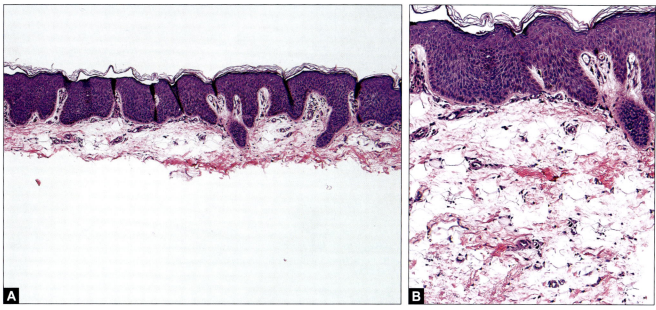

Figs 1.24A and B: (A) Low powered view of Goltz's syndrome. Notice attenuated dermis; (B) High power fat cells within the dermis

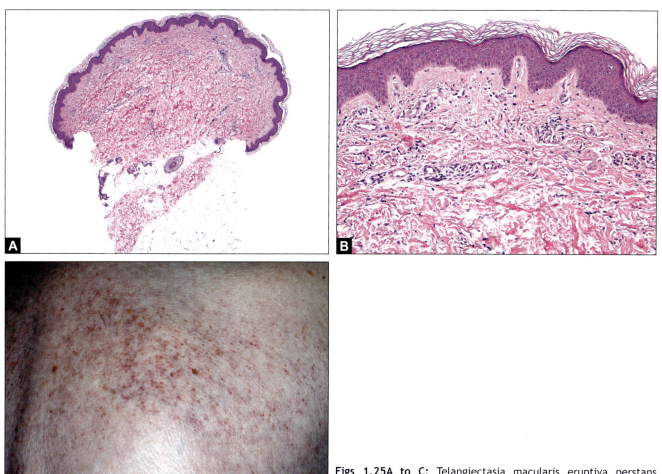

Figs 1.25A to C: Telangiectasia macularis eruptiva perstans (A) Lower power; (B) Higher power: telangiectatic blood vessels with surrounding mast cells; (C) Clinical figure.

Color Atlas of Differential Diagnosis of Dermatopathology

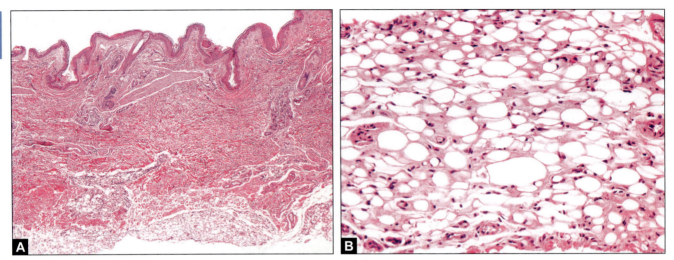

Figs 1.26A and B: Localized/involutional lipodystrophy.

Disorders Involving Subcutaneous Tissue

- Fat decreased in amount:
  - Lipodystrophy
- *Fat cells hyalinized*: Localized lipodystrophy (Figs 1.26A and B)
- Fat increased in amount in biopsy from scalp; lipedematous alopecia.

BIBLIOGRAPHY

1. Farmer ER, Hood AF. Pathology of the Skin, 2nd edition. New York: McGraw-Hill; 2000.
2. McKee PH, Calonje E, Granter SR. Pathology of the Skin with Clinical Correlations. Mosby: Elsevier; 2005.
3. Weedon D. Weedon's Skin Pathology, 3rd edition. Churchill Livingstone: Elsevier; 2010.

CHAPTER 2

The Spongiotic and Psoriasiform Patterns

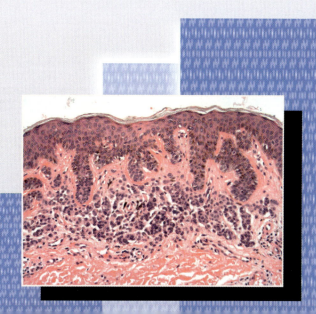

THE SPONGIOTIC PATTERN

The common spongiotic (eczematous) dermatitides are contact dermatitis, nummular dermatitis, seborrheic dermatitis, atopic dermatitis, photodermatitis, xerotic (asteatotic) dermatitis, dyshidrotic dermatitis and stasis dermatitis. Histopathology cannot reliably differentiate among these in most instances. The specific type of dermatitis must be determined clinically. Biopsies are performed to help eliminate simulators of dermatitis, such as dermatophytosis, pityriasis rosea, insect bite reactions, erythema annulare centrifugum, Gianotti-Crosti syndrome, Grover's disease, drug eruptions and cutaneous T-cell lymphoma (mycosis fungoides in particular), all of which may exhibit some degree of spongiosis (Table 2.1).

Common Types of Spongiotic Dermatitis

Contact Dermatitis

Contact dermatitis can be subdivided into two types. The most common is the irritant type, in which skin exposed to an irritant, such as a strong soap becomes edematous, red and scaly. The allergic type requires prior sensitization and is specific immunological reaction to an allergen, such as rhus (poison ivy), preservatives and fragrances. Histopathology of allergic contact dermatitis and irritant type of contact dermatitis are usually indistinguishable except in early lesions of irritant type of contact where there may be superficial epidermal necrosis (Figs 2.1A to E).

■ *Criteria for diagnosis*

- Spongiotic dermatitis plus clinical history of exposure to irritant or allergen, and/or a positive patch test for allergic contact dermatitis
- Early lesions of irritant contact dermatitis may demonstrate superficial epidermal necrosis.

■ *Differential diagnosis*

- Other forms of spongiotic dermatitis and simulators of dermatitis, particularly spongiotic drug eruptions, mycosis fungoides, dermatophytosis and viral exanthems (Table 2.1). Rarely, the urticarial phase of bullous pemphigoid may mimic contact dermatitis (Fig. 2.1C).

■ *Pitfalls*

- Spongiosis occasionally occurs in psoriasis, mycosis fungoides and other typically "nonspongiotic" disorders.

■ *Pearls*

- The intraepidermal vesicles in spongiotic dermatitis have a "vase-like" shape and open to the epidermal surface, while genuine Pautrier microabscesses of mycosis fungoides are round and rarely connect to the epidermal surface (Fig. 2.1B). The lymphocytes in Pautrier microabscess are hyperchromatic and contain little cytoplasm in contrast to more prominent cytoplasm in exocytosis
- In pityriasis rosea, spongiosis is focal and small parakeratotic mounds without serum occupy the overlying stratum corneum (Fig. 2.8D).

Table 2.1: Spongiotic dermatitis and simulators	
Types of Dermatitis	**Dermatitis Simulators**
Atopic dermatitis	Dermatophytosis/tinea
Allergic contact dermatitis	Id reaction
Irritant contact dermatitis	Insect bite reaction
Nummular dermatitis	Erythema annulare centrifugum (Chapter 3)
Seborrheic dermatitis	Pityriasis rosea (Pityriasiform dermatitis Chapter 3)
Dyshidrotic dermatitis	Gianotti-Crosti syndrome
Xerotic (Asteatotic) dermatitis	Parapsoriasis and mycosis fungoides
Stasis dermatitis	Grover's disease (spongiotic type)
	Spongiotic drug eruption
	Polymorphous light eruption
	Pruritic urticarial papules and plaques of pregnancy (polymorphous eruption of pregnancy)
	Spongiotic phase of bullous pemphigoid/pemphigus

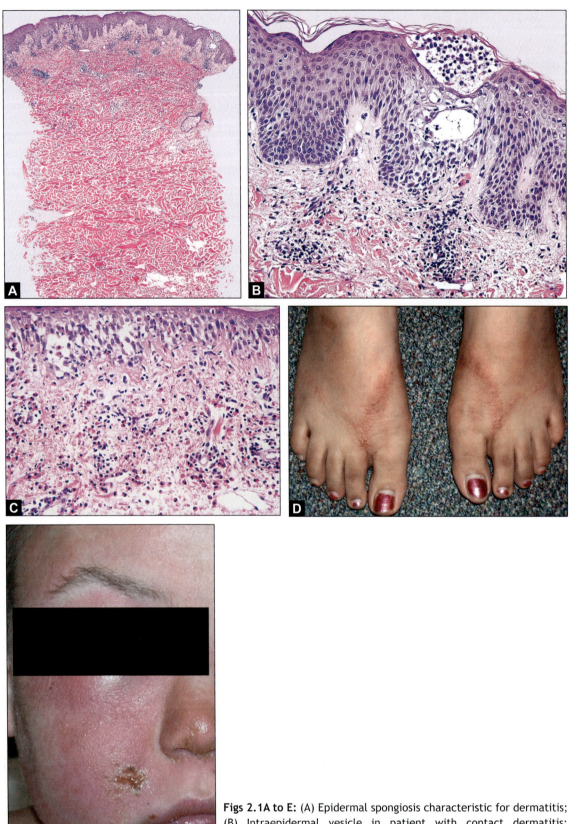

Figs 2.1A to E: (A) Epidermal spongiosis characteristic for dermatitis; (B) Intraepidermal vesicle in patient with contact dermatitis; (C) Spongiotic bullous pemphigoid. Unlike allergic contact dermatitis eosinophils predominate; (D) Allergic contact dermatitis secondary to sandals; (E) Allergic contact dermatitis secondary to poison ivy.

Atopic Dermatitis (Figs 2.2A to C)

▪ Criteria for diagnosis

- Chronic dermatitis, usually in a flexural distribution, with a family or personal history of asthma and/or allergies (atopy)
- Specific diagnosis cannot be made on histopathologic examination alone. Clinical correlation is required.

▪ Differential diagnosis

- Other forms of spongiotic dermatitis and dermatitis simulators
- Pityriasis alba (hypopigmented patches on the face of children with dark skin) is a variant of atopic dermatitis.

▪ Pitfalls

- Excoriation may produce an inflammatory infiltrate indistinguishable from other spongiotic and psoriasiform disorders

- Atopic dermatitis frequently can become secondary impetiginized with Staphylococcus aureus, and occasionally herpes virus (kaposiform varicelliform eruption) (Fig. 2.2C)
- Early lesions of mycosis fungoides/parapsoriasis can be difficult to distinguish.

▪ Pearls

- Spongiosis of follicular epithelium is more common in atopic dermatitis than other spongiotic disorders
- Inflammation is often less pronounced than other spongiotic dermatitides (unless impetiginized)
- Sclerotic collagen bundles and stellate fibroblasts within dermis suggest chronicity and rubbing (Fig. 2.2A).

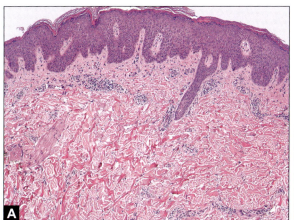

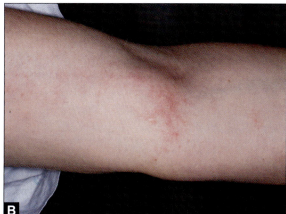

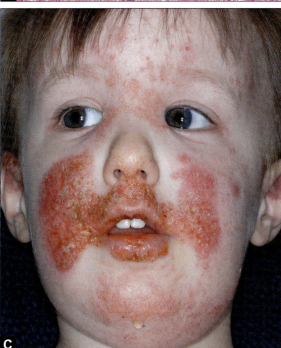

Figs 2.2A to C: Atopic dermatitis. (A) Epidermal hyperplasia from chronic rubbing; (B) Scaly patches in antecubital fossa; (C) Impetiginized atopic dermatitis.

Nummular Dermatitis

■ *Criteria for diagnosis*

- Erythematous plaques that are approximately the size and shape of coins (Fig. 2.3A)
- Histology if performed:
  - Spongiotic dermatitis
  - Frequently psoriasiform epidermal hyperplasia (Fig. 2.3B)
  - Eosinophils usually conspicuous (Fig. 2.3C).

■ *Pitfalls*

- Eosinophils are frequently present and not reliable feature in distinguishing contact dermatitis from nummular dermatitis.

■ *Pearls*

- Of all the dermatoses, nummular dermatitis most commonly exhibits psoriasiform pattern.

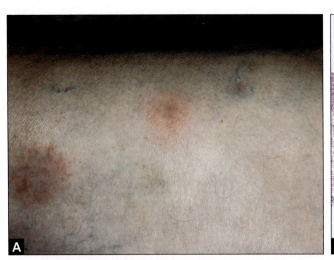

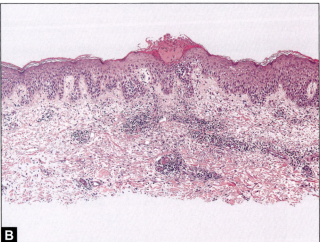

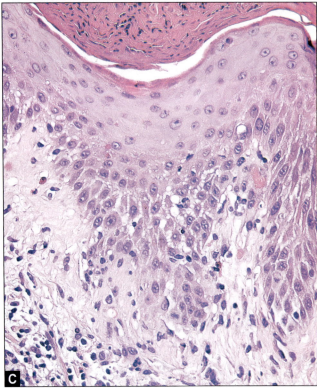

Figs 2.3A to C: Nummular (A) Round coin sized scaly plaques; (B) Psoriasiform epidermal hyperplasia associated with spongiosis; (C) Parakeratotic mound with neuts but also eosinophils and spongiosis.

Seborrheic Dermatitis

■ *Criteria for diagnosis*

- Clinical history of scaly plaques on scalp, ears, eyebrows, nasolabial folds and upper trunk (Figs 2.4A and B)
- Axilla or groin occasionally affected.

■ *Histology if performed*

- Parakeratosis and spongiosis most pronounced around follicular ostia (Figs 2.4C to E)
- Pityrosporum yeast spores often present in the stratum corneum.

■ *Differential diagnosis*

- Other spongiotic dermatitides and simulators
- Psoriasis
- Dermatophytosis (tinea facie, tinea capitis).

■ *Pitfalls*

- Neutrophils and "squirting papilla" (neutrophils extending into epidermis) can be seen in both psoriasis and seborrheic dermatitis.

■ *Pearls*

- Necrotic keratinocytes can be seen in seborrheic dermatitis associated with HIV disease
- Sebaceous glands can be shrunken in seborrheic dermatitis involving the scalp
- Seborrheic dermatitis is more common in patients with Parkinson's disease, patients with systemic diseases and hospitalized patients
- Seborrheic dermatitis like rash can be seen in riboflavine and zinc deficiency.

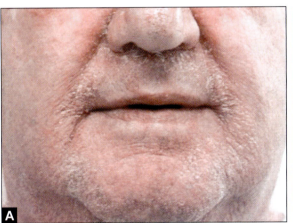
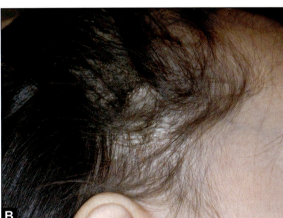
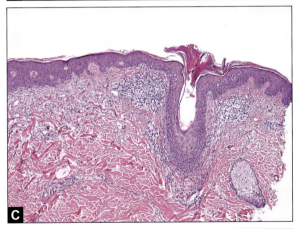
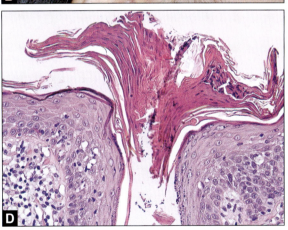
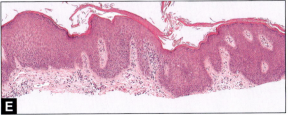

Figs 2.4A to E: Seborrheic dermatitis. (A) Note prominent scaling around eyes and nasolabial folds; (B) Scaling behind ears; (C and E) Psoriasiform epidermal hyperplasia with spongiosis; (D) Parakeratotic mounds around follicular infundibuli clue to diagnosis.

Dyshidrotic Dermatitis (Pompholyx)
(Figs 2.5A to C)

■ *Criteria for diagnosis*

- Spongiotic dermatitis on hands and sides of fingers with vesicle formation
- Histology reveals dermatitis.

■ *Differential diagnosis*

- Vesiculobullous dermatophytosis
- Contact dermatitis of the hands.

■ *Pitfalls*

- Palmoplantar psoriasis may exhibit significant spongiosis and vesicle formation (see Fig. 2.16F).

■ *Pearls*

- Parakeratotic mounds in palmoplantar psoriasis are frequently tiered (see Fig. 2.16G).

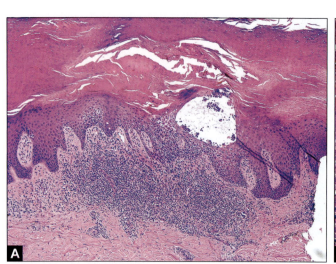

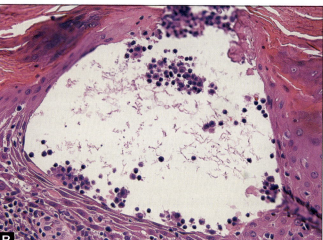

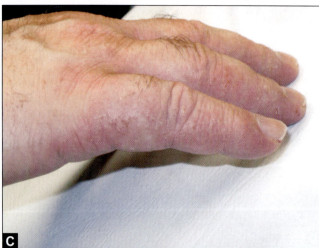

Figs 2.5A to C: Dyshidrotic dermatitis. (A and B) Bx from acral skin with prominent spongiosis; (C) Vesicles on sides of fingers are characteristic.

Stasis Dermatitis (Figs 2.6A to D)

■ *Criteria for diagnosis*

- Edematous red legs with pitting edema, prominent varicose veins and hemosiderin deposition.

■ *Histology*

- Spongiotic dermatitis plus increased density of dermal blood vessels (Fig. 2.6A)
- Hemosiderin and fibrosis within dermis (Fig. 2.6B)
- Dermal mucin deposition in some cases
- Subcutaneous tissue may exhibit lipomembranous changes.

■ *Differential diagnosis*

- Psoriasis
- Dermatitis
- Pretibial myxedema.

■ *Pitfalls*

- Stasis dermatitis may predispose to allergic contact dermatitis
- Dermal mucin may be mistaken for pretibial myxedema.

■ *Pearls*

- Unlike pretibial myxedema, stasis dermatitis exhibits a grenz zone of papillary dermal collagen that is devoid of mucin
- Clinicians can misdiagnose stasis dermatitis as cellulitis.

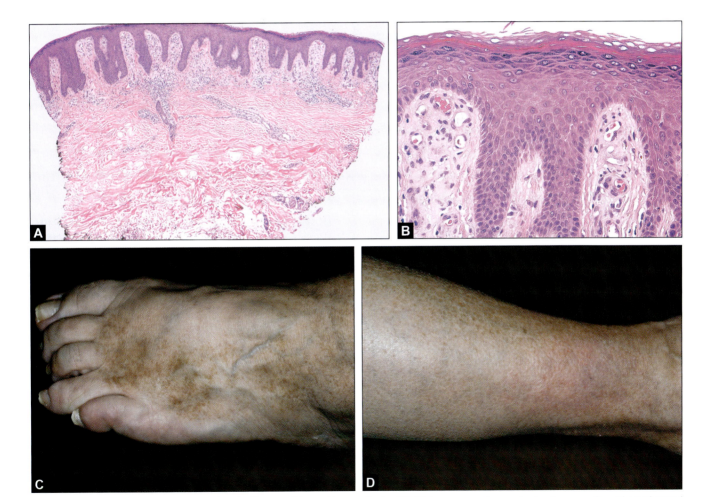

Figs 2.6A to D: Stasis dermatitis. (A) Psoriasiform epidermal hyperplasia; (B) Higher power demonstrates increased number of round blood vessels within the dermis; (C) Yellow brown patches due to hemosiderin deposition usually appreciated clinically; (D) Erythema resembling cellulitis may be present.

Xerotic (Asteatotic) Dermatitis

▪ *Criteria for diagnosis*

- Dry, cracked or fissured red patches and plaques
- Histology if performed:
  - Hyperkeratosis, slight epidermal acanthosis, spongiosis and sparse inflammatory infiltrate (Fig. 2.7).

▪ *Pitfalls*

- Confusing xerosis from ichthyosis. Most ichthyosis start during childhood, but acquired ichthyosis due to medications, systemic diseases or malignancies can occur.

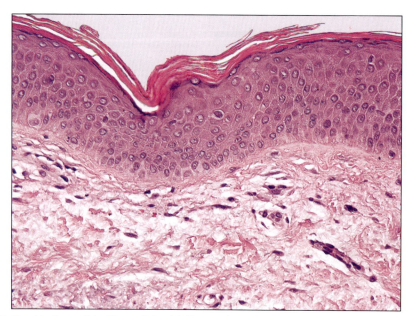

Fig. 2.7: Xerotic dermatitis. Note minimal inflammation, slight parakeratosis and hyperkeratosis.

Pityriasis Rosea (Figs 2.8A to D)

Criteria for diagnosis

- Oval red to pink papules, patches, or plaques with peripheral scale predominantly involving the trunk (Fig. 2.8A)
- Histology if biopsied:
  - Focal spongiosis, extravasated erythrocytes, exocytosis of lymphocytes and discrete parakeratotic mounds (Figs 2.8B and C).

Differential diagnosis

- Erythema annulare centrifugum (see "pitfalls" below)
- Spongiotic dermatitis and simulators, particularly nummular dermatitis
- Secondary syphilis
- Other disorders exhibiting the "pityriasiform" pattern, particularly drug eruptions, viral exanthems and small plaque parapsoriasis.

Pitfalls

- Histopathologically pityriasis rosea is indistinguishable from the superficial form of erythema annulare centrifugum and small plaque parapsoriasis

- The herald patch of pityriasis rosea exhibits psoriasiform epidermal hyperplasia.

Pearls

- Presence of plasma cells and/or lichenoid inflammation should raise consideration of secondary syphilis
- In contrast to genuine spongiotic dermatitis, spongiosis and parakeratosis, pityriasis rosea is confined to small, discrete foci
- Extravasated red blood cells are often present in the papillary dermis or epidermis
- Pityriasis rosea generally resolves within 6–10 weeks; if lesions persists for more than 20 weeks, nummular dermatitis or small plaque parapsoriasis should be considered
- Pityriasis rosea in darker complected patients may involve the face.

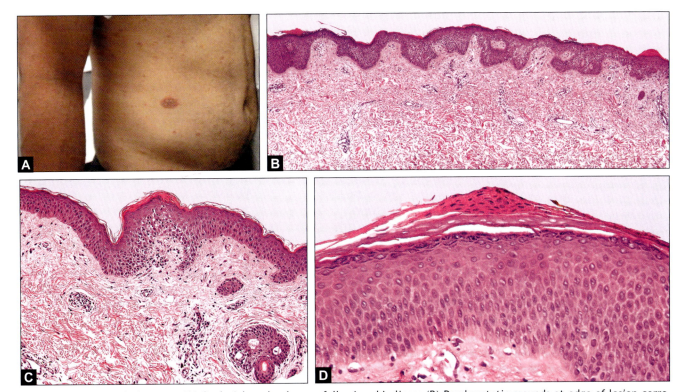

Figs 2.8A to D: Pityriasis rosea. (A) Oval pink scaly plaques following skin lines; (B) Parakeratotic mounds at edge of lesion corresponds to collarette of scale seen clinically; (C) Focal spongiosis with inflammation and extravasated erythrocytes; (D) Pityriasis rosea with dry mounds.

Insect Bite Reaction

■ *Criteria for diagnosis*

- Wedge shaped infiltrate (Fig. 2.9A)
- Eosinophiles in interstitium between collagen bundles
- Basophilic material/fibrin between collagen bundles
- Centrally located spongiotic vesicle or epidermal perforation
- In scabies:
  - Occasional mites or eggs within stratum corneum
- In tick bites:
  - Occasional mouth parts within dermis associated with granulomatous infiltrate (Fig. 2.9B)
  - Occluded blood vessels due to tick bite associated cryoglubulinemia.

■ *Differential diagnosis*

- Lymphomatoid papulosis (LyP)

■ *Pitfalls*

- Large CD30+ cells are characteristic of LyP and other types of lymphoma but are often seen in insect bite reactions, as well as numerous other reactive inflammatory conditions (Fig. 2.9C).

■ *Pearls*

- Patients are usually not aware that they are being bitten so clinical history is often noncontributory.

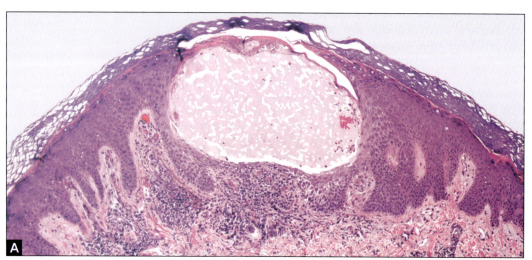

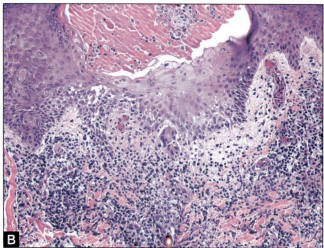
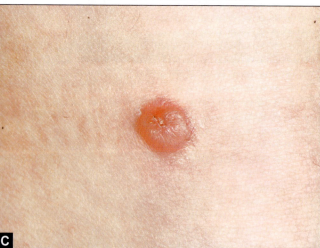

Figs 2.9A to C: Insect bite reaction. (A) Spongiosis with underlying wedge shaped infiltrate; (B) Occasionally granulomatous inflammation due to insect parts can be seen; (C) Bullous insect bite.

Polymorphous Light Eruption

■ *Criteria for diagnosis*

- Perivascular inflammatory cell infiltrate with papillary dermal edema and sometimes spongiosis plus a clinical history of a photo distributed (face, neck, arms, dorsal hands) eruption of papules, plaques or papulovesicles after light exposure.

■ *Differential diagnosis*

- Lupus erythematosus should have interface changes
- Dermatitis
- Drug eruption.

■ *Pitfalls*

- Polymorphous light eruption (PMLE) can occur anytime of the year since patients may travel

- Insect bite can resemble PMLE with papillary dermal edema, but eosinophils are not prominent in PMLE (Figs 2.10A and B).

■ *Pearls*

- The term "polymorphous" refers to the variability in the lesions between patients; within a given patient, the rash is generally monomorphous
- Edematous papules and plaques are the most common.

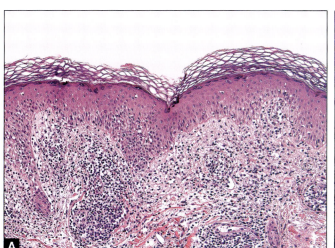 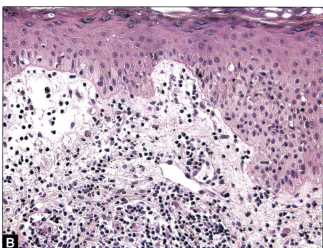

Figs 2.10A and B: Polymorphous light eruption. (A) Lymphocytic infiltrate with lack of parakeratosis; (B) Papillary dermal edema clue to diagnosis.

Pruritic Urticarial Papules and Plaques of Pregnancy/Polymorphous Eruption of Pregnancy

■ *Criteria for diagnosis*

- Superficial and deep perivascular and interstitial inflammatory infiltrate containing eosinophils
- Mild papillary dermal edema (Fig. 2.11A) and slight spongiosis
- Clinical history of a pregnant female (usually primigravida) near term
- Urticarial papules and plaques on the trunk, accentuated in striae.

■ *Pitfalls*

- Early lesions of herpes gestationis can resemble PMLE, but blisters will eventually appear, and direct immunofluorescence will be positive for linear staining along basement membrane zone with C3.

■ *Pearls*

- The dermatoses of pregnancy usually start during the third trimester.

■ *Differential diagnosis*

- Dermatitis (Fig. 2.11B)
- Insect bites
- Herpes gestation.

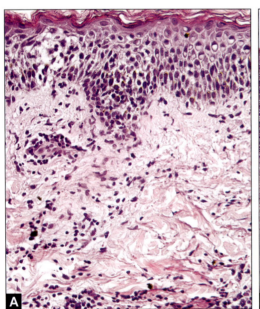 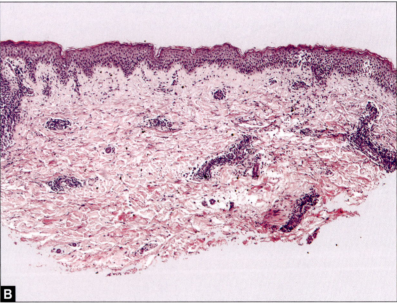

Figs 2.11A and B: Pruritic urticarial papules and plaques of pregnancy. (A) Papillary dermal edema is clue to diagnosis; (B) Lack of scale is clue to dermatitis simulator.

Dermatophytosis (Tinea) (Figs 2.12A to D)

■ *Criteria for diagnosis*

- Spores, hyphae and neutrophils within a stratum corneum occupied by compact orthokeratosis (Figs 2.12A and B).

■ *Differential diagnosis*

- Spongiotic dermatitis, particularly dyshidrotic, contact, seborrheic or atopic dermatitis (depending on anatomic site)
- Candidiasis
- Psoriasis
- Erythrasma (for tinea pedis) (see Figs 1.2A to C)
- Tinea versicolor (a superficial fungal infection caused by Pityrosporum ovale/Malassezia furfur).

■ *Pitfalls*

- A blistering form of dermatophytosis (bullous tinea) may occur on the hands and feet, and simulate an autoimmune vesiculobullous disorder or dyshidrotic dermatitis

- Partially treated dermatophytosis may appear unusual clinically and biopsies may contain only small numbers of organisms.

■ *Pearls*

- The "sandwich sign" is particularly characteristic of dermatophytosis (fungi between normal orthokeratotic stratum corneum on the surface and underlying compact orthokeratotic or parakeratotic layers)
- Neutrophils within stratum corneum are clue to tinea infection, and the histology of psoriasis and tinea can be identical.

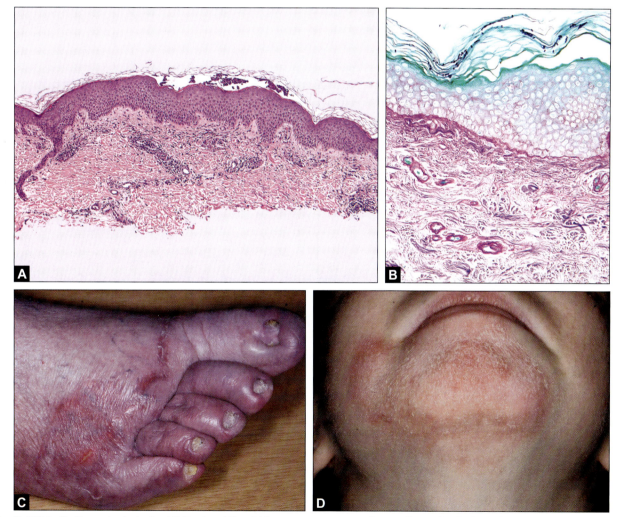

Figs 2.12A to D: Dermatophytosis. (A) Neutrophils within stratum corneum clue to diagnosis; (B) Periodic acid-Schiff stain demonstrates hyphae; (C) Tinea pedis and onychomycosis; (D) Tinea faciei.

Grover's Disease (Transient Acantholytic Dermatosis)

■ *Criteria for diagnosis*

- Itchy rash with nondescriptured macules and papules on trunk
- Histology polymorphous:
  - Sine qua non is focal acantholysis
  - The acantholysis can be associated with spongiosis (Figs 2.13A and B):
    - Dyskeratosis
    - Corps ronds
    - Corps grains.

■ *Pitfalls*

- Due to polymorphous nature of histology Grover's disease can be misdiagnosed as dermatitis or other acantholytic diseases, such as pemphigus and Darier's disease
- Focal acantholysis can also be seen as an incidental finding and is not diagnostic for Grover's disease.

■ *Pearls*

- Step sections or recuts through the block are often necessary to find the characteristic histological findings
- Acantholysis in association with acrosyringium is clue to diagnosis.

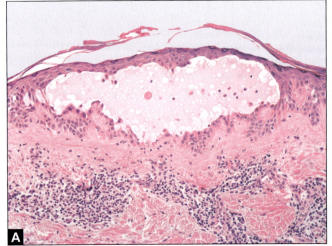 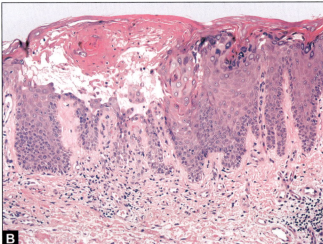

Figs 2.13A and B: Grover's disease. (A) Spongiosis may be prominent; (B) Acantholysis associated with spongiosis clue to diagnosis.

Gianotti-Crosti Syndrome (Papular Acral Dermatitis of Childhood)

Gianotti-Crosti is a type of exanthem caused by a number of different viruses.

■ *Criteria for diagnosis*

- Acute symmetrical papular/papulovesicular eruption involving face, limbs, elbows and knees (Fig. 2.14A)
- Trunk and mucous membranes are spared
- Most common in children between 2 years and 6 years
- Occasional lymph node involvement.

■ *Histology: (Fig. 2.14B)*

- Spongiosis
- Papillary dermal edema
- Superficial perivascular and somewhat lichenoid infiltrate (Fig. 2.14C).

■ *Pitfalls*

- Misdiagnosing Gianotti-Crosti syndrome as a dermatitis.

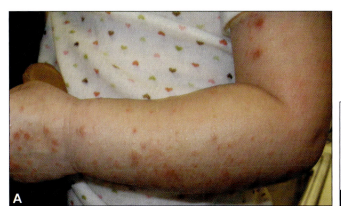

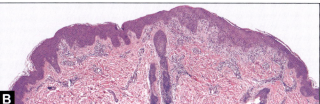

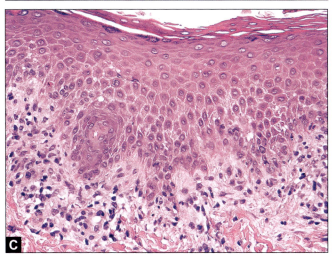

Figs 2.14A to C: Gianotti-Crosti syndrome. (A) Symmetrical papulovesicular eruption on extremities; (B) Histology reveals small lesion with lack of scale; (C) Lichenoid inflammation frequently present.

Parapsoriasis and Mycosis Fungoides

Parapsoriasis is a term introduced by Brocq in 1902 to describe a group of dermatoses that like psoriasis were chronic, idiopathic and difficult to treat. Clinically, parapsoriasis has been categorized as large plaque or small plaque based on the size of the lesions. Many cases of so-called large plaque parapsoriasis are indistinguishable from early lesions of mycosis fungoides. Small plaque parapsoriasis typically behaves as an inflammatory disorder rather than a neoplastic one, but evolution into mycosis fungoides has been documented.

Since parapsoriasis and early mycosis fungoides may be indistinguishable from inflammatory diseases, clinical-pathologic correlation is essential, and additional biopsies are prudent if a presumed dermatitis fails to respond to treatment. Not uncommonly, multiple biopsies performed over a period of several months or years are required before a diagnosis of mycosis fungoides can be confidently established.

▣ *Criteria for diagnosis*

- *Clinical*: Chronic patches and plaques with fine scale and atrophic and wrinkled appearance (Figs 2.15A and D).

▣ *Histology*

- Lichenoid/band like infiltrate (Fig. 2.15B)
- Epidermotropism
- Lymphocytes lining along basal layers of epidermis (Fig. 2.15C)
- Lymphocytes extending into granular cell layer

- Haloed lymphocytes within epidermis
- Epidermal lymphocytes larger then dermal
- Cerebriform lymphocytes
- Sclerotic collagen bundles within papillary dermis.

▣ *Differential diagnosis*

- Dermatitis
- Drug eruption
- Lymphomatoid papulosis
- Actinic reticuloid.

▣ *Pitfalls*

- Mycosis fungoides has numerous variants that can easily be missed without a high incidence of suspicion
    - Hypopigmented mycosis fungoides
    - Purpuric mycosis fungoides
    - Granulomatous slack Skin
    - Folliculo-adnexotropic mycosis fungoides
    - Mycosis fungoides associated with follicular mucinosis
    - Woringer-Kolopp (localized plaque)
    - Erythrodermic mycosis fungoides
    - Sézary syndrome (leukemic variant).

▣ *Pearls*

- Spongiosis, papillary dermal edema or eosinophils are typically absent in parapsoriasis and suggest spongiotic dermatitis instead.

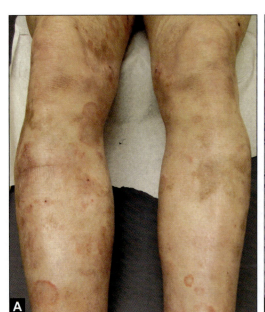

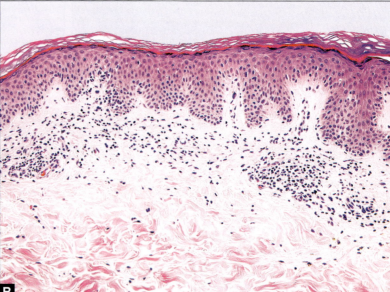

Figs 2.15A and B

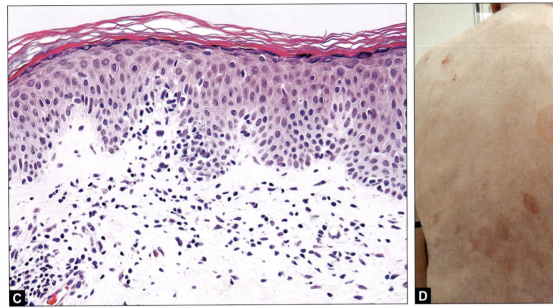

Figs 2.15A to D: Mycosis fungoides. (A) Scaly figurate plaques; (B) Psoriasiform lichenoid pattern militates against the diagnosis of dermatitis; (C) Note minimal scale and lymphocytes lining up along basal layers of epidermis; (D) Clinical picture of mycosis fungoides.

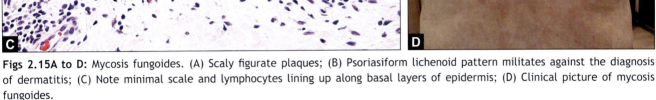

THE PSORIASIFORM PATTERN

When dermatitis becomes chronic the epidermis becomes thickened in a manner typical of psoriasis. The psoriasiform pattern should prompt consideration of specific differential diagnostic considerations (Box 2.1).

Box 2.1: Differential diagnosis of the psoriasiform pattern

- Psoriasis
- Pityriasiform dermatoses (see Chapter 3)
- Acute generalized exanthematous pustulosis
- Chronic spongiotic dermatitis
- Clear cell acanthoma
- Epidermal nevus/inflammatory linear verrucous epidermal nevus
- Glucagonoma syndrome (necrolytic migratory erythema)
- Lichen simplex chronicus/prurigo nodularis
- Nutritional deficiency dermatosis
- Pityriasis rubra pilaris
- Psoriasiform keratosis
- Tinea/candidiasis
- Psoriasiform lichenoid pattern (see Chapter 3)

Psoriasis (Figs 2.16A to J)

Psoriasis has many different clinical variants from guttate, plaque, pustular, inverse, rupoid, linear, erythrodermic, impetigo herpetiformis (psoriasis of pregnancy) and acrodermatitis continua of Hallopeau. The histology of all these variants has common features enabling accurate diagnosis (Fig. 2.16A).

Histological criteria for diagnosis

- Psoriasiform epidermal hyperplasia (regularly elongated rete) (Fig. 2.16B) with hypogranulosis, dilated papillary dermal blood vessels and neutrophils within a parakeratotic stratum corneum plus a clinical history of circumscribed scaly erythematous plaques (Fig. 2.16C)
- Aggregates of neutrophils within the epidermis (Munro's microabscesses and spongiform pustules of Kogoj-figures) are common in the guttate and pustular forms of psoriasis (Figs 2.16D and E).

Differential diagnosis

- Box 2.1

■ *Pitfalls*

- Spongiosis and edema may be seen in acute forms of psoriasis and in lesions on the palms and soles, causing confusion with spongiotic dermatitis (Fig. 2.16F)
- Pustule formation may simulate an infectious disease.

■ *Pearls*

- In contrast to psoriasis, chronic spongiotic dermatitis has an intact or accentuated granular layer, and rete elongation is less regular
- Eosinophils are usually inconspicuous or altogether absent in psoriasis

- Serum within the stratum corneum is more characteristic of chronic spongiotic dermatitis (except in palmoplantar psoriasis)
- Dilated tortuous blood vessels within the papillary dermis often remain when all other features of psoriasis have resolved (Figs 2.16G and H)
- Suprabasilar mitotic figures can be clue to diagnosis (Fig. 2.16E).
- Inflammatory linear epidermal nevus has alternating columns of parakeratosis with intervening areas of orthokeratosis (Fig. 2.16J)
- Acute generalized exanthematous pustulosis has eosinophils and occasionally exhibits vasculitis.

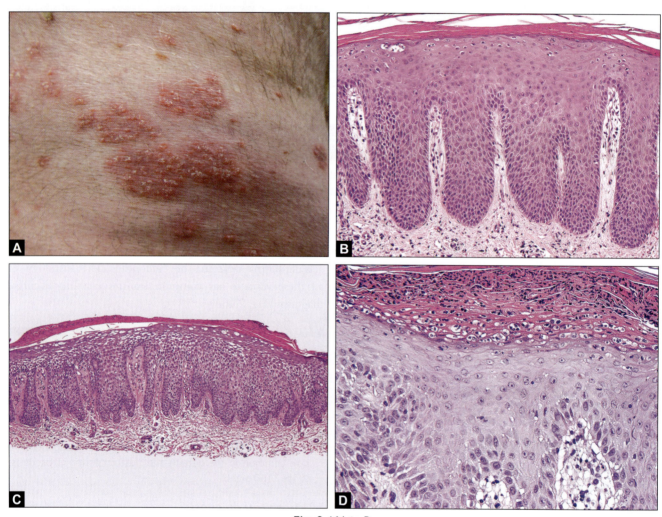

Figs 2.16A to D

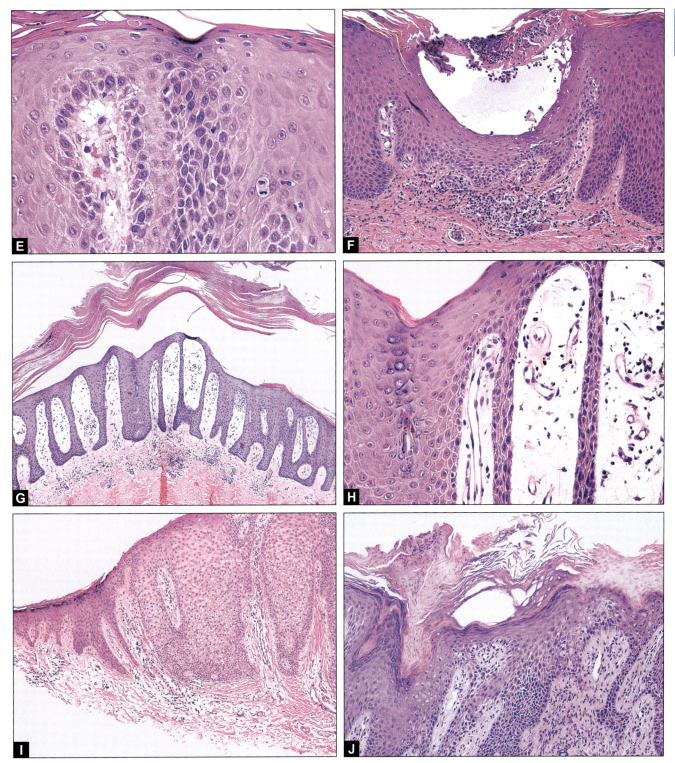

Figs 2.16A to J: Psoriasis. (A) Psoriasis :red plaques with silvery scale; (B) Uniform lengths of rete ridges clue to diagnosis; (C) Spongiosis may be present especially in erythrodermic patients; (D) Psoriasis: Monroe microabscess (neutrophils within statum corneum clue to diagnosis); (E) Suprabasilar mitotic figure clue to diagnosis of psoriasis (F) Palmoplantar plantar psoriasis with large pustule; (G) Psoriasis: Tortuous blood vessels in papillary dermis clue to diagnosis; (H) Close up of tortuous blood vessels in papillary dermis; (I) Histological differential: clear cell acanthoma. Sharp demarcation of clear cell acanthoma from surrounding epidermis clue to diagnosis;(J) Histological differential: inflammatory linear epidermal nevus. Staggared parakeratotic columns clue to diagnosis.

Pityriasis Rubra Pilaris

■ *Criteria for diagnosis*

- Epidermal acanthosis with hypergranulosis, alternating horizontal and vertical zones of parakeratosis (checkerboard parakeratosis), follicular hyperkeratosis (follicular plugs) and rarely acantholysis with a clinical history of red-orange follicular papules that coalesce into plaques with islands of sparing (Fig. 2.17A).

■ *Differential diagnosis*

- Psoriasis
- Chronic spongiotic dermatitis
- Acantholytic dermatoses (rarely).

■ *Pitfalls*

- The histopathologic features of pityriasis rubra pilaris (PRP), particularly in an evolving lesion are quite variable
- Acantholysis, dyskeratosis and lichenoid inflammation can be seen.

■ *Pearls*

- In contrast to psoriasis, PRP exhibits irregularly elongated rete, a preserved granular layer and follicular plugs; neutrophils and pustules are not seen (Fig. 2.17B)
- Clinical features of PRP are often necessary to make a definitive diagnosis.

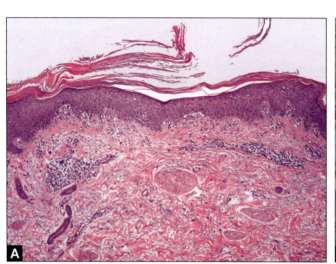 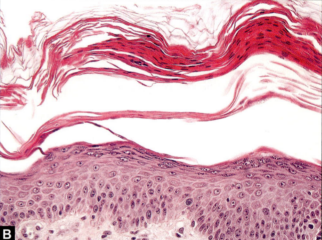

Figs 2.17A and B: Pityriasis rubra pilaris. (A) Notice "checkerboard" like appearance of parakeratotic cells; (B) Unlike psoriasis retained granular cell layer.

Nutritional Deficiency Dermatoses and Glucagonoma Syndrome

■ **Criteria for diagnosis**

- Psoriasiform epidermal hyperplasia
- Confluent parakeratosis (Fig. 2.18A)
- Superficial epidermal necrosis or pallor (Fig. 2.18B)
- Neutrophils within stratum corneum.

■ **Differential diagnosis**

- Other psoriasiform dermatoses.

■ **Pitfalls**

- Nutritional deficiency dermatoses and glucagonoma syndrome cannot be distinguished histopathologically; clinical confirmation is necessary

- Necrolytic acral erythema has identical histology but usually associated with hepatitis C infection.

■ **Pearls**

- Confluent parakeratosis is clue to diagnosis
- Multiple biopsies may be necessary
- Bullous lesions have been reported.

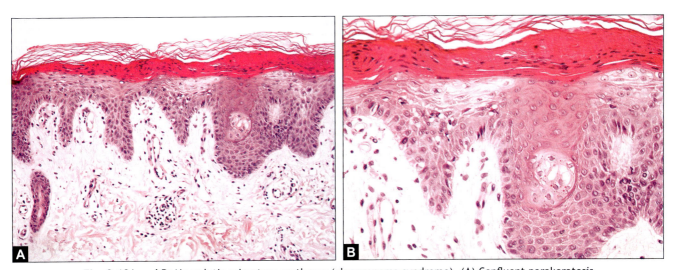

Figs 2.18A and B: Necrolytic migratory erythema (glucagonoma syndrome). (A) Confluent parakeratosis may be seen; (B) Pallor in upper portion of epidermis is characteristic.

Prurigo Nodule/Lichen Simplex Chronicus

◼ *Criteria for diagnosis*

- Lichen simplex chronicus
  - *Clinically*: Chronic pruritic lichenified plaque usually on ankle or nape of neck (Fig. 2.19A)
- Prurigo nodularis
  - Multiple symmetrical lichenified papules and plaques most commonly on extremities and legs.

◼ *Histology*

- Psoriasiform epidermal hyperplasia
- Compact orthokeratosis
- Vertical streaking of collagen bundles within papillary dermis (Figs 2.19B and C)
- Sparse inflammatory infiltrate.

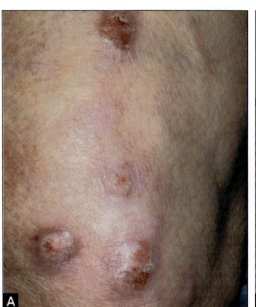

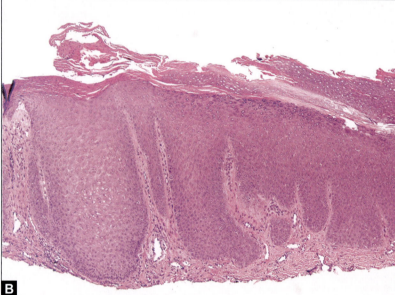

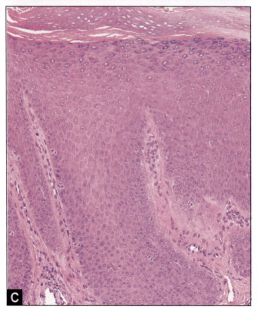

Figs 2.19A to C: Prurigo nodularis. (A) Clinical picture of prurigo nodularis; (B and C) Epidermal acanthosis, hypergranulosis and vertical streaking of collagen bundles in papillary dermis.

BIBLIOGRAPHY

1. Ackerman AB, Denianke K, Sceppa J, et al. Mycosis Fungoides: Perspective Historical Allied with Critique Methodical for the Purpose of Illumination Maximal Atlas and Text. New York: Ardor Scribendi; 2008.

2. Antley CM, Carrington PR, Mrak RE, et al. Grover's disease (transient acantholytic dermatosis): relationship of acantholysis to acrosyringia. J Cutan Pathol. 1998. 25(10):545-9.

3. Gonzalez JR, Botet MV, Sanchez JL. The histopathology of acrodermatitis enteropathica. Am J Dermatopathol. 1982;4(4):303-11.

4. Gottleib GJ, Ackerman AB. The "sandwich sign" of dermatophytosis. Am J Dermatopathol 1986; 8: 347-50.

5. Kardaun SH, Kuiper H, Fidler V, et al. The histopathological spectrum of acute generalized exanthematous pustulosis (AGEP) and its differentiation from generalized pustular psoriasis. J Cutan Pathol. 2010;37(12):1220-9.

6. Kheir SM, Omura EF, Grizzle WE, et al. Histologic variation in the skin lesions of the glucagonoma syndrome. Am J Surg Pathol. 1986;10(7):445-53.

7. Lee WJ, Kim CH, Won CH, et al. Bullous acrodermatitis enteropathica with interface dermatitis. J Cutan Pathol. 2010; 37(9):1013-5.

8. Panizzon R, Bloch PH. Histopathology of pityriasis rosea Gibert. Qualitative and quantitative light-microscopic study of 62 biopsies of 40 patients. Dermatologica. 1982;165(6):551-8.

9. Smith KJ, Skelton H. Histopathologic features seen in Gianotti-Crosti syndrome secondary to Epstein-Barr virus. J Am Acad Dermatol. 2000;43(6): 1076-9.

10. Soeprono FF, Histologic criteria for the diagnosis of pityriasis rubra pilaris. Am J Dermatopathol. 1986;8(4):277-83.

11. Streit M, Braathen LR. Contact dermatitis: clinics and pathology. Acta Odontol Scand. 2001;59(5):309-14.

12. White CR Jr. Histopathology of exogenous and systemic contact eczema. Semin Dermatol. 1990;9(3):226-9.

CHAPTER 3

The Interface and Perivascular/Periadnexal Patterns

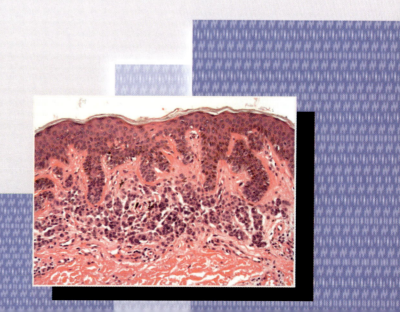

INTRODUCTION

The interface pattern or interface dermatitis refers to an infiltrate of leukocytes, mostly lymphocytes, distributed along the dermoepidermal junction. Many diseases with an interface infiltrate also contain inflammation around blood vessels and occasionally, adnexal structures (perivascular/periadnexal pattern).

Interface reactions can be categorized into four patterns:
1. The vacuolar pattern (Fig. 3.1)
2. The lichenoid pattern (Fig. 3.2)
3. The pityriasiform pattern (Fig. 3.3)
4. The interface and perivascular/periadnexal pattern (Fig. 3.4).

Many disorders often exhibit two or more of these subtypes simultaneously or at various points during their course. Moreover, which of these patterns predominates may differ among variants of a disease. For example, systemic lupus erythematosus (SLE) usually demonstrates vacuolar interface dermatitis, while discoid lupus often contains perivascular and periadnexal inflammation as well. Patterns also vary depending on the stage of the disease. The lichenoid pattern is characteristic of established lichen planus but resolving lesions may appear more vacuolar. Nevertheless, by identifying the subtype of interface reaction, a dermatopathologist can often narrow a differential diagnosis or arrive at a specific diagnosis.

As with most inflammatory diseases of the skin, this potential for overlap and variation in the histopathologic features means that assessment of the entire constellation of findings combined with careful consideration of clinical information is essential to reach a correct diagnosis.

THE VACUOLAR PATTERN

The vacuolar pattern is an interface reaction in which a relatively sparse collection of mostly lymphocytes occupies the dermoepidermal junction and the epidermis exhibits basal layer keratinocytes that contain intracytoplasmic vacuoles (vacuolar degeneration) and/or numerous necrotic keratinocytes (Fig. 3.1). Note that the dermoepidermal junction is not obscured by inflammation but the damaged basement membrane zone and basal layer keratinocytes make it indistinct. Diseases that frequently exhibit vacuolar pattern are given in Box 3.1.

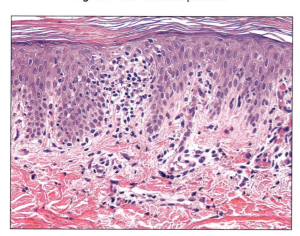

Fig. 3.1: The vacuolar pattern.

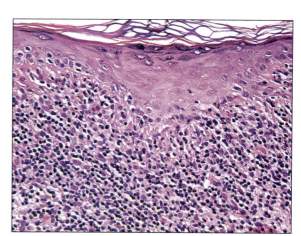

Fig. 3.2: The lichenoid pattern.

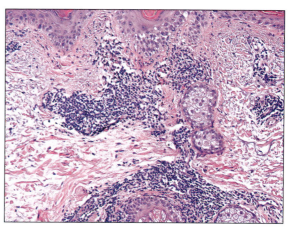

Fig. 3.3: The pityriasiform pattern.

Fig. 3.4: The interface and perivascular/periadnexal pattern.

Box 3.1: Diseases that frequently exhibit the vacuolar pattern

- Erythema multiforme
- Toxic epidermal necrolysis
- Lupus erythematosus (especially systemic lupus erythematosus and subacute cutaneous lupus erythematosus)
- Dermatomyositis
- Graft-versus-host disease (acute phase)
- Fixed drug eruption
- Erythema dyschromicum perstans (ashy dermatosis)
- Atrophic lichen planus (and other resolving lichenoid diseases)
- Interface drug eruptions
- Viral exanthems
- Lichen sclerosus

Erythema Multiforme (EM) (Figs 3.5A to E)

Criteria for diagnosis

- Vacuolar interface dermatitis with conspicuous keratinocyte necrosis, often with perivascular dermatitis of the superficial vascular plexus, and a clinical appearance that characteristically manifests as discrete "targetoid" papules with a predilection for acral skin and involvement of oral or ocular mucosa as well.

Differential diagnosis

- Toxic epidermal necrolysis (TEN), acute graft-versus-host disease (GVHD), fixed drug eruption, pityriasis lichenoides chronica (PLC), urticarial phase bullous pemphigoid, viral exanthems [including herpes simplex virus (HSV)], SLE and dermatomyositis, coma bulla, paraneoplastic pemphigus.

Pitfalls

- Acute graft-versus-host disease and drug eruptions are often impossible to reliably differentiate from EM on histopathology alone; clinical information is required
- Urticarial phase bullous pemphigoid may simulate EM clinically and occasionally, EM may contain eosinophils in the inflammatory infiltrate causing some overlap histopathologically as well.

Pearls

- Inflammation of follicular epithelium is more common in GVHD; however, clinical information should be sought to differentiate GVHD from EM. (The eruption of GVHD is often more generalized, lacks targetoid papules and may be associated with hepatic and gastrointestinal involvement)

- Staphylococcal scalded skin syndrome (SSSS) may simulate early TEN clinically in some cases but in EM, necrotic keratinocytes are distributed throughout the full thickness of the epidermis, while SSSS exhibits acantholysis limited to the granular layer or complete sloughing of the stratum corneum
- A fixed drug eruption generally contains more melanophages, more neutrophils and more eosinophils than EM, and the infiltrate more often involves the deep dermis in a perivascular distribution. Lesions are usually fewer in number in fixed drug eruptions than in EM
- Pityriasis lichenoides usually has superficial and deep perivascular inflammation in addition to interface inflammation and typically has at least a focally parakeratotic stratum corneum containing granulocytes
- Eosinophils are occasionally seen in EM (particularly in those cases that are caused by drugs); however, numerous eosinophils aligned along the dermoepidermal junction favors urticarial bullous pemphigoid
- Viral exanthems including those due to HSV may be histologically indistinguishable from EM if characteristic viral inclusions are not evident
- Connective tissue diseases, such as lupus and dermatomyositis typically have hyperkeratosis, follicular keratin 'plugs' [in discoid lupus erythematosus (DLE)] and epidermal atrophy
- Unlike EM, coma bulla characteristically exhibit necrosis of eccrine glands in addition to interface change
- Paraneoplastic pemphigus may resemble EM but usually has a greater density of inflammatory cells.

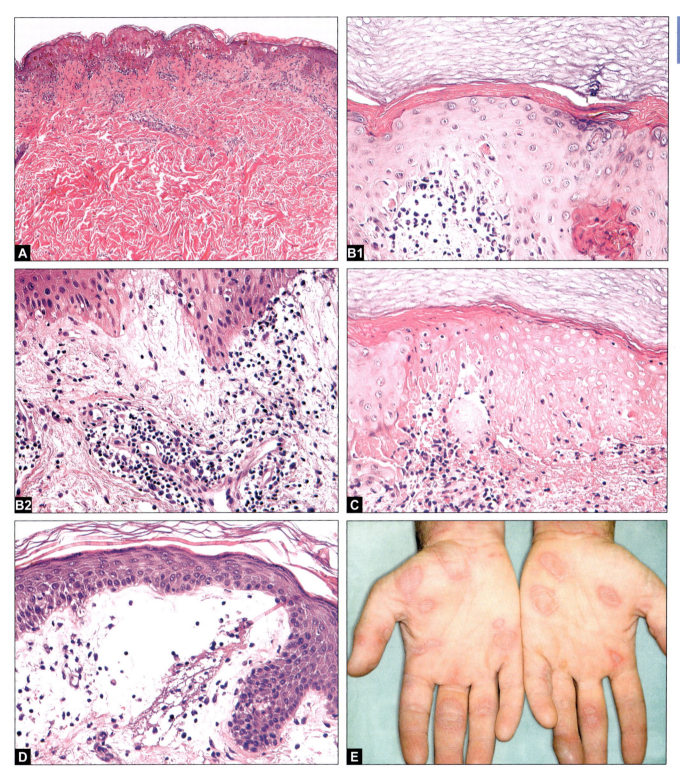

Figs 3.5A to E: Erythema multiforme. (A) The inflammation is typically interface and also surrounds the vessels of the superficial vascular plexus; (B) A vacuolar pattern is common and the infiltrate is composed almost entirely of lymphocytes. Note that the stratum corneum is unaltered reflecting the acute onset; (C) Necrotic keratinocytes increase in number as the lesions develop and a blister may develop. Erythrocytes often fill the papillary dermis and the blister cavity; (D) In some instances, keratinocyte destruction and spongiosis are severe and result in blisters that resemble those of bullous pemphigoid and other vesiculobullous diseases; (E) Clinically, lesions may vary greatly but target lesions are characteristic.
Courtesy: Dr Jeffrey Miller

Toxic Epidermal Necrolysis (Figs 3.6A and B)

■ *Criteria for diagnosis*

- Extensive epidermal necrosis with minimal inflammation; diffuse erythematous patches and involvement of mucosa and conjunctiva clinically.

■ *Differential diagnosis*

- Erythema multiforme, fixed drug eruption.

■ *Pitfalls*

- Erythema multiforme can be difficult (or impossible in some cases) to differentiate from TEN (and some consider them to be a spectrum of the same process).

■ *Pearls*

- Erythema multiforme typically contains a much more conspicuous inflammatory cell infiltrate; necrotic keratinocytes are more common than full thickness epidermal necrosis
- Clinically, TEN may occasionally be confused with SSSS since both may cause rapid sloughing of skin and pathologists may be asked to differentiate the two by frozen sections of blistered or sloughed skin
- Histopathologically, SSSS is typified by acantholysis in the granular layer or complete separation of the stratum corneum, not the full thickness epidermal necrosis of TEN.

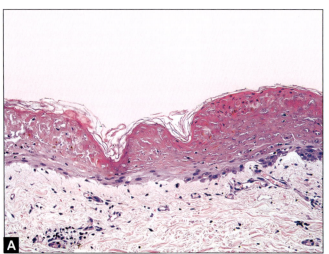 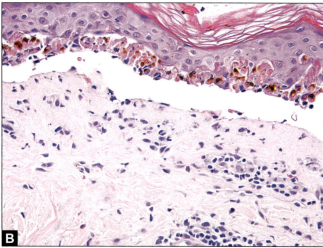

Figs 3.6A and B: Toxic epidermal necrolysis. (A) Early lesions often have features similar to those of erythema multiforme. In this case, rapid basal layer keratinocyte destruction is causing subepidermal clefting, a commonly encountered feature; (B) Established lesions are characterized by areas of keratinocyte necrosis involving full thickness of the epidermis. Inflammation is usually minimal.

Systemic Lupus Erythematosus (Figs 3.7A to C)

■ Criteria for diagnosis

- Vacuolar interface dermatitis, often with epidermal atrophy and dilated vessels occurring primarily in sun-exposed skin and a clinical history compatible with lupus erythematosus.

■ Differential diagnosis

- There are many subtypes of lupus erythematosus and specification of the subtype is generally impossible based on histopathology alone
- Lupus erythematosus, especially SLE, is often indistinguishable from dermatomyositis; other simulators include GVHD and EM.

■ Pitfalls

- Since cutaneous lupus erythematosus can vary so greatly in appearance, the differential may be broad

- Attempts to classify the subtype of lupus erythematosus on histopathology alone should be avoided since the histopathologic pattern does not always correlate with the clinical type.

■ Pearls

- A diagnosis of "connective tissue disease consistent with lupus erythematosus" is more accurate and usually adequate for clinical purposes
- Increased deposition of dermal ground substance (dermal "mucin") supports a diagnosis of connective tissue disease, particularly lupus erythematosus.

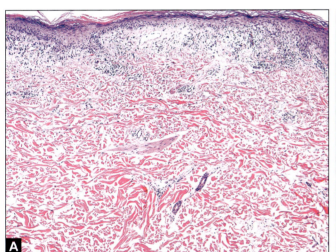

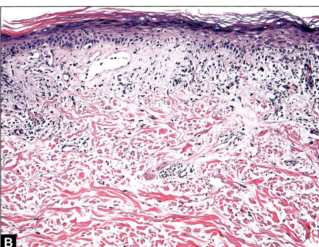

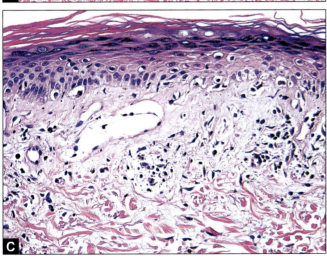

Figs 3.7A to C: Systemic lupus erythematosus. (A) The inflammatory infiltrate is often sparse and is usually confined to the dermoepidermal junction. The reticular dermis is often uninvolved; (B) Commonly, there is epidermal atrophy, mild dermal edema and dilated vessels; (C) Vacuolar change is subtle in some instances, but in most cases basal keratinocytes with clear cytoplasm are apparent.

Subacute Cutaneous Lupus Erythematosus (SCLE) (Figs 3.8A to E)

■ *Criteria for diagnosis*

- Interface inflammation (lichenoid or vacuolar in type) with epidermal atrophy, dermal edema and dermal mucin within the context of clinical features of SCLE including recurrent photo distributed, often annular, erythematous scaling papules and plaques.

■ *Differential diagnosis*

- Other forms of lupus erythematosus, dermatomyositis, lupus-like drug eruption and EM.

■ *Pitfalls*

- As with other forms of lupus erythematosus, the histopathologic features do not correlate reliably with the clinical subtype.

■ *Pearls*

- As with other types of lupus, overly specific diagnoses should be avoided since the histopathologic pattern does not always reflect the clinical features.

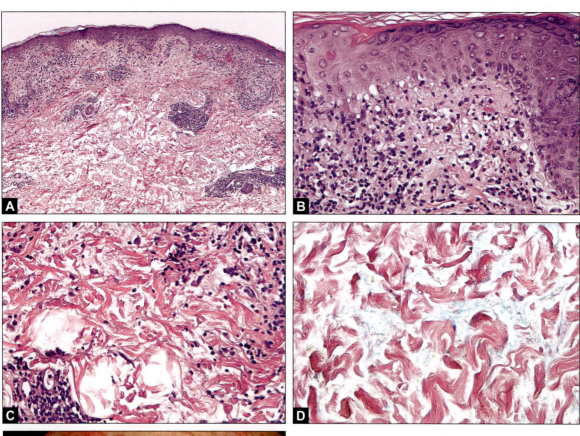

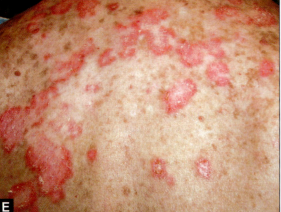

Figs 3.8A to E: Subacute cutaneous lupus erythematosus. (A) The features of subacute cutaneous lupus erythematosus overlap with both discoid lupus erythematosus and systemic lupus erythematosus, but interface inflammation is common to all the three forms; (B) By comparison to systemic lupus erythematosus, the infiltrate is usually of greater density. Subacute cutaneous lupus erythematosus tends to have some epidermal atrophy but hyperkeratosis and follicular plugging are less common than in DLE; (C) In addition to deep dermal perivascular and periadnexal inflammation, the dermis often contains increased ground substance; (D) Mucin stains, such as this colloidal iron preparation, are sometimes useful for demonstrating the increased ground substance; (E) A typical clinical presentation is annular, erythematous scaling papules and plaques.

Dermatomyositis (Figs 3.9A to E)

■ *Criteria for diagnosis*

- Vacuolar interface dermatitis, usually with epidermal atrophy, increased ground substance (dermal "mucin"), dilated vessels and a clinical history compatible with dermatomyositis. Violet-pink poikilodermatous patches on the eyelids (the heliotrope rash), upper chest and back, as well as Gottron's papules, erythema of the skin over joints (Gottron's sign) and psoriasis-like scalp dermatitis are among the common cutaneous clinical findings
- Edema may be prominent within the tissue from the periorbital "heliotrope" rash
- Tissue from Gottron's papules usually shows vacuolar change but the epidermis may be atrophic, hypertrophic or normal in thickness.

■ *Differential diagnosis*

- Lupus erythematosus may be indistinguishable from dermatomyositis histopathologically
- Interface drug eruptions may closely mimic dermatomyositis.

■ *Pearls*

- Unlike lupus erythematosus, the infiltrate in dermatomyositis may occasionally contain eosinophils
- As is the case for lupus erythematosus, the presence of increased dermal ground substances ("mucin") is a clue to the diagnosis of a connective tissue disease.

■ *Pitfalls*

- Some authors claim that dermatomyositis may be differentiated from lupus by various histopathologic features but clinical features and serologic data are usually more reliable methods of distinguishing the two
- As is the case for lupus erythematosus, an overly-definitive "line diagnosis" is not advisable and usually not necessary.

The Interface and Perivascular/Periadnexal Patterns

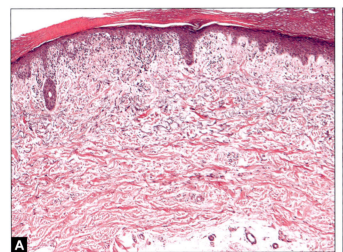
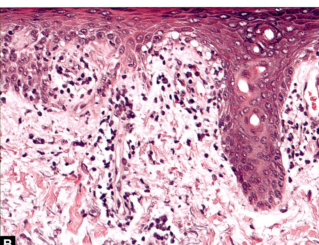

Figs 3.9A and B

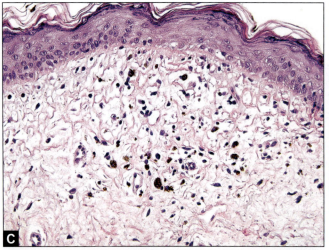

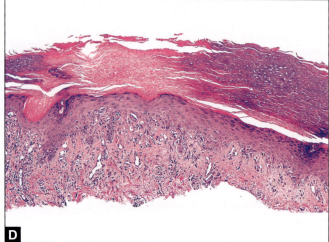

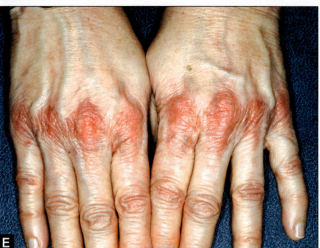

Figs 3.9A to E: Dermatomyositis. (A) As in systemic lupus erythematosus, epidermal atrophy is common in dermatomyositis; (B) Vacuolar interface dermatitis is characteristic. Necrotic keratinocytes are usually not a prominent feature; (C) Rete are diminished or absent. Pigment incontinence may be prominent; (D) Vacuolar interface dermatitis is evident in this biopsy of erythematous skin from the knuckle (Gottron's sign). Epidermal atrophy is not as apparent since it is acral skin; (E) Erythema of the skin over joints (Gottron's sign) is characteristic of dermatomyositis.

INTERFACE DRUG ERUPTION
(FIGS 3.10A TO C)

■ *Criteria for diagnosis*

- Vacuolar infiltrate with onset after introduction of a medication or other clinical features that support a drug as the etiologic agent.

■ *Differential diagnosis*

- Virtually, any vacuolar disease may be a differential diagnostic consideration, but the differential may include diseases with other inflammatory patterns since drug eruptions commonly show combinations of inflammatory patterns.

■ *Pitfalls*

- Interface drug eruptions commonly exhibit the vacuolar pattern but may also show a lichenoid pattern or a combination of the two (see below). Both clinically and histopathologically, differential from connective tissue disease may be difficult. Eosinophils within the infiltrate favor a drug reaction over lupus erythematosus but eosinophils may be seen in dermatomyositis so definitive diagnosis requires correlation with clinical data.

■ *Pearls*

- The clinical features vary but many interface drug eruptions are described as morbilliform or similar to an autoimmune connective tissue disease
- Parakeratosis, necrotic keratinocytes above the basal layer, the presence of eosinophils and plasma cells in the infiltrate and the presence of some perivascular inflammation in the deeper dermis are all clues that favor a drug eruption over lichen planus and most connective tissue diseases.

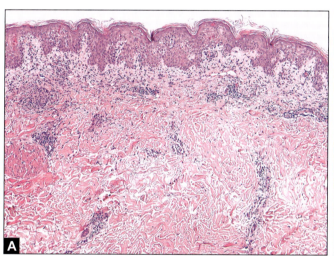

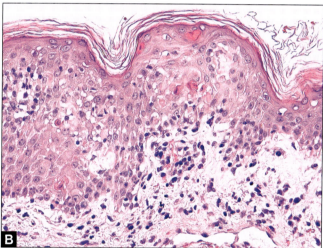

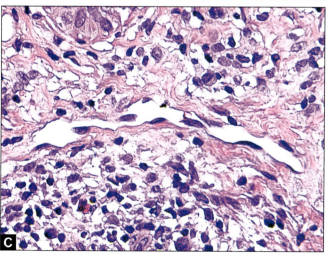

Figs 3.10A to C: Interface drug eruption. (A) There is an interface dermatitis, as well as some inflammation around the superficial vasculature; (B) Vacuolar change is present and necrotic keratinocytes are conspicuous with many scattered throughout the spinous layer of the epidermis; (C) In addition to lymphocytes, the infiltrate often contains at least a few eosinophils and plasma cells.

Fixed Drug Eruption (Figs 3.11A and B)

■ *Criteria for diagnosis*

- Vacuolar (or sometimes lichenoid) pattern with conspicuous necrotic keratinocytes and dermal melanophages
- A clinical history indicating one or more red-violet plaques that recur at the same anatomic site with each exposure to a certain drug and that resolve with prominent postinflammatory hyperpigmentation.

■ *Differential diagnosis*

- If the biopsy is accompanied by the clinical history described above, there is little else to consider. If not however, many vacuolar or lichenoid diseases enter the differential.

■ *Pitfalls*

- The first occurrences of a fixed drug eruption may not show numerous melanophages; they tend to accumulate with repeated exposures.

■ *Pearls*

- Melanophages within the dermis are a helpful clue to the diagnosis since they indicate that inflammation has occurred at this site previously. They are not specific, however, since lichenoid keratosis and other localized interface processes commonly feature them.

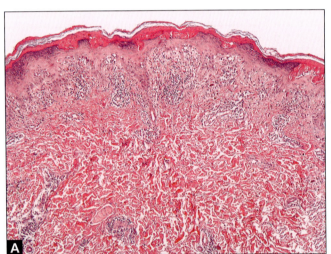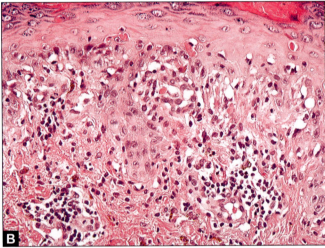

Figs 3.11A and B: Fixed drug eruption. (A) Vacuolar interface dermatitis is present along with hyperparakeratosis; (B) As is often the case in drug eruptions, necrotic keratinocytes are a prominent feature. Melanophages within the dermal infiltrate are a clue to the repetitive nature of the inflammation.

Acute Graft-Versus-Host Disease (GVHD)
(Figs 3.12A to C)

▪ *Criteria for diagnosis*

- An interface dermatitis usually vacuolar type, that evolves within 100 days of engraftment after transplantation (usually bone marrow). The likelihood and severity of GVHD correlates with the degree of human leucocyte antigen disparity between donor and recipient.

▪ *Differential diagnosis*

- Interface drug eruptions may be identical to GVHD; other considerations include viral exanthems and other vacuolar processes.

▪ *Pitfalls*

- There is no histopathologic feature that allows reliable distinction of GVHD from EM. Without a clinical description of the rash or additional information about symptoms, no definitive diagnosis can be made
- Biopsies may show seemingly normal skin if performed early in the evolution of the disorder.

▪ *Pearls*

- Erythema multiforme is less likely to involve adnexal epithelium than is acute GVHD
- Clinical history trumps histopathologic findings in any case, and pathologists should not feel compelled to render a definitive diagnosis of GVHD regardless of the pressure by clinicians to do so.

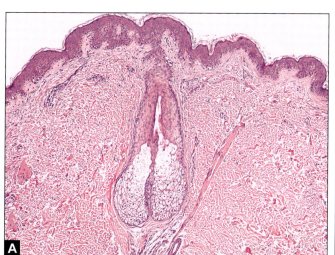

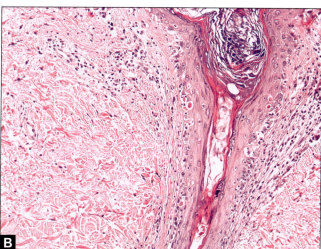

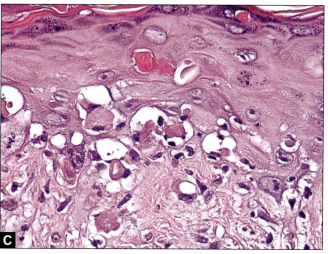

Figs 3.12A to C: Acute graft-versus-host disease. (A) Biopsies may show virtually normal-appearing skin early in the evolution of the disorder. Examination of multiple levels may reveal an occasional necrotic keratinocyte, but this does not differentiate acute graft-versus-host disease from a drug eruption; (B) Extension of the interface dermatitis along the epithelium of hair follicles is a common (albeit nonspecific) feature of acute graft-versus-host disease; (C) In this established lesion, numerous necrotic keratinocytes are the dominant findings. Intraepidermal lymphocytes directly adjacent to necrotic keratinocytes (so-called "satellite cell necrosis") is a common finding in acute graft-versus-host disease.

THE LICHENOID PATTERN

The lichenoid reaction pattern is a type of interface dermatitis in which the inflammatory infiltrate is sufficiently dense that it obscures portions of the dermoepidermal junction. Vacuolar degeneration may be present but is usually inconspicuous by comparison to the density of the inflammation.

Lichenoid inflammation is probably the most common reaction pattern in the skin and in addition to "lichenoid dermatitides" it frequently accompanies neoplasms and other inflammatory disorders. Diseases exhibiting a lichenoid pattern are given in Box 3.2.

Box 3.2: Diseases frequently exhibiting the lichenoid pattern

- Lichen planus (and variants)
- Lichenoid keratosis
- Lichenoid reactions to neoplasms
- Lichen striatus
- Lichen nitidus
- Interface drug eruptions
- Porokeratosis
- Paraneoplastic pemphigus
- Lichenoid pigmented purpuric eruption (Gougerot and Blum)
- Mycosis fungoides
- Lichenoid reactions to tattoos
- Lichenoid viral exanthems

Lichen Planus (Figs 3.13A to G)

■ *Criteria for diagnosis*

- Lichenoid and superficial perivascular infiltrate that at least focally obscures the dermoepidermal junction with a history of pruritic violaceous or erythematous papules and plaques
- Stratum corneum is normal in early lesions but compact hyperorthokeratosis often develops with time.

■ *Differential diagnosis*

- Lichenoid keratosis, lichenoid drug eruption, DLE, porokeratosis.

■ *Pitfalls*

- Variants of lichen planus are numerous with many different clinical and histopathologic appearances (Table 3.1).

■ *Pearls*

- The wedge-shaped hypergranulosis of lichen planus is uncommon in most of its mimics.

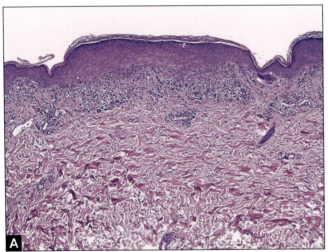
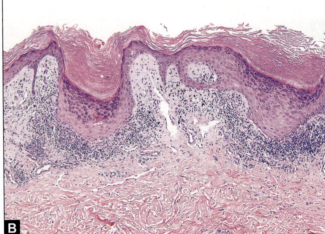

Figs 3.13A and B

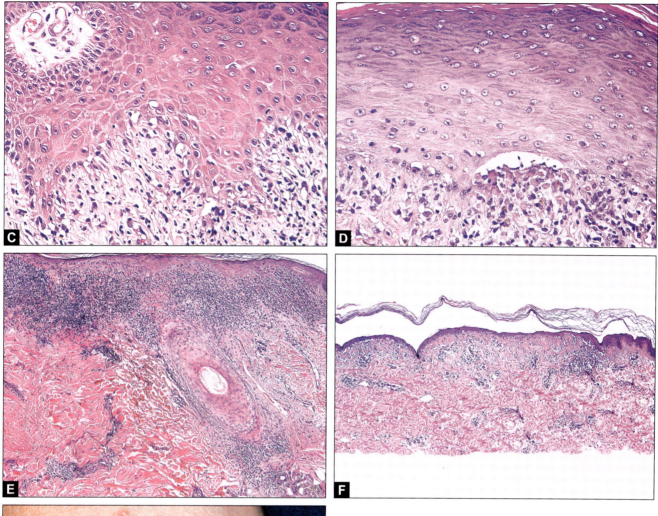

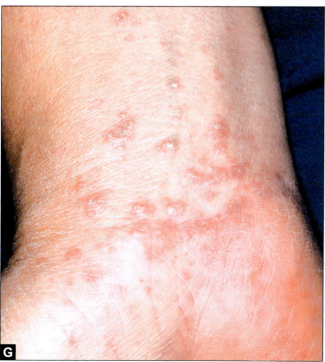

Figs 3.13A to G: Lichen planus. (A) In this fully evolved lesion, lymphocytes form a band along the dermoepidermal junction; (B) Lymphocytes may also collect in a patchy distributions along the junction. The epidermis is acanthotic and there is hyper-granulosis with a wedge-shaped pattern, a feature helpful in distinguishing lichen planus from simulators; (C) The rete tips are angular (saw tooth acanthosis) and the dermoepidermal junction is obscured; (D) Colloid bodies (necrotic keratinocytes) are common within the lower epidermis and the papillary dermis. Clefts between the epidermis and dermis may form in areas of extensive damage (Max Joseph spaces); (E) In this variant, the inflammation also surrounds follicular epithelium. The follicular infundibula may expand and develop a bulbous shape; (F) Resolving lesions may have an atrophic epidermis, a sparse residual inflammatory infiltrate (that often appears more vacuolar than lichenoid) and sclerotic papillary dermal collagen; (G) Pruritic papules and plaques are the most frequent clinical presentation of established lesions.

Table 3.1: Variants of lichen planus

Variant	Clinical Features	Histopathologic Features
Actinic lichen planus	Precipitated by sunlight	Typical lichen planus
Lichen planus hypertrophicus	Thick hyperkeratotic plaques on shins	Marked epidermal hyperplasia (hyperplastic lichen planus)
Annular lichen planus	Lesion arranged in an annular pattern; most common in groin or oral mucosa	Typical lichen planus
Ulcerative lichen planus	Most commonly affects oral mucosa, anogenital area or soles	Ulcers superimposed on otherwise typical lichen planus
Bullous lichen planus	Sudden eruption of vesicles	Subepidermal blisters with papillary dermal edema, less inflammation, minimally altered epidermis and stratum corneum (except for hypergranulosis)
Oral lichen planus	Painful erosions and white reticulated patches	Oral mucosa with lichenoid infiltrate
Lichen planopilaris	Keratotic follicular lesions that may result in follicular scarring alopecia	A lichenoid reaction involving the epithelium of hair follicles, especially the infundubilum and isthmus
Graham-Little-Piccardi syndrome	Keratotic follicular papules scarring alopecia of scalp; sometimes groin and axillary alopecia	Same as lichen planopilaris
Atrophic lichen planus		The interface infiltrate is sparse and may appear more vacuolar than lichenoid; the papillary dermal collagen may appear sclerotic

Lichenoid Keratosis (Lichen Planus-Like Keratosis) (Figs 3.14A to E)

■ *Criteria for diagnosis*

- Interface lichenoid infiltrate with epidermal hyperplasia or atrophy, hyperkeratosis, colloid bodies and often, features of a solar lentigo or seborrheic keratosis at the periphery, along with a clinical history of a solitary lesion.

■ *Differential diagnosis*

- Lichenoid keratoses most closely simulate lichen planus histopathologically but portions of a solar lentigo at the periphery of the infiltrate are often apparent
- Lichenoid keratoses usually develop on sun-exposed skin. Basal cell carcinoma or melanocytic nevus is often the clinical impression and typically they are solitary.

■ *Pitfalls*

- A largely regressed melanoma in situ may closely mimic lichen planus on rare occasions
- Differentiating between lichenoid keratosis and an actinic keratosis with a lichenoid infiltrate can be challenging in some cases.

Pearls

- The clinical history is usually that of a solitary lesion on sun-exposed skin with a clinical differential that includes basal cell carcinoma
- Finding portions of a solar lentigo or seborrheic keratosis at the periphery of the infiltrate is a clue to the diagnosis of lichenoid keratosis
- Extensive solar elastosis should prompt careful examination of the cytologic atypia to exclude the possibility that the lesion is actually a lichenoid actinic keratosis
- Histopathologic clues that favor lichenoid keratosis include parakeratosis that is irregular, patchy basilar pigmentation (since most LKs are regressing solar lentigos) and rete that vary in length and are bulbous (lentigo-like) rather than the regular, angular, "saw-tooth" acanthosis of lichen planus.

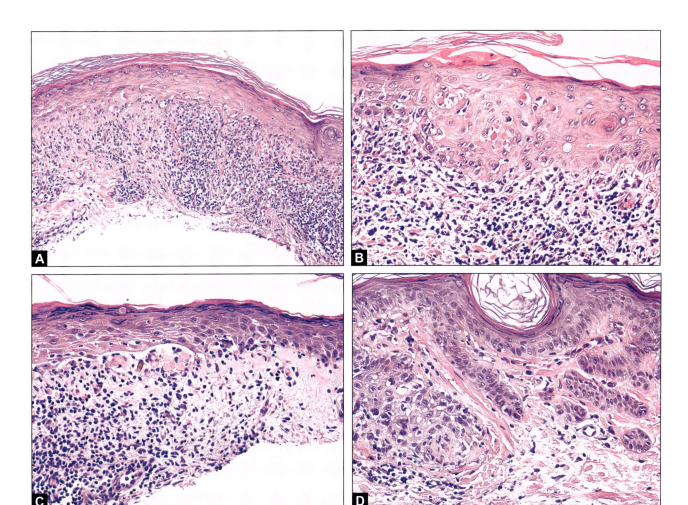

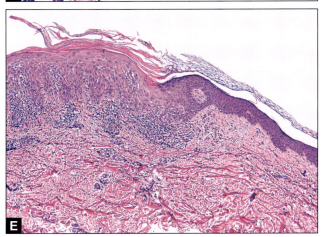

Figs 3.14A to E: Lichenoid keratosis. (A) There is a lichenoid interface infiltrate, necrotic keratinocytes and some angulated rete, features characteristic of lichen planus; (B) Unlike lichen planus, the stratum corneum of a lichenoid keratosis is often altered by areas of parakeratosis; (C) Colloid bodies are conspicuous; (D) In many instances, the remnants of a solar lentigo can be seen at the edge of the interface infiltrate; (E) The epidermal keratinocytes often have reactive atypia but pleomorphism and architectural disorder of the degree seen in actinic keratoses or squamous cell carcinomas should not be present.

Lichenoid Reactions to Neoplasms
(Figs 3.15A to D)

■ *Criteria for diagnosis*

- Lichenoid interface inflammation in combination with a neoplasm.

■ *Differential diagnosis*

- Neoplasms with lichenoid infiltrates most closely mimic lichenoid keratoses both clinically and histopathologically, but they may be mistaken for virtually any interface process.

■ *Pitfalls*

- Overlooking the evidence of potentially serious neoplasm, such as melanoma, is clearly the most significant danger; if there is any doubt, additional sections of a biopsy should be examined and immunohistochemical markers for melanoma may be helpful

- Regressing melanomas (and nevi) may develop "pseudonests", which are collections of melanocytes that form secondary to the necrosis of adjacent keratinocytes. Careful examination of the entire breadth of the lesion (and in some cases, multiple additional levels) may be necessary to differentiate these from the 'genuine' melanocytic nests of a nevus or melanoma.

■ *Pearls*

- Immunohistochemistry for melanocytic markers is helpful in excluding an occult melanoma or nevus; markers, such as microphthalmia-associated transcription factor, that targets nuclear antigens may be particularly helpful when attempting to identify melanocytes obscured by inflammation

- Colloid bodies are not reliable evidences that a lichenoid lesion is a lichenoid keratosis rather than a regressing nevus or melanoma; they may be seen in all of these conditions and in inflammatory conditions as well.

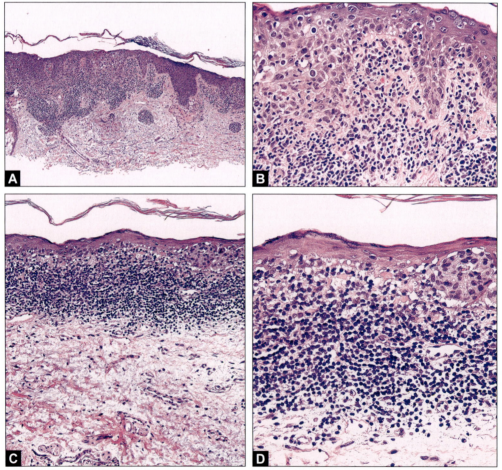

Figs 3.15A to D: Lichenoid actinic keratosis. (A) These may simulate lichenoid keratoses clinically and histopathologically; (B) The disordered maturation and keratinocyte pleomorphism are beyond the mild reactive atypia of a lichenoid keratosis; (C) Regressing melanoma. The dense lichenoid infiltrate obscures much of the regressing melanoma and simulates a lichenoid keratosis; (D) On close examination, a large nest of melanocytes is evident within the right side of the field. Additional sections of the biopsy revealed definitive evidence of melanoma.

Lichen Striatus (Figs 3.16A to C)

▮ *Criteria for diagnosis*

- A lichenoid interface infiltrate in conjunction with a clinical appearance of numerous tiny papules following the lines of Blaschko in a segmental distribution, most often in children.

▮ *Differential diagnosis*

- Clinically and histopathologically, linear lichen planus and inflammatory linear verrucous epidermal nevus (ILVEN) may simulate lichen striatus but lichen striatus is notorious for mimicking many inflammatory conditions and on occasion may even simulate mycosis fungoides.

▮ *Pitfalls*

- Clinical features of the lesions are crucial to diagnosis since histopathologic features vary.

▮ *Pearls*

- Lymphocytes within and around eccrine coils strongly favors lichen striatus over most other lichenoid disorders; the inflammation often surrounds follicular epithelium as well
- Parakeratosis and spongiosis favor lichen striatus over lichen planus and lichen nitidus
- Lichen striatus usually lacks the verrucous or psoriasiform epidermal hyperplasia of ILVEN.

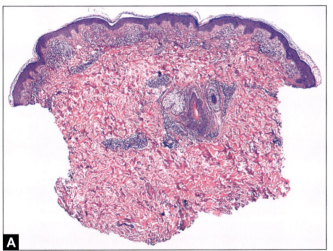

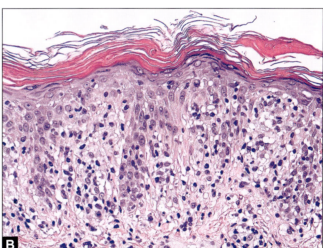

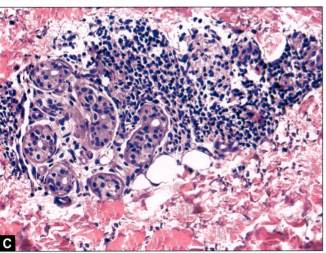

Figs 3.16A to C: Lichen striatus. (A) A lichenoid interface is present but inflammation is also evident within the deep dermis; (B) Spongiosis and dyskeratosis are sometimes features of lichen striatus. These features are rarely seen in lichen nitidus and lichen planus; (C) Inflammation around eccrine glands is particularly common in lichen striatus and is not seen in most of its histopathologic simulators.

Lichen Nitidus (Figs 3.17A to D)

■ *Criteria for diagnosis*

- A focal, circumscribed lichenoid interface infiltrate that confined to one or two dermal papillae in conjunction with a clinical appearance of numerous closely set flesh-colored papules of 1–2 mm in diameter
- Children and adolescents are most commonly involved; the distribution and extent are variable; genital skin and acral skin are most commonly involved.

■ *Differential diagnosis*

- Lichen planus, lichen striatus.

■ *Pitfalls*

- The characteristic 'ball-and-claw' is small and may be easily missed in an incompletely sectioned biopsy
- Occasionally, lichen striatus and lichen planus may very closely resemble lichen nitidus.

■ *Pearls*

- Serial sections should be considered if a biopsy of suspected lichen nitidus fails to show the characteristic histopathologic findings
- A lichenoid infiltrate containing macrophages, especially multinucleated giant cells is not a feature of lichen planus
- Unlike lichen striatus, the infiltrate in lichen nitidus does not involve the deeper dermis or eccrine coils
- The clinical appearance of lichen nitidus is quite distinctive and is rarely confused with either lichen planus or lichen striatus; rarely however, lichen nitidus and lichen planus appear concomitantly in the same patient.

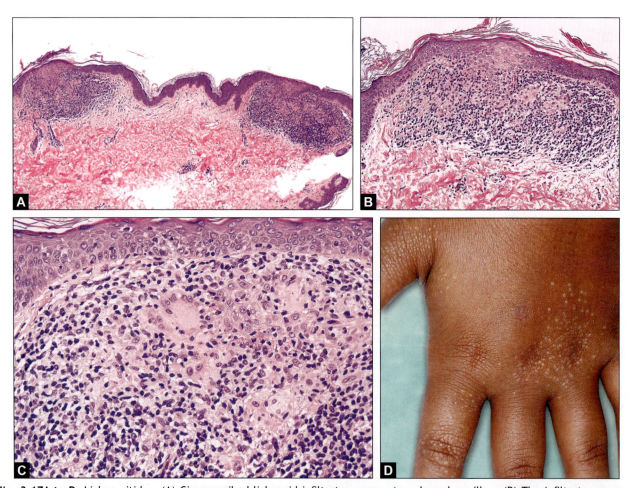

Figs 3.17A to D: Lichen nitidus. (A) Circumscribed lichenoid infiltrates occupy two dermal papillae; (B) The infiltrate appears to expand dermal papilla. The epidermal rete on either side may elongate forming a collarette around the aggregate (the so-called ball-and-claw sign); (C) In the early phases, lymphocytes predominate but in established lesions they are joined by macrophages including some that are multinucleated; (D) Closely set tiny flesh-colored papules are the characteristic clinical presentation.

Chronic Graft-Versus-Host Disease* (GVHD) (Figs 3.18A to C)

*See discussion of acute GVHD above.

■ Criteria for diagnosis

- An interface dermatitis, usually lichenoid type that typically evolves more than 100 days after bone marrow transplantation
- Interface inflammatory infiltrate, usually of the lichenoid type, typically evolving more than 30 days after transplantation with a predilection for distal extremities and hyperpigmentation.

■ Differential diagnosis

- Lichenoid drug eruptions, lichen planus and rarely, viral exanthems may be identical to chronic GVHD histopathologically.

■ Pitfalls

- Chronic GVHD cannot be reliably distinguished from lichenoid drug eruptions and viral exanthems and without clinical information, and definitive diagnosis is rarely possible since many patients with GVHD are on medications and may be at increased risk of viral infections
- Histopathologic grading may not correlate with clinical severity.

■ Pearls

- The lichenoid infiltrate of GVHD is more likely to contain eosinophils and plasma cells than lichen planus
- Elevated bilirubin and alkaline phosphatase levels are often present in GVHD.

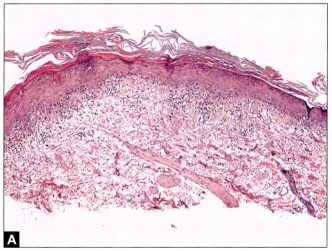

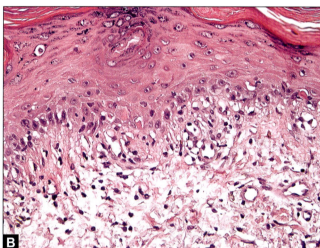

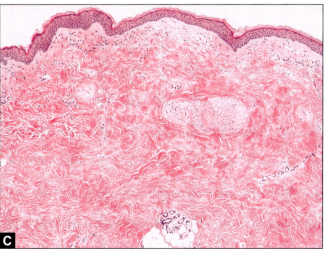

Figs 3.18A to C: Chronic graft-versus-host disease. (A) By comparison to the acute phase, the infiltrate of chronic graft-versus-host disease is typically lichenoid rather than vacuolar; (B) In this established lesion, the lichenoid infiltrate and epidermal hyperplasia are virtually identical to lichen planus; (C) In some cases, a morphea/scleroderma appearance eventually evolves ("sclerodermoid graft-versus-host disease").

Porokeratosis (Figs 3.19A to C)

■ *Criteria for diagnosis*

- An epidermis containing one or more cornoid lamella in association with a clinical history of a pink papule with a collarette of scale
- Keratinocyte atypia may or may not be present. When evident, it is usually of the degree seen in early actinic keratosis.

■ *Differential diagnosis*

- Actinic keratosis, lichenoid keratosis.

■ *Pitfalls*

- Cornoid lamella is often focal; examination of additional levels may be necessary to identify them, they may not be sampled in narrow shave biopsies
- Cornoid lamella may vary greatly in appearance

- Epidermal "dysplasia" and squamous cell carcinoma may develop in porokeratosis
- Specifying the variant of porokeratosis cannot be done on histopathologic grounds and requires clinical correlation.

■ *Pearls*

- Well formed cornoid lamella is nearly pathognomonic of porokeratosis.

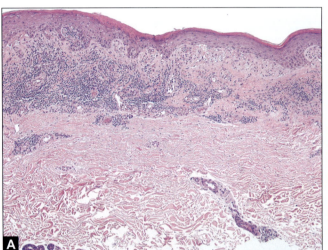
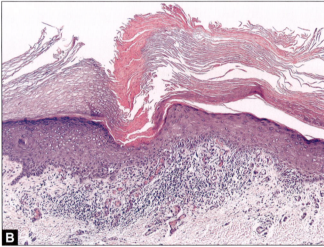
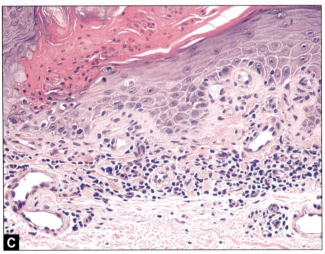

Figs 3.19A to C: Porokeratosis. (A) In some sections, the features may be a nonspecific lichenoid interface infiltrate; (B) However, other sections show angled parakeratotic tiers overlying a granular cell layer that is diminished or absent; cornoid lamella that are the key to identifying porokeratosis; (C) The changes can also simulate actinic keratoses and cornoid lamella-like structures may occasionally be seen in actinic keratoses. The distribution and clinical appearance usually differentiates the two, however.

Paraneoplastic Pemphigus (Figs 3.20A and B)

Criteria for diagnosis

- An interface infiltrate, sometimes with intraepidermal acantholysis and/or subepidermal clefting within the clinical context of hemorrhagic oral erosions along with cutaneous erosion or lichen planus-like papules.

Differential diagnosis

- Histopathologically and clinically paraneoplastic pemphigus may closely resemble EM, however, the differential diagnosis is broad and includes many interface disorders.

Pitfalls

- Paraneoplastic pemphigus may closely mimic EM both clinically and histopathologically
- Immunofluorescence studies are necessary to confirm the diagnosis.

Pearls

- The infiltrate in paraneoplastic pemphigus is often of greater density than that of EM
- Most common associations are hematologic malignancies, thymomas and Castleman's disease but can occur in association with virtually any malignancy.

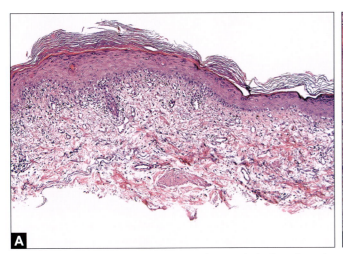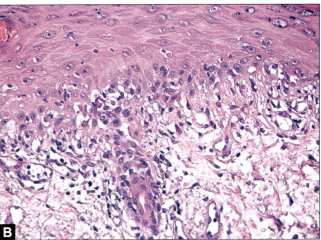

Figs 3.20A and B: Paraneoplastic pemphigus. (A) An interface dermatitis, usually of the lichenoid type is characteristic; (B) Necrotic keratinocytes may be seen. Intraepidermal acantholysis and subepidermal blister formation may sometimes occur, but interface dermatitis is probably the most common manifestation.

Lichenoid Pigmented Purpuric Eruption (Gougerot and Blum) (Figs 3.21A and B)

▪ *Criteria for diagnosis*

- An interface infiltrate accompanied by perivascular inflammation and extravasation of erythrocytes (but no leukocytoclastic vasculitis) in the clinical context of erythematous patches and bronze pigmentation typical of pigmented purpuric dermatitis.

▪ *Differential diagnosis*

- Other variants of pigmented purpuric dermatitis, pityriasis lichenoides, other types of "lymphocytic vasculitis"; some forms of mycosis fungoides.

▪ *Pitfalls*

- Extravasated erythrocytes may be focal and therefore easily missed in early lesions
- Early lesions of pityriasis lichenoides may exhibit extensive overlapping features histopathologically.

▪ *Pearls*

- Lichenoid pigmented purpura can usually be distinguished from pityriasis lichenoides chronic on clinical examination.

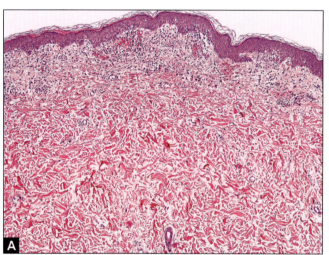 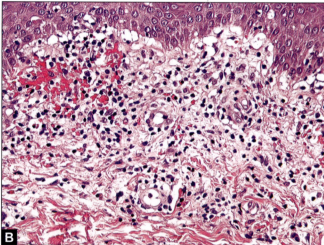

Figs 3.21A and B: Lichenoid pigmented purpuric eruption. (A) An interface infiltrate is present along with multiple foci of hemorrhage; (B) The extravasated erythrocytes are admixed with lymphocytes within the papillary dermis. The infiltrate does not usually involve the deeper dermis.

Lichen Sclerosus (Figs 3.22A and B)

■ *Criteria for diagnosis*

- An interface infiltrate accompanied by sclerosis/homogenization of dermal collagen that is loose and edematous appearing at first, with gradual evolution into hyalinized-appearing sclerotic collagen; clinical features that include erythematous plaques of variable size and distribution that eventually develop white centers.

■ *Differential diagnosis*

- Lupus erythematosus; chronic radiation dermatitis; morphea/scleroderma.

■ *Pitfalls*

- Early lesions (or the advancing border of established lesions) may not show the characteristic collagen homogenization

- Despite the formerly used term (lichen sclerosus et atrophicus), epidermal atrophy is variable and the epidermis may be of normal thickness, especially in early lesions
- Some cases may be indistinguishable from morphea/scleroderma and cases with overlapping features occasionally occur.

■ *Pearls*

- Chronic radiation dermatitis generally lacks an interface infiltrate and contains atypical fibroblasts and endothelial cells, which are not seen in lichen sclerosus
- In general, the sclerosing fibrosis of lichen sclerosus is initially most prominent within the papillary dermis, while that of morphea/scleroderma involves the reticular dermis.

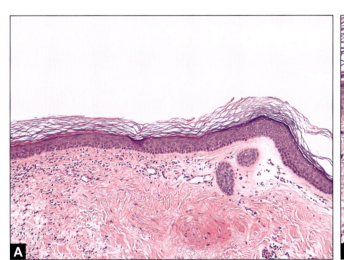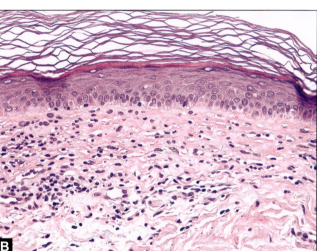

Figs 3.22A and B: Lichen sclerosus. (A) The interface infiltrate does not have distinctive qualities but careful examination will usually reveal the characteristic sclerosis of papillary dermal collagen (right side of the field); (B) In early lesions or at the advancing border of a lesion, the interface inflammatory infiltrate may lack any specific features but there may be some subtle homogenization of the papillary dermal collagen.

THE PITYRIASIFORM PATTERN

The pityriasiform pattern is a third subtype in which there is an interface infiltrate along with exocytosis of lymphocytes into the middle and upper epidermis, focal epidermal spongiosis accompanied by zones of parakeratosis and (sometimes) extravasated red blood cells (see Fig. 3.3). Because spongiosis and psoriasiform hyperplasia may be present, some classify pityriasiform disorders as spongiotic rather than interface. Regardless of the category in which one chooses to place it, its recognition may narrow a differential diagnosis considerably in certain instances (Box 3.3).

Box 3.3: Diseases frequently exhibiting the pityriasiform pattern

- Pityriasis lichenoides
  - Pityriasis lichenoides chronica
  - Pityriasis lichenoides et varioliform acuta
- Pityriasis rosea (late-stage lesions)
- Erythema annulare centrifugum
- Pityriasiform drug eruption
- Secondary syphilis
- Dermatophytosis
- Mycosis fungoides

Pityriasis Lichenoides Chronica (Figs 3.23A to D)

■ *Criteria for diagnosis*

- Interface dermatitis, usually with pityriasiform features (focal spongiosis with exocytosis of lymphocytes, parakeratotic scale, and extravasated erythrocytes) with clinical features including chronic, generalized, small, crusted papules that resolve with postinflammatory pigmentary alteration.

■ *Differential diagnosis*

- Other pityriasiform disorders, especially pityriasis rosea and syphilis, connective tissue diseases, drug eruptions, viral exanthems, pigmented purpuric dermatitis, parapsoriasis, mycosis fungoides and guttate psoriasis.

■ *Pitfalls*

- In some cases, spongiosis is minimal and the findings may closely simulate mycosis fungoides.

■ *Pearls*

- Pityriasis rosea is usually very distinct from pityriasis lichenoides clinically and typically shows more spongiosis and lacks the compact confluent parakeratosis of PLC
- Pityriasis lichenoides chronica may overlap with pityriasis lichenoides et varioliformis acuta (PLEVA) both clinically and histopathologically.

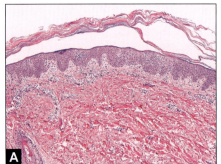
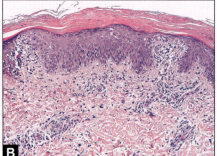
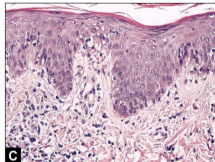
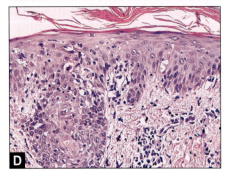

Figs 3.23A to D: Pityriaisis lichenoides chronica. (A) There is exocytosis along with broad zones of hyperkeratosis; (B) Close inspection typically reveals vacuolar interface change in addition to exocytosis that is sometimes focal, as it is here (resembling pityriasis rosea); (C) Exocytosis of lymphocytes may be extensive and is often accompanied by extravasated erythrocytes; (D) Necrotic keratinocytes often accompany the vacuolar change.

Pityriasis Lichenoides et Varioliformis Acuta (Figs 3.24A to C)

▪ *Criteria for diagnosis*

- Interface dermatitis, usually with pityriasiform features (focal spongiosis with exocytosis of lymphocytes, parakeratotic scale and extravasated erythrocytes) and necrotic epidermal keratinocytes.

▪ *Differential diagnosis*

- Other pityriasiform disorders, especially pityriasis rosea and lymphomatoid papulosis (LyP).

▪ *Pitfalls*

- Lymphomatoid papulosis has some overlapping clinical and histopathologic features; it is characterized by an infiltrate containing CD30+ cells but these cells may be present in PLEVA and many other inflammatory conditions as well.

▪ *Pearls*

- Lymphomatoid papulosis typically contains numerous large, "transformed-appearing" lymphocytes that express CD30; PLEVA may also contain similar cells but typically not in the numbers seen in LyP
- Pityriasis lichenoides chronica may overlap with PLEVA both clinically and histopathologically and many authors consider them to represent a continuum of the same disorder.

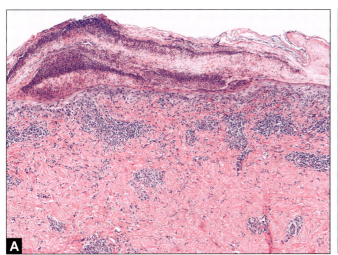
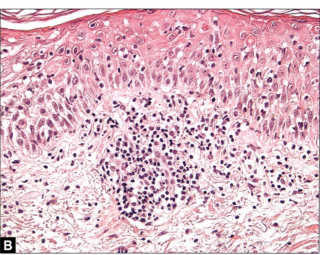
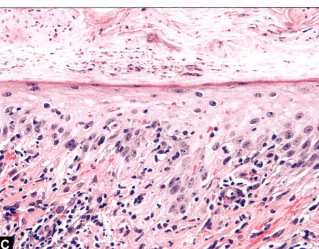

Figs 3.24A to C: Pityriasis lichenoides et varioliform acuta. (A) An interface infiltrate with perivascular involvement is common, and the stratum corneum is often occupied by necroinflammatory debris in established lesions; (B) As with other pityriasiform diseases, exocytosis of lymphocytes is typical and necrotic keratinocytes are characteristic; (C) Erythrocytes may also extend into the epidermis. Note again the necrotic keratinocytes.

THE INTERFACE AND PERIVASCULAR/ PERIADNEXAL PATTERN

Any of the patterns described above may be accompanied by an inflammatory cell infiltrate around blood vessels and/or adnexal structures within the reticular dermis. This can be called the interface and perivascular/periadnexal pattern (see Fig. 3.4). The infiltrate may surround only the vessels of the superficial dermis or it may be both superficial and deep. The diseases that exhibit the interface and perivascular/periadnexal pattern are shown in Box 3.4.

> **Box 3.4: Diseases frequently exhibiting the interface and perivascular/periadnexal pattern**
>
> - Lupus erythematosus (especially the discoid and subacute forms)
> - Polymorphous light eruption
> - Phototoxic dermatitis
> - Lichen striatus
> - Pernio
> - Arthropod bite reaction
> - Erythema migrans (Borreliosis/Lyme disease)
> - Secondary syphilis
> - Erythema annulare centrifugum
> - Drug eruptions

Discoid Lupus Erythematosus (Figs 3.25A to E)

■ *Criteria for diagnosis*

- Interface inflammation (lichenoid or vacuolar in type), often with inflammatory cells around adnexa and vessels within the deep dermis, and clinical findings of DLE, typically well-demarcated erythematous scaly plaques with hyperpigmented borders and central atrophy, depigmentation and alopecia.

■ *Differential diagnosis*

- Other forms of lupus erythematosus, particularly SCLE; lupus-like drug eruption.

■ *Pitfalls*

- As mentioned previously, the histopathologic features of lupus erythematosus do not necessarily correlate with the clinical features
- In rare cases, epidermal hypertrophy may be so severe as to mimic squamous cell carcinoma; rarely, carcinoma may develop in lesions of DLE.

■ *Pearls*

- Other than on the face, necrotic keratinocytes are usually more numerous than in other forms of lupus and dermatomyositis
- Hypertrophic DLE may present with marked epidermal hyperplasia, including verrucous hyperplasia (verrucous DLE).

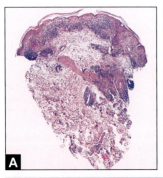
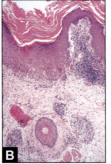
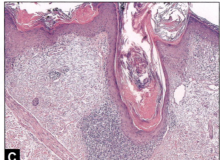
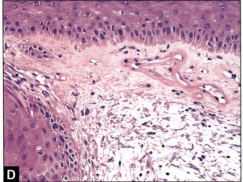
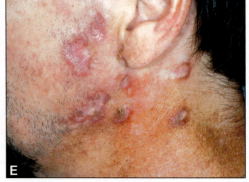

Figs 3.25A to E: Discoid lupus erythematosus. (A) The presence of interface inflammation is usually accompanied by perifollicular and perivascular infiltrates; (B) Except for lesions on the face, which may resemble SLE or SCLE, DLE often exhibits epidermal hyperplasia and hyperkeratosis; (C) Dense perifollicular inflammation and follicular hyperkeratosis (follicular plugging) are characteristic features; (D) The prolonged interface inflammation may produce an apparent thickening or hyalinization of the basement membrane zone; (E) Well-demarcated erythematous scaly plaques with hyperpigmented borders are the most common clinical findings.

Secondary Syphilis (Figs 3.26A to C)

■ *Criteria for diagnosis*

- Interface, pityriasiform or interface and perivascular infiltrates, typically lymphocytes with many plasma cells but also other inflammatory cells types, including macrophages
- Numerous clinical manifestations; often pink scaly patches resembling pityriasis rosea (common clinical differential diagnosis); some cases may show pink papules with collarettes of scale; condylomata lata appear as grayish moist papules or nodules on the genital mucosa.

■ *Differential diagnosis*

- Pityriasis lichenoides, mycosis fungoides, Borreliosis and many other inflammatory conditions.

■ *Pitfalls*

- The histopathologic appearance is so variable that the histopathologic differential diagnosis is quite broad and includes entities that exhibit the psoriasiform, interface and nodular/diffuse patterns, among others.

■ *Pearls*

- Epidermal hyperplasia (often somewhat psoriasiform) with a dense lichenoid infiltrate that includes plasma cells, macrophages, eosinophils and neutrophils should raise strong suspicion for secondary syphilis
- Serologic tests, such as the rapid plasma reagin assay, Venereal Disease Research Laboratory and fluorescent treponemal antibody absorption remain the gold standard for the confirmation of diagnosis
- Immunohistochemical stains specific for Treponema pallidum are now commercially available and allow identification of the spirochetes in many cases.

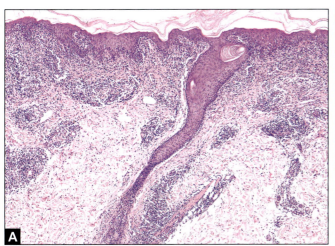

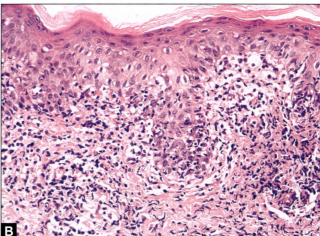

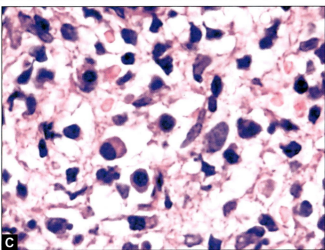

Figs 3.26A to C: Secondary syphilis. (A) A variably dense interface dermatitis is typically present, but dermal inflammation is usually heavy as well; (B) There is often exocytosis of lymphocytes and erythrocytes into the epidermis in a manner similar to pityriasis lichenoides. Epidermal hyperplasia may be evident and is sometimes psoriasiform; (C) Plasma cells are usually a prominent component of the inflammatory infiltrate.

Pernio (Figs 3.27A to D)

Criteria for diagnosis

- Papillary dermal edema and interface and perivascular infiltrate, sometimes with blistering, erosion or ulceration. Clinical features include red to purple macules or papules on acral skin (especially the dorsal surfaces of the toes) following exposure to cold and damp conditions.

Differential diagnosis

- Polymorphous light eruption, lupus erythematosus (particularly DLE and chilblain lupus), lichen striatus.

Pitfalls

- Chilblain lupus may be impossible to differentiate from pernio histopathologically.

Pearls

- Since fingers and toes are most commonly affected, papillary dermal edema with an interface and perivascular infiltrate on acral skin should always raise the possibility of pernio, particularly in cold damp climates
- Clinical history is required to differentiate pernio from chilblain lupus erythematosus.

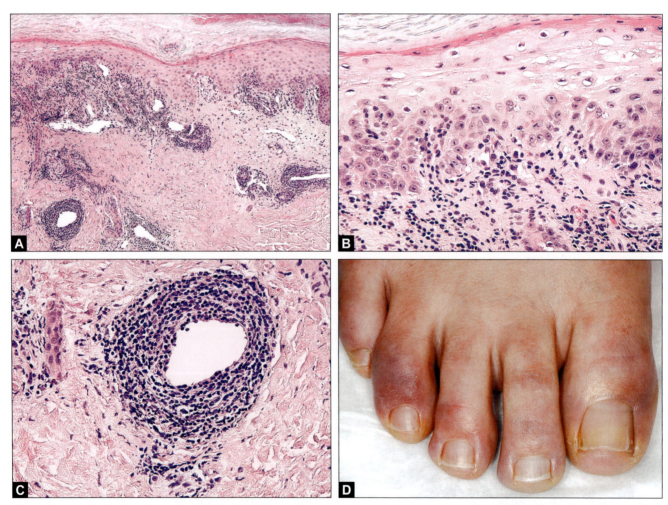

Figs 3.27A to D: Pernio. (A) A superficial and deep perivascular lymphocytic infiltrate predominates. The inflammation may be prominent around eccrine coils as well. Edema of the papillary dermis is common in established lesions; (B) Although subtle, interface change is often present; (C) Dermal vessels may show a dense transmural lymphocytic infiltrate; (D) The most common clinical presentation is red to purple macules or papules on acral skin (especially the dorsal surfaces of the toes) following exposure to cold and damp conditions.

■ Criteria for diagnosis

- If the annular border is sampled, a superficial and deep perivascular infiltrate composed primarily of lymphocytes with rare plasma cells, is characteristic; biopsies from skin within the vicinity of the tick bite will demonstrate spongiosis, variable epidermal necrosis (and sometimes tick mouth parts) and a mixed infiltrate including eosinophils (typical of an arthropod bite reaction).

■ Differential diagnosis

- Erythema annulare centrifugum (particularly the so-called "deep variant" that lacks epidermal involvement); tumid lupus erythematosus, drug eruptions (which may also contain plasma cells), other superficial and deep perivascular processes.

■ Pitfalls

- As noted, the features may vary dramatically depending on where a lesion is biopsied
- Stains for microorganisms (such as, Warthin-Starry and Steiner preparations) may occasionally allow identification of Borrelia burgdorferi within biopsies, but an absence of their detection does not exclude the diagnosis, and care must be taken not to overinterpret these stains.

■ Pearls

- Serologic tests (i.e. serum titers of antibodies to B. burgdorferi) are usually necessary for definitive diagnosis
- The lack of dermal mucin can help differentiate it from tumid lupus erythematosus in many cases.

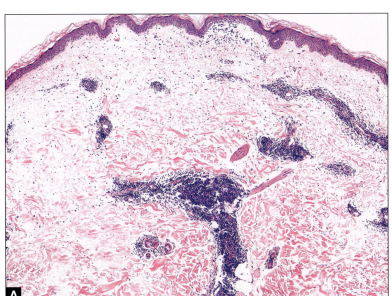

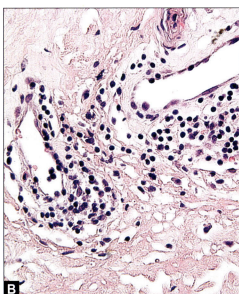

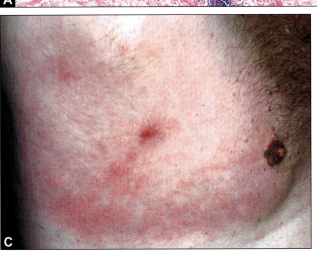

Figs 3.28A to C: Erythema migrans. (A) Inflammation is usually most conspicuous around the dermal vasculature. Interface change is often absent but occasionally a small focus, such as that depicted here, is evident; (B) The infiltrate is usually sparse and composed predominantly of lymphocytes. The lack of dermal mucin can help differentiate it from tumid lupus erythematosus in many cases. Plasma cells are often identified if sought, but they are not present to the degree that is typically seen in secondary syphilis; (C) An expanding annular patch is the characteristic clinical feature. In this lesion, the central tick bite site is evident.

Chronic Actinic Dermatitis/Actinic Reticuloid (Figs 3.29A to D)

■ *Criteria for diagnosis*

- Spongiotic, interface and/or superficial and deep perivascular inflammation within the clinical context of lesions exacerbated by light exposure.

■ *Differential diagnosis*

- Neurodermatitis or other nonspecific forms of dermatitis may enter the differential of most forms of phototoxic dermatitis
- Actinic reticuloid may be mistaken for other forms of interface dermatitis and mycosis fungoides; it shares features of mycosis fungoides both clinically and histopathologically.

■ *Pitfalls*

- Pruritus is common in photodermatitis and excoriation or prurigo changes may dominate the histopathologic picture in some cases

- The histopathologic and clinical features of actinic reticuloid may overlap extensively with mycosis fungoides or other types of cutaneous T-cell lymphoma.

■ *Pearls*

- The intraepidermal lymphocytes in actinic reticuloid (chronic actinic dermatitis) are predominantly CD8+, while in most cases (but not all) of mycosis fungoides, CD4+ cells predominate
- Clinical history is necessary to establish these diagnoses.

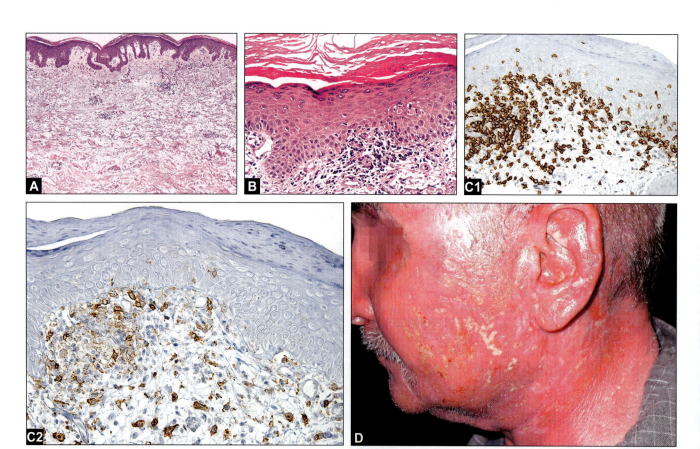

Figs 3.29A to D: Chronic actinic dermatitis. (A) Chronic photosensitivity occasionally occurs in the absence of a recognizable sensitizer or may persist after discontinuation of a suspected photosensitizer. The histopathologic features vary but often a sparse interface/superficial and deep perivascular infiltrate is present; (B) Actinic reticuloid. A more significant lichenoid interface dermatitis is present in some forms of chronic actinic dermatitis and this variant is often referred to as actinic reticuloid. Exocytosis is prominent in some cases and the condition may closely mimic mycosis fungoides histopathologically and clinically; (C) The lymphocytic population in actinic reticuloid often contains an increased number of T-cells expressing CD8 (a) as compared to those expressing CD4 (b). The opposite is true; (D) In this severe case, erythroderma has developed.

Other Conditions with an Interface Pattern

Mycosis Fungoides

Figures 3.30A to C show mycosis fungoides.

(See Chapter 15 for additional details about mycosis fungoides and other lymphomas that may exhibit an interface pattern)

Lichen Amyloidosis

Figure 3.31 shows lichen amyloidosis.

(See Chapters 1 and 10 for additional images of lichen amyloidosis)

Interface/Lichenoid Reactions to Tattoo

Figures 3.32A and B show interface/lichenoid reactions to tattoo.

Polymorphous Light Eruption

Figures 3.33A and B show polymorphous light eruption (PMLE).

(See Chapter 2 for additional images of PMLE)

Dermatophytosis/Tinea

Figures 3.34A and B show dermatophytosis/tinea.

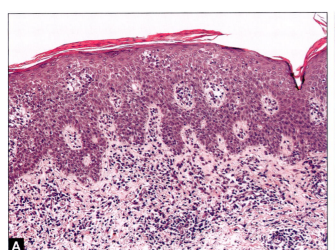

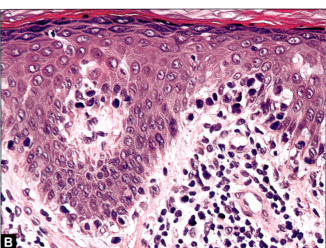

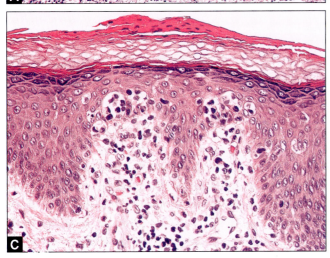

Figs 3.30A to C: Mycosis fungoides. (A) Frequently exhibits an interface pattern, especially in early patch and plaque stage lesions, and can be very difficult to differentiate from other interface disorders; (B) Careful examination may provide clues to the diagnosis, such as intraepidermal lymphocytes, that are larger than those in the underlying dermis; (C) Pautrier microabscess formation is one of the most specific features of mycosis fungoides but is relatively uncommon, especially in early lesions.

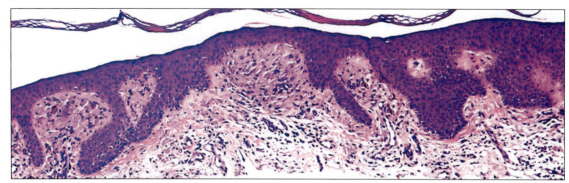

Fig. 3.31: Lichen amyloidosis. While the first impression is often that of the normal skin pattern or a depositional disorder, occasionally lichen amyloidosis and macular amyloidosis present with patchy inflammation in the papillary dermis and dermoepidermal junction.

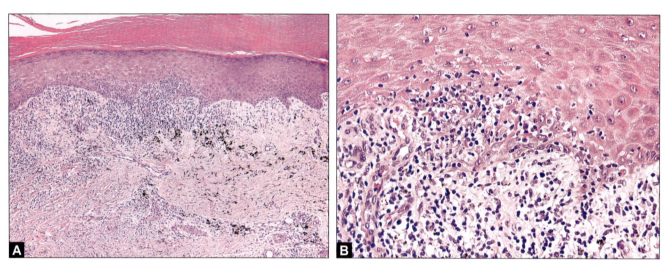

Figs 3.32A and B: Interface/lichenoid reactions to tattoo. (A) An interface reaction, usually of the lichenoid type is not an uncommon response to tattoos; (B) The features resemble lichen planus, but obvious exogenous pigment is evident in the dermis.

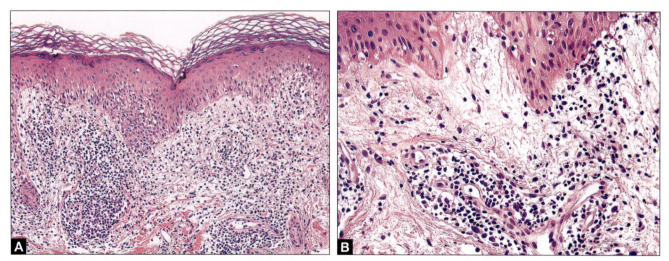

Figs 3.33A and B: Polymorphous light eruption. (A) May be confused with other conditions that have an interface and perivascular inflammation in cases with less spongiosis and edema; (B) The characteristic edema and spongiosis are usually evident in at least some foci within a given sample, however.

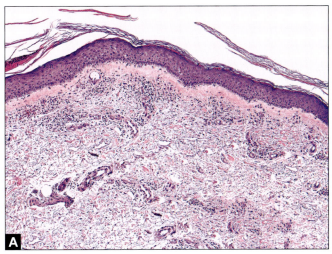 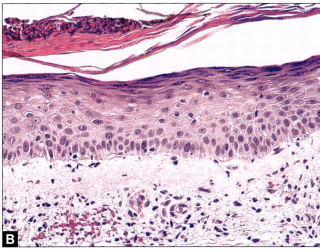

Figs 3.34A and B: Dermatophytosis/tinea. (A) Occasionally, the inflammatory cell infiltrate in dermatophytosis may have a predominantly interface distribution; (B) There is subtle vacuolar change but the parakeratotic scale containing neutrophils should always prompt the consideration of dermatophytosis/tinea.

BIBLIOGRAPHY

1. Ackerman AB, Guo A, Vitale PA. Clues to diagnosis in Dermatopathology II. Hong Kong: ASCP Press; 1992.
2. Crowson AN, Magro CM, Mihm MC. Interface Dermatitis. Arch Pathol Lab Med. 2008;132:652-66.
3. Farmer ER, Hood AF. Pathology of the Skin, 2nd edition. New York: McGraw-Hill USA. 2000. pp. 611-33.
4. French LE. Toxic epidermal necrolysis and Stevens Johnson syndrome: our current understanding. Allergo Int. 2006; 55:9-16.
5. Gravante C, Delogu D, Marianetti M, et al. Toxic epidermal necrolysis and Stevens Johnson syndrome: 11 years experience and outcome. Eur Rev Med Pharmacol Sci. 2007;11:119-27.
6. Helm KF, Peters MS. Deposition of membrane attack complex in cutaneous lesions of lupus erythematosus. J Am Acad Dermatol. 1993;28:687-91.
7. Horn TD. Interface Dermatitis. In: Barnhill RL, Crowson AN (Eds). Textbook of Dermatopathology, 2nd edition. New York: McGraw-Hill Companies; 2004. pp. 35-60.
8. Jerdan MS, Hood AF, Moore GW, et al. Histopathologic comparison of the subsets of lupus erythematosus. Arch Dermatol. 1990;126:52-5.
9. Magro CM, Morrison C, Kovatich A, et al. Pityriasis Lichenoides is a Cutaneous T-Cell Dyscrasia: a clinical, genotypic, and phenotypic study. Hum Pathol. 2002;33:788-95.
10. McKee PH, Calonje E, Granter SR. Pathology of the skin with clinical correlations. Mosby: Elsevier; 2005.
11. Ragaz A, Ackerman AB. Evolution, maturation, and regression of lesions of lichen planus. New observations and correlations of clinical and histologic findings. Am J Dermatopathol. 1981;3:5-25.
12. Weedon D. Weedon's Skin Pathology, 3rd edition. Churchill Livingstone: Elsevier; 2010.

CHAPTER 4

The Blistering and Acantholytic Patterns

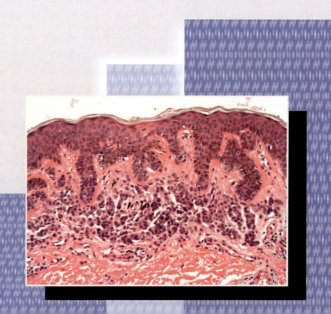

INTRODUCTION

Like most of the other reaction patterns of the skin, blistering and acantholyis of the epidermis may have a wide array of etiologies, ranging from congenital diseases (Hailey-Hailey disease) to autoimmune disorders (bullous pemphigoid) to infections (herpes virus). The clinical history (if supplied) usually allows the differential to be narrowed substantially, but the authors advise adhering to the pattern analysis method and considering the full spectrum of processes that can produce these findings histopathologically before attempting to correlate with the clinical information.

In order to narrow the differential diagnosis, blistering diseases can be subclassified by first identifying the apparent mechanism and then the histologic plane of separation (Table 4.1).

- Severe spongiosis may cause intraepidermal blistering as a result of intercellular edema that becomes so pronounced that it separates keratinocytes, a common example being contact dermatitis (Fig. 4.1A)
- Ballooning degeneration may appear similar at first except that the edema is intracellular and the blister develops as a result of cell death. Herpes virus infection often causes this type of blister formation (Fig. 4.1B)
- Acantholysis is loss of keratinocyte cell adhesion (in the absence of pronounced spongiosis). Hailey-Hailey disease, Darier's disease and pemphigus vulgaris are the best examples of this phenomenon (Fig. 4.1C)
- Basal layer keratinocyte destruction by an interface inflammatory infiltrate is a common cause of blister formation that may be encountered with virtually any interface dermatosis, including lichen planus and erythema multiforme (EM) (Fig. 4.1D)
- Basement membrane zone destruction is the hallmark of the subepidermal blistering diseases, most commonly epidermolysis bullosa acquisita (EBA) and bullous pemphigoid (Fig. 4.1E)
- Finally, destruction of papillary dermal structural components (dermolysis) may lead to blister formation.

Examples include blisters over scars, bullous amyloidosis and bullous lichen sclerosis (Fig. 4.1F).

While it is not always possible to determine the exact mechanism by light microscopy, this is the first step in narrowing the differential diagnosis.

At the same time, the histologic plane of separation should be assessed. In general, this is best accomplished by distinguishing between intraepidermal and subepidermal blistering. Intraepidermal blisters may then be subclassified by whether they are primarily intracorneal or subcorneal, intraepidermal or suprabasilar.

Finally, no blistering disease can be diagnosed definitively without clinical correlation. Clinical clues to diagnosis include the following:

- *Site and distribution of the lesions*: For example, Hailey-Hailey disease usually affects intertriginous areas, while Darier's disease has a predilection for the face, postauricular area, scalp, chest and back (the "seborrheic" distribution)
- *Arrangement of the blisters*: Grouped blisters are typical of dermatitis herpetiformis, while those of immunoglobulin A (IgA) bullous dermatosis commonly have an annular pattern
- *Presence of inflammation*: Bullous pemphigoid blisters usually have an erythematous base. Epidermolysis bullosa acquisita and porphyria cutanea tarda typically occur on noninflamed skin
- *Age*: Bullous pemphigoid has a marked predilection for the elderly, while EBA tends to occur in middle-aged adults
- *Medical history*: If the patient has a known malignancy, paraneoplastic pemphigus becomes a consideration. If the eruption has occurred after a new medication has been started, one must consider pseudoporphyria, drug-induced IgA bullous dermatosis or drug-induced pemphigus.

Table 4.1: Mechanisms of blistering diseases		
Category	*Mechanism*	*Diseases*
Spongiotic	Intercellular edema	Contact dermatitis
Ballooning degeneration	Intracellular edema	Herpes virus infections
Acantholysis	Loss of cell adhesion due to desmosome destruction (autoimmune-mediated or direct damage)	Pemphigus
		Darier's disease
		Hailey-Hailey disease
		Staphylococcal scalded skin syndrome
		Bullous impetigo
		Bullous tinea

Contd...

Category	Mechanism	Diseases
Basal layer keratinocyte damage	Basal layer keratinocyte destruction by an interface inflammatory infiltrate	Bullous erythema multiforme
		Bullous lichen planus
Basement membrane zone damage		Bullous pemphigoid
		Epidermolysis bullosa acquisita
Dermolysis	Destruction of papillary dermal structural components	Bullous lichen sclerosus
		Bullous amyloidosis
		Blisters over scars
		Bullous leukocytoclastic vasculitis

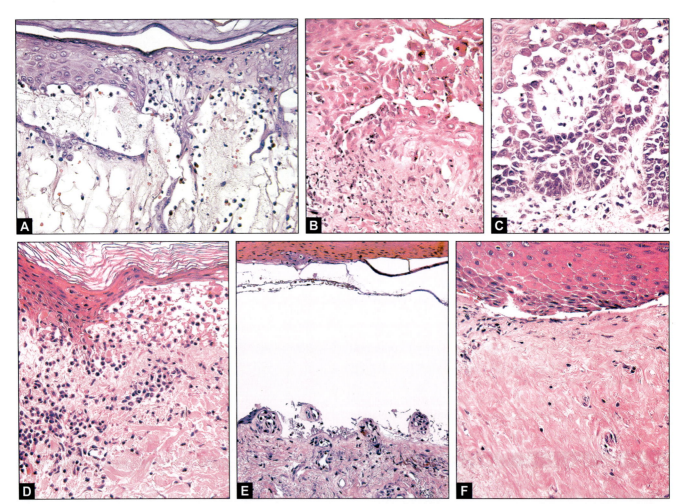

Figs 4.1A to F: (A) In this case of acute contact dermatitis, severe edema and spongiosis has produced vesiculation and blister formation; (B) Ballooning degeneration in herpes virus infection. There is acantholysis in the center of the blister, but also note that the enlarged cells with pale cytoplasm at the periphery; (C) Acantholysis in a case of Hailey-Hailey disease; (D) Blister formation as a result of severe interface damage in a case of bullous erythema multiforme; (E) This subepidermal blister in a case of epidermolysis bullosa acquisita is the result of basement membrane zone destruction; (F) In this severe case of lichen sclerosus, blisters have developed over areas of extreme dermal sclerosis.

Impetigo and Bullous Impetigo (Figs 4.2A to C)

■ *Criteria for diagnosis*

- Shallow erosions with honey colored crusts, occasionally with pustules (intact blisters rare)
- Subcorneal neutrophils with focal acantholysis
- Bacteria (Gram-positive cocci) may be identified in stratum corneum by Gram stain but are often absent (and are not required for diagnosis).

■ *Differential diagnosis*

- Secondarily impetiginized spongiotic dermatitis
- Staphylococcal scalded skin syndrome (SSSS).

■ *Pitfalls*

- Despite the name, 'bullae' are rarely seen in bullous impetigo since their superficial location makes them prone to excoriation and rupture.

■ *Pearls*

- Impetigo can occur in almost any anatomic site and age group
- Vast majority of bullous cases occur in infants and children
- Face is the most common site but may also involve buttocks, trunk and perineum
- Intact blisters (seen only occasionally) are flaccid and contain clear yellow fluid that becomes dark and turbid
- Lesions may resolve spontaneously or ulcerate (ecthyma)
- "Secondary" impetigo may occur in any dermatitis, particularly eczematous dermatitis, especially excoriated atopic dermatitis
- Conventional impetigo is usually caused by group A *streptococci*
- Bullous impetigo is almost invariably caused by *Staphylococcus aureus* phage group 2 type 71 [the same organism responsible for SSSS; (Figs 4.3A to C)].

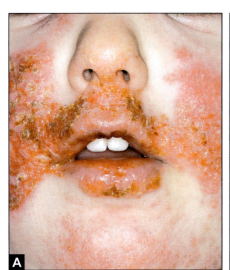 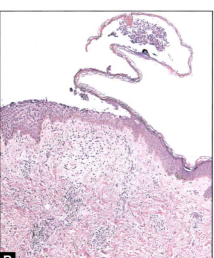 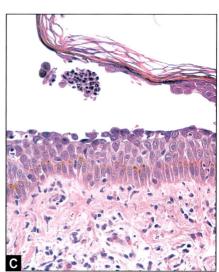

Figs 4.2A to C: Impetigo. (A) Eroded pink patches with "honey-colored" crusts appeared on the cheeks of this patient with atopic dermatitis; Bullous impetigo. (B) Acantholysis within the granular cell layer has produced this blister. An intact blister "roof" such as this is rarely present; (C) Collections of neutrophils are present in the blister cavity.

Staphylococcal Scalded Skin Syndrome
(Figs 4.3A to C)

■ *Criteria for diagnosis*

- Tender erythematous orange-tinted rash evolving to desquamating patches involving intertriginous and periorificial skin in an ill-appearing infant or child (fewer than 50 cases have occurred in adults)
- Subcorneal collections of neutrophils with minimal acantholysis and no dyskeratosis; only sparse dermal inflammation.

■ *Differential diagnosis*

- Impetigo
- Bullous tinea/dermatophytosis.

■ *Pitfalls*

- Fully evolved lesions may develop neutrophilic infiltrates creating an appearance that is histopathologically indistinguishable from impetigo
- Bacteria are almost never identified within biopsy specimens.

■ *Pearls*

- Most common in young children or adults with renal disease
- Staphylococci infection by group II phage type 71 is the most common cause
- Staphylococci produce toxins that destroy desmoglein 1
- Toxins disseminate systemically, but the bacteria often remain localized to the site of infection, thus cultures of skin lesions are usually negative for staphylococcus organisms and organisms are almost never seen within biopsies
- Most adults have antibodies that neutralize the toxins and therefore rapidly clear them; neonates and infants lack these antibodies.

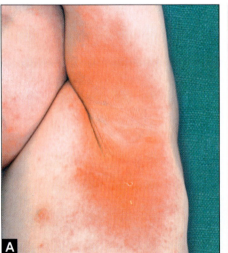

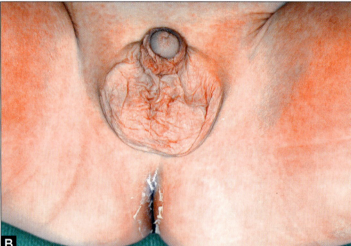

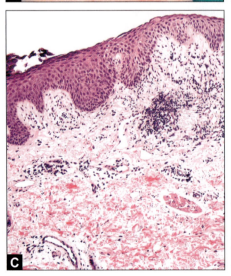

Figs 4.3A to C: Staphylococcal scalded skin syndrome. (A) Desquamating red patch in the axilla of an infant; (B) Red patches in the groin. Note the perianal desquamation; (C) An intact blister is seldom seen, and often the epidermis simply lacks the stratum corneum. Inflammation may be minimal or there may be collections of neutrophils on the surface of the remaining epidermis.

Bullous Tinea/Bullous Dermatophytosis
(Figs 4.4A to C)

■ *Criteria for diagnosis*

- Scaly pink patches
- Vesicles, bulla or pustules
- Fungal organisms present (confirmed with periodic acid-Schiff and/or Grocott methenamine silver stains, if necessary).

■ *Differential diagnosis*

- Autoimmune blistering diseases
- Other bullous infectious diseases.

■ *Pitfalls*

- In rare cases, the clinician may have.

■ *Pearls*

- Blisters are an uncommon presentation of tinea/dermato-phytosis
- Mostly occur on the feet
- Scaly patches typical of ordinary tinea are usually present around the blisters, a helpful clinical clue
- Onychomyosis is commonly present.

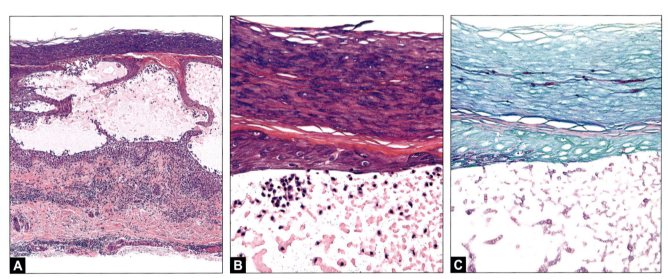

Figs 4.4A to C: Bullous tinea/dermatophytosis. (A) An intraepidermal multiloculated blister containing a mixed inflammatory cell infiltrate is present in the biopsy of this patient with a suspected autoimmune blistering disorder; (B) Close inspection may suggest the presence of fungal elements in the stratum corneum or the blister cavity; (C) On periodic acid-Schiff stain, the fungal elements are obvious.

Immunoglobulin A Pemphigus

■ *Criteria for diagnosis*

- Flaccid blisters and pustules on an erythematous base
- Subcorneal or intraepidermal pustules
- Direct immunofluorescence demonstrating intercellular epidermal deposition of IgA
- Microorganisms must be absent (confirmed with fungal and Gram stains if necessary).

■ *Differential diagnosis*

- Other pemphigus variants
- Impetigo
- Staphylococcal scalded skin syndrome
- Pustular drug eruption/acute generalized exanthematous pustulosis (AGEP)
- Pustular psoriasis
- Subcorneal pustular dermatosis (see below).

■ *Pitfalls*

- Without confirmation by direct immunofluorescence (DIF), definitive diagnosis cannot be made since the disease may be otherwise identical to subcorneal pustular dermatosis (Sneddon-Wilkinson disease)
- Even DIF findings may not be entirely specific, since some cases have reportedly shown IgG in addition to IgA.

■ *Pearls*

- Some cases of subcorneal pustular dermatosis (Sneddon-Wilkinson disease) may represent IgA pemphigus not confirmed by DIF examination (Figs 4.5A and B)
- Definitive diagnosis requires confirmation of intercellular IgA by DIF
- A monoclonal gammopathy is occasionally associated with IgA pemphigus.

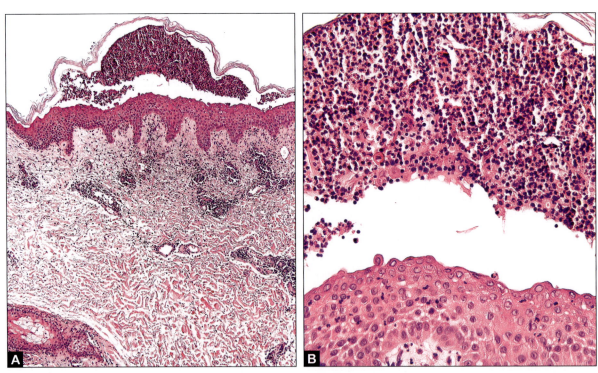

Figs 4.5A and B: Subcorneal pustular dermatosis. (A) Subcorneal blister filled with neutrophils is characteristic. The dermis contains a mixed infiltrate that includes lymphocytes, as well as neutrophils; (B) There is acantholysis within the superficial layers of the epidermis.

Subcorneal Pustular Dermatosis (Sneddon-Wilkinson disease)

■ *Criteria for diagnosis*

- Recurrent flaccid pustules, most often on the flexures and abdomen
- Subcorneal collections of neutrophils with focal acantholysis
- Absence of intraepidermal microabscess or spongiform pustule formation (unlike pustular psoriasis)
- Microorganisms must be absent (confirmed with fungal and Gram stains)
- Negative DIF.

■ *Differential diagnosis*

- IgA pemphigus (see above)
- Other pemphigus variants, especially pemphigus foliaceous and pemphigus erythematosus
- Impetigo
- Staphylococcal scalded skin syndrome
- Pustular drug eruption/AGEP
- Pustular psoriasis.

■ *Pitfalls*

- Again, without DIF, exclusion of IgA pemphigus is impossible.

■ *Pearls*

- IgA pemphigus (and other pemphigus variants) must be excluded by DIF
- Unlike pustular psoriasis, intraepidermal microabscesses and spongiform pustules are absent
- Acute generalized exanthematous pustulosis usually has smaller pustules, but cannot always be reliably distinguished.

Infantile Acropustulosis

■ *Criteria for diagnosis*

- Recurrent crops of pruritic pustules and blisters presenting in the first year of life on feet and hands (Fig. 4.6)
- Spongiosis and focal epidermal necrosis early, followed by subcorneal pustules containing neutrophils and eosinophils
- Microorganisms must be absent (confirmed with fungal and Gram stains)
- Scabies must be excluded.

■ *Differential diagnosis*

- Impetigo
- Pustular drug eruption/AGEP
- Pustular psoriasis
- Subcorneal pustular dermatosis.

■ *Pitfalls*

- Scabies must be excluded.

■ *Pearls*

- Predilection for black infants
- Resolves within 2 years in most of the cases
- Association with scabies infestation or atopic dermatitis reported in some cases.

The Blistering and Acantholytic Patterns

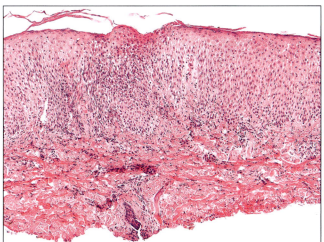

Fig. 4.6: This biopsy of an early lesion from the foot of an infant shows infiltration of the epidermis by neutrophils and a few eosinophils. Pustules and vesicles developed soon afterward.

Bullous Diabetocorum

■ *Criteria for diagnosis*

- Large blisters arising spontaneously on legs, feet or hands in patients with chronic diabetes mellitus
- Subcorneal, intraepidermal or subepidermal blisters
- Microorganisms are absent (confirmed with fungal and Gram stains)
- Negative DIF (Fig. 4.7).

■ *Differential diagnosis*

- Blistering diseases of virtually all types (including bullous stasis)
- Bullous insect bite reactions.

■ *Pitfalls*

- Since histopathologically, the clefting/blistering may occur at any level within the epidermis, clinical correlation is necessary and DIF studies may be necessary.

■ *Pearls*

- The inflammatory infiltrate is usually sparse and inflammation is usually limited to perivascular lymphocytes and macrophages
- Capillary wall thickening may be present
- Blisters may heal spontaneously but tend to recur.

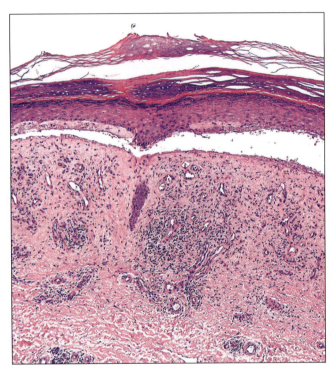

Fig. 4.7: This subepidermal blister was one of several that developed on the shins of a patient with diabetes mellitus. Direct immunofluorescence studies were negative. There is stasis change, and since the majority of cases occur on the distal lower extremities, a vascular mechanism may be responsible. Stasis dermatitis itself may be blister, but usually there is more inflammation and edema.

Pemphigus Foliaceus (Figs 4.8A to D)

▪ *Criteria for diagnosis*

- Pink scaly patches, crusted erosions; intact blisters rare
- No mucosal involvement
- Subcorneal blister with acantholytic keratinocytes and some dyskeratotic cells in granular layer
- Intercellular deposition of IgG (with or without C on DIF; pattern may be indistinguishable from other forms of pemphigus but is sometimes confined to the superficial epidermis).

▪ *Differential diagnosis*

- Pemphigus vulgaris
- Impetigo (especially when eroded lesions develop superimposed bacterial infection)
- Staphylococcal scalded skin syndrome (usually easily excluded on clinical grounds)
- IgA pemphigus
- Subcorneal pustular dermatosis.

▪ *Pitfalls*

- May be mistaken clinically and histopathologically for an ulcerated and/or acantholytic actinic keratosis or excoriated dermatitis
- Early lesions may show only eosinophilic spongiosis and abscesses without acantholysis and dyskeratosis
- Cleavage plane may extend below granular layer and can even be suprabasilar in some areas, simulating pemphigus vulgaris.

▪ *Pearls*

- Middle-aged and elderly patients
- Seborrheic dermatitis or actinic keratosis is common clinical simulator
- Head and neck, trunk, proximal extremities and intertriginous areas are the most common sites.

Pemphigus Erythematosus

▪ *Criteria for diagnosis*

- Lesions similar to pemphigus foliaceous (patches, crusted erosions, rare intact blisters) but with predilection for face and upper chest (sun-exposed areas), often with a lupus-like appearance and serologic and/or direct immunofluorescence findings of lupus (Figs 4.8E and F)
- No mucosal involvement
- Subcorneal blister with acantholytic keratinocytes, often with dyskeratotic cells in granular layers
- Direct immunofluorescence: Linear or granular IgG and sometimes C3 along basement membrane zone.

▪ *Differential diagnosis*

- Pemphigus vulgaris
- Impetigo (especially when eroded lesions develop superimposed bacterial infection)
- Staphylococcal scalded skin syndrome (usually easily excluded on clinical grounds)
- IgA pemphigus
- Subcorneal pustular dermatosis.

▪ *Pitfalls*

- Paraneoplastic pemphigus may simulate pemphigus erythematosus (an interface infiltrate and, occasionally, a similar pattern on direct immunofluorescence).

▪ *Pearls*

- Considered by many to be a variant of pemphigus foliaceus that favors sun-exposed skin
- Face and upper chest are most common sites
- Antinuclear antibodies, dsDNA, Sjögren's syndrome A and Sjögren's syndrome B may be positive
- Interface dermatitis similar to that of lupus erythematosus is sometimes present.

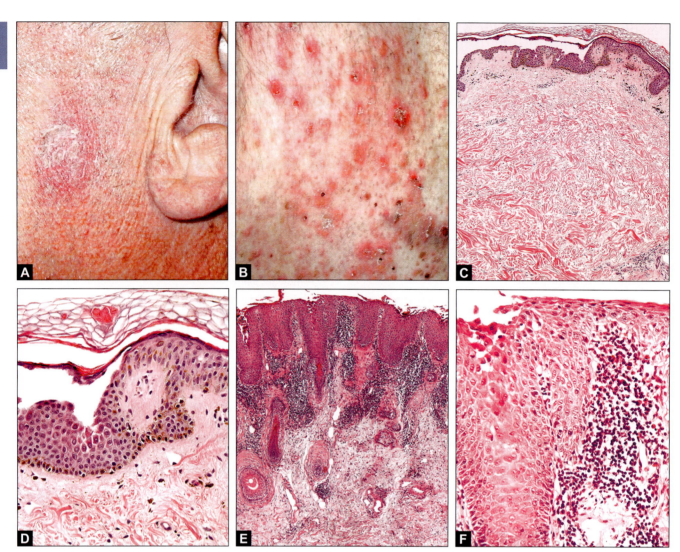

Figs 4.8A to F: Pemphigus foliaceus. (A) Erosions without visible blisters are common, as seen here. This patient's lesions were initially localized to the head and neck and thought to be actinic keratosis; (B) Scaly or crusted erosions are the predominant feature in some cases; (C) The blister is subcorneal or within the granular cell layer. Obtaining an intact blister, such as this, is uncommon since they are so fragile; (D) The blister is evolving due to acantholysis within the granular layer. Dyskeratotic cells are not present. New lesions, such as this usually lack inflammation, but some become impetiginized rapidly and contain neutrophils and other inflammatory cells; (E) Pemphigus erythematosus. There is superficial acantholysis that is virtually identical to that of pemphigus foliaceus, but the dermis contains a dense inflammatory cell infiltrate; (F) Closer examination reveals numerous lymphocytes and eosinophils that approximate the dermoepidermal junction. Vacuoles are evident within the basement membrane region in a few areas.

Hailey-Hailey Disease (Figs 4.9A to D)

■ *Criteria for diagnosis*

- Sharply marginated scaly macerated or crusted patches or blisters on intertriginous skin
- Epidermal acantholysis and acanthosis, with or without mild dyskeratosis
- No patterned immunoreactant deposition on direct immuno-fluorescence.

■ *Differential diagnosis*

- Clinical differential often includes intertrigo, candidiasis, contact dermatitis, inverse psoriasis or dermatophytosis
- Darier's disease, Grover's disease, pemphigus vulgaris, acantholytic dermatosis of the genitocrural region.

■ *Pitfalls*

- Acantholysis of pemphigus vulgaris occasionally appears to extend into stratum spinosum, particularly if some regions are sectioned tangentially
- Hailey-Hailey disease is histopathologically identical to some cases of "acantholytic dermatosis of the genitocrural region" (see below).

■ *Pearls*

- Clinically, macerated or crusted patches are more common than intact blisters
- Secondary bacterial infection of lesions produces odor
- Autosomal dominant inheritance but often presents in adulthood
- Unlike pemphigus, the acantholysis involves entire stratum spinosum
- Unlike Darier's disease, dyskeratotic cells are usually few in number
- Acantholytic dermatosis of the genitocrural region is a rare disorder that presents with scaly papules and plaques in the genital, perianal and inguinal regions; it is histopathologically identical to Hailey-Hailey disease but has no familial association and very rarely produces clinically appreciable blisters.

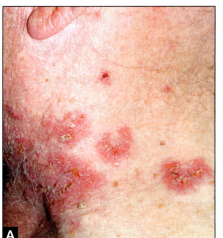
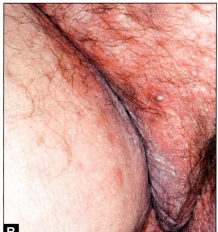
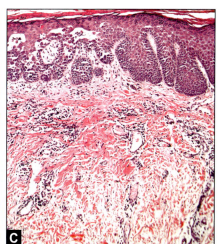
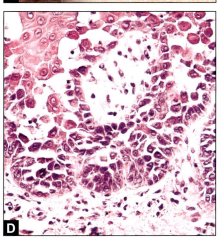

Figs 4.9A to D: Hailey-Hailey disease. (A) Lesions have a predilection for flexural and/or intertriginous skin. The neck, as shown here, is a favored site; (B) The groin and axilla are commonly involved. The lesions seem to be induced by friction or minor trauma; (C) There is usually acantholysis throughout the stratum corneum. Acanthosis and hyper-parakeratosis are common; (D) The acantholysis is often likened to a "dilapidated brick wall". Dyskeratosis is minimal by comparison to Darier's disease.

Darier's Disease (Figs 4.10A to E)

■ *Criteria for diagnosis*

- Patches of small, rough, pink-brown papules involving the seborrheic areas (central chest, neck, back and upper arms) (Fig. 4.10A)
- Acantholytic dyskeratosis with suprabasal cleavage
- Autosomal dominant inheritance.

■ *Differential diagnosis*

- Hailey-Hailey disease
- Grover's disease
- Pemphigus vulgaris
- Acantholytic dyskeratotic acanthoma
- Herpes virus infection.

■ *Pitfalls*

- Without clinical history, reliable distinction from Grover's disease, Hailey-Hailey disease and other acantholytic disorders is not possible.

■ *Pearls*

- Disease usually manifests in late childhood or early adulthood
- Secondary infection or colonization by bacteria and yeast is common
- Plaques with a "cobblestone" appearance are often seen on oral mucosa
- Acanthosis, papillomatosis and hyperparakeratosis are common
- Acantholytic dyskeratosis is the most prominent within dells between epidermal papilla
- Dyskeratotic cells are more numerous than in Hailey-Hailey disease
- Lacunae filled with dyskeratotic cells often develop.

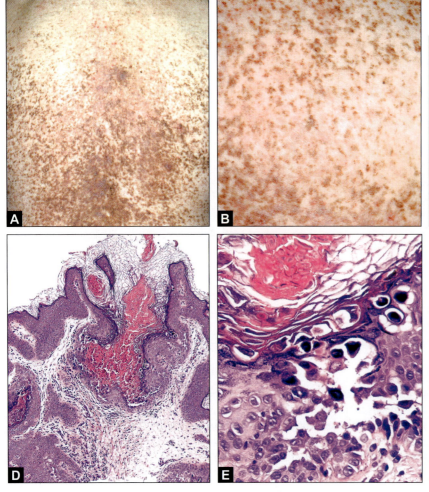

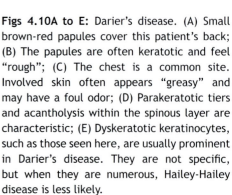

Figs 4.10A to E: Darier's disease. (A) Small brown-red papules cover this patient's back; (B) The papules are often keratotic and feel "rough"; (C) The chest is a common site. Involved skin often appears "greasy" and may have a foul odor; (D) Parakeratotic tiers and acantholysis within the spinous layer are characteristic; (E) Dyskeratotic keratinocytes, such as those seen here, are usually prominent in Darier's disease. They are not specific, but when they are numerous, Hailey-Hailey disease is less likely.

Grover's Disease (Focal Transient Acantholytis Dyskeratosis) (Figs 4.11A to D)

Criteria for diagnosis

- Numerous small pruritic pink papules, often with superficial crusts
- Foci of acantholytic dyskeratosis with intervening areas of nonacantholytic or normal epidermis.

Differential diagnosis

- Darier's disease, Hailey-Hailey disease, pemphigus vulgaris and pemphigus foliaceous
- Spongiotic dermatitis.

Pitfalls

- Lesions are often excoriated obscuring the acantholysis
- Occasional cases are histopathologically similar to pemphigus vulgaris, pemphigus foliaceous, Hailey-Hailey disease and Darier's disease
- The acantholysis may be subtle and focal and not apparent in every section.

Pearls

- Strong predilection for males, usually the trunk and proximal extremities
- The condition is often exacerbated by heat or exercise
- Since the acantholysis is sometimes subtle and focal, multiple levels may be helpful in its identification
- Given the potential for overlapping histopathologic features, clinical correlation is often necessary for definitive diagnosis
- The presence of more than one pattern of acantholysis is a clue to Grover's disease (e.g. a resemblance to pemphigus foliaceous in one area, Darier's in another)
- Acantholytic zones are usually much smaller in Grover's than in other acantholytic diseases
- Spongiosis either within acantholytic regions or between them is a clue to Grover's disease.

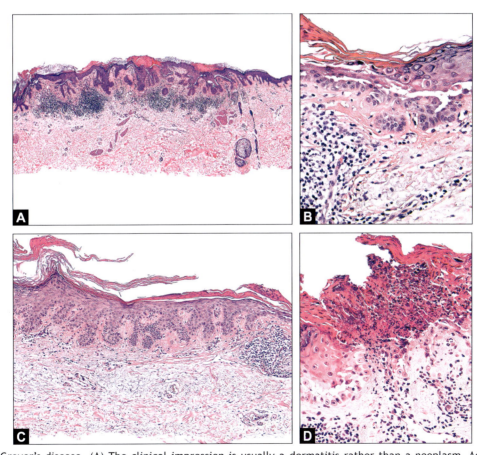

Figs 4.11A to D: Grover's disease. (A) The clinical impression is usually a dermatitis rather than a neoplasm. Acantholytic zones are usually smaller or focal in Grover's than in other acantholytic diseases; (B) The acantholysis is usually suprabasilar but can be intraspinous or superficial as well. Note the inflammation and parakeratosis; (C) In some cases there is very little acantholysis and the major finding is changes that resemble lichen simplex chronicus/prurigo; (D) Since it is usually pruritic, areas of excoriation, such as this are a common finding.

Warty Dyskeratoma

■ *Criteria for diagnosis*

- Solitary papule
- Epidermal invagination (or dilated follicular infundibulum) containing acantholytic and dyskeratotic keratinocytes
- Acanthosis, often with papillomatous or verrucous architecture around central invagination (Fig. 4.12A)
- No cytologic atypia of the degree encountered in squamous cell carcinomas or actinic keratosis (Fig. 4.12B).

■ *Differential diagnosis*

- Acantholytic squamous cell carcinoma/acantholytic actinic keratosis
- Acantholytic dyskeratotic acanthoma
- Acantholytic dermatoses.

■ *Pitfalls*

- Reactive cytologic atypia may simulate acantholytic squamous cell carcinomas and actinic keratosis

- Depending on the plane of section, acantholysis may appear multifocal, simulating acantholytic dermatoses.

■ *Pearls*

- Clinical impression is often basal cell carcinoma, seborrheic keratosis or wart
- Absence of solar elastosis may help exclude actinic keratosis and squamous cell carcinomas
- Early lesions may show only a hyperkeratotic plug within a dilated infundibulum lined by dyskeratotic cells
- Unlike acantholytic squamous cell carcinomas and actinic keratoses, warty dyskeratomas lack significant nuclear atypia, nuclear crowding, mitotic figures and keratotic whorls ("horn pearls").

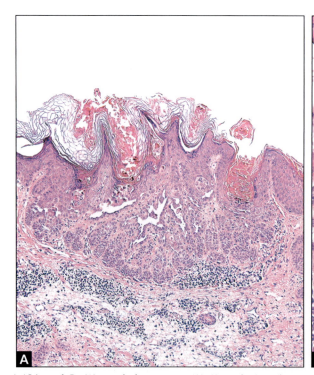
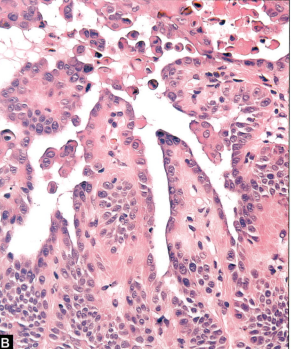

Figs 4.12A and B: Warty dyskeratoma. (A) Many lesions have verrucous or papillomatous hyperplasia surrounding the central invagination; (B) The acantholysis may be either suprabasal or intraepidermal. Dyskeratotic keratinocytes are always present but the cytologic atypia of an actinic keratosis or squamous cell carcinoma is absent.

Acantholytic Dyskeratotic Acanthoma
(Figs 4.13A and B)

■ Criteria for diagnosis

- A papule with confluent acantholysis and dyskeratosis
- No atypia of the degree seen in actinic keratosis or squamous cell carcinomas
- Not centered on a follicular infundibulum and no endophytic invagination.

■ Differential diagnosis

- Warty dyskeratoma
- A single lesion of Darier's disease, Grover's disease or other acantholytic and dyskeratotic dermatosis.

■ Pitfalls

- Without knowledge of the anatomic site and number of lesions, the features are nonspecific, and acantholytic disorders, such as Grover's disease cannot be excluded.

■ Pearls

- Lesions may occur at any site but genital lesions usually represent other acantholytic entities
- A solitary papule on the trunk is the most common presentation
- Considered a type of benign keratosis
- The lesions are broad and predominantly exophytic; the absence of an endophytic invagination or involvement of a follicular infundibulum helps exclude a warty dyskeratoma.

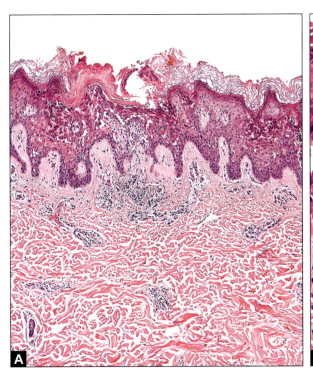 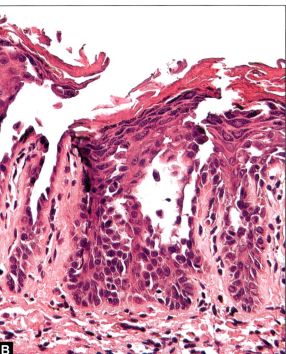

Figs 4.13A and B: Acantholytic dyskeratotic acanthoma. (A) Most lesions are predominantly exophytic and broad by comparison to warty dyskeratomas and they lack a central invagination; (B) The acantholysis and dyskeratosis is very similar to that of a warty dyskeratoma.

Herpes Virus Infection (Figs 4.14A to D)

■ *Criteria for diagnosis*

- Tense vesicles, blisters or small ulcers on an erythematous base
- Keratinocytes with herpes viral cytopathic effect, defined as one or more of the following:
  - Multinucleation with molding of nuclei
  - Intranuclear or intracytoplasmic inclusions
  - Pale gray or blue nuclei ("steel gray nuclei").

■ *Differential diagnosis*

- Other acantholytic blistering diseases
- Other viral infections including early lesions of Orf and Hand-Foot-and-Mouth disease
- Nonspecific causes of ulcers, including excoriation

■ *Pitfalls*

- Definitive diagnosis requires unequivocal identification of herpes viral cytopathic effect, which may be focal or altogether absent in some cases
- Herpes virus infection may induce a secondary necrotizing vasculitis at the site of the lesion.

■ *Pearls*

- If herpes virus infection is suspected but definitive viral cytopathic effect is not evident, serial sections or additional levels may reveal it
- Dyskeratotic cells within adnexal epithelium are sometimes seen in addition to the epidermal changes; occasionally, only the adnexal epithelium is involved
- Unlike cytomegalovirus (which typically infects endothelial cells or fibroblasts), herpes virus infects keratinocytes
- The herpes viral cytopathic effect is relatively characteristic and more pronounced than other viral diseases that may produce inclusion bodies (e.g. Orf).

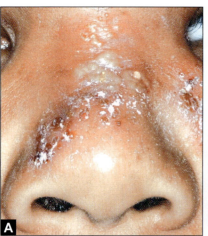

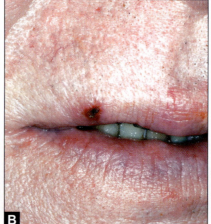

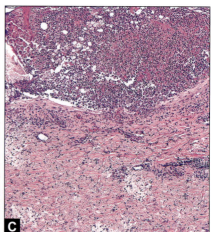

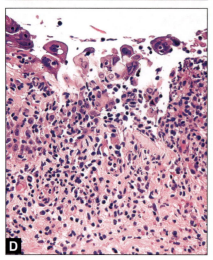

Figs 4.14A to D: (A) Herpes (HSV 1). Grouped vesicles and hemorrhagic crusts are typical; (B) Herpes labialis (HSV 1). On the mucosa, the vesicles tend to rupture early in their course leaving crusted ulcers; (C) Herpes virus infection. An intraepidermal vesicle filled with neutrophils and degenerating keratinocytes with large virocytes is at the left; (D) Even in extensively ulcerated lesions, characteristic virocytes may be seen at the periphery. Note the multinucleated cells with nuclear molding.

Pemphigus Vulgaris (Figs 4.15A to G)

■ *Criteria for diagnosis*

- Oral erosions and ulcers in all cases
- Flaccid bulla and erosions on skin
- Suprabasal acantholysis and separation
- *Direct immunofluorescence*: Intercellular deposition of IgG and sometimes C3.

■ *Differential diagnosis*

- Other forms of pemphigus (including paraneoplastic pemphigus)
- Hailey-Hailey disease
- Grover's disease
- Acantholytic dyskeratotic acanthoma
- Acantholytic actinic keratosis
- Herpes virus infections.

■ *Pitfalls*

- Early lesions and skin adjacent to blisters may only show nonspecific eosinophilic spongiosis and lack the characteristic suprabasilar acantholysis

- Acantholysis may occasionally extend beyond the suprabasilar epidermis (an appearance that may be due to tangential sectioning), simulating other acantholytic diseases.

■ *Pearls*

- Unlike pemphigus vulgaris:
  - The acantholytic area is broad and confluent
  - Parakeratosis is usually absent
  - The epidermis above the acantholytic zone is usually intact
  - Dyskeratotic cells are usually few in number
  - Spongiosis is minimal
  - Acanthosis is absent.

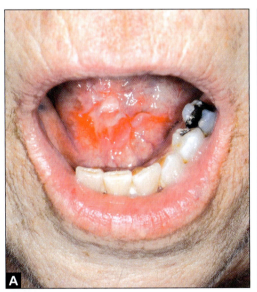

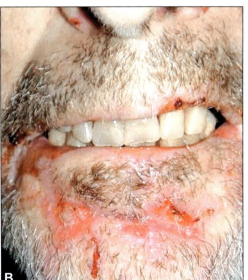

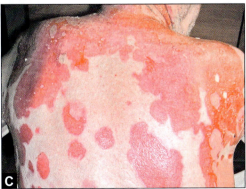

Figs 4.15A to C

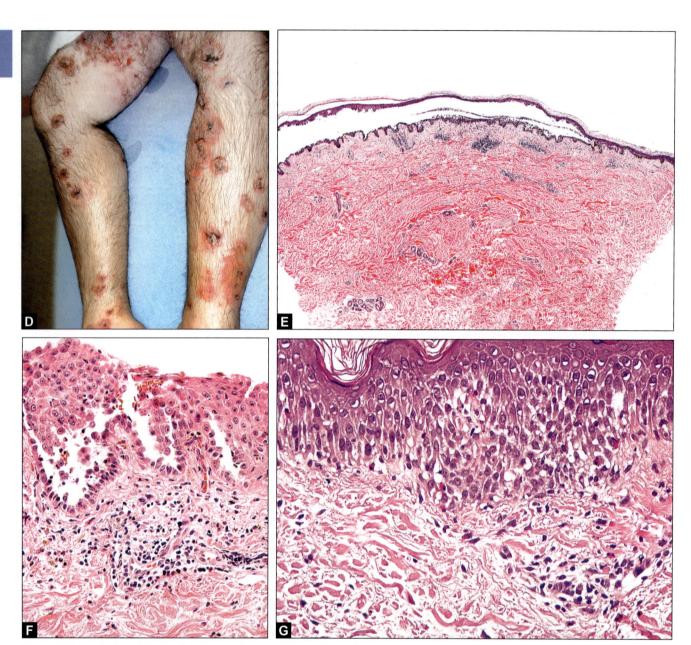

Figs 4.15A to G: Pemphigus vulgaris. (A) The disease usually presents first with painful erosions or blisters within the mouth; (B) The blisters and erosions spread to involve the skin, usually within a few weeks or months; (C) The blisters are fragile, flaccid and easily ruptured, leaving painful red erosions; (D) Several small intact blisters are present, mostly on this patient's upper inner right thigh. The erosions are the site of ruptured blisters; (E) The acantholysis usually involves broad, contiguous areas of the epidermis, which differentiates it from most other conditions that have suprabasilar acantholysis. The stratum corneum is usually unaltered; (F) The plane of acantholysis is almost completely restricted to the suprabasal keratinocyte layer, imparting the so-called "tombstone" appearance that refers to the presence of individual basal keratinocytes that remain anchored to the basement membrane zone; (G) In early lesions or at the periphery of blisters or erosions, there is often eosinophilic spongiosis.

Pemphigus Vegetans

■ *Criteria for diagnosis*

- Flaccid bulla, pustules or erosions that develop into verrucous lesions within intertriginous areas
- *Direct immunofluorescence*: Intercellular deposition of IgG and sometimes C3.

■ *Differential diagnosis*

- Other verrucous and/or pseudoeiptheliomatous processes, such as blastomycosis and iododermas (Fig. 4.16A)
- Other forms of pemphigus (including paraneoplastic pemphigus).

■ *Pitfalls*

- Early lesions and skin adjacent to blisters may only show nonspecific eosinophilic spongiosis and lack the characteristic suprabasilar acantholysis (Fig. 4.16B)

- Acantholysis may occasionally extend beyond the suprabasilar epidermis (an appearance that may be due to tangential sectioning) simulating other acantholytic diseases.

■ *Pearls*

- Confirmation of the diagnosis requires DIF showing intercellular deposition of IgG and/or C3 (identical to pemphigus vulgaris)
- Best considered a variant of pemphigus
- Some cases are virtually identical to pemphigus vulgaris in their presentation (oral lesions) and their progression to skin involvement, but the erosions evolve into vegetation (the Neumann variant)
- In others, the lesions start as pustules that develop into verrucous plaques (the Hallopeau variant); this type is usually less aggressive.

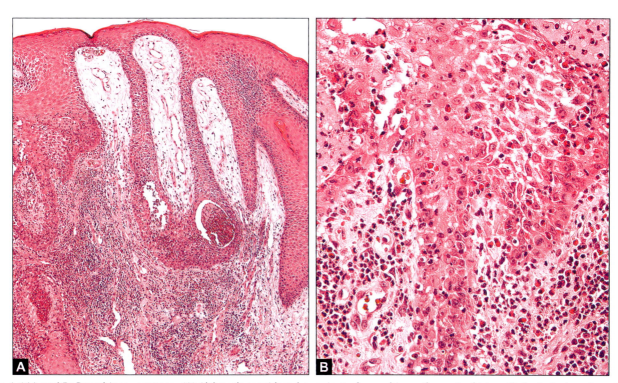

Figs 4.16A and B: Pemphigus vegetans. (A) Although considered a variant of pemphigus, the major histopathologic feature is marked epidermal hyperplasia, often with "pseudoepitheliomaotus" architecture. The microabscesses within the elongated epidermal tongues are composed mostly of eosinophils; (B) There is acantholysis, but it is usually much more limited than in pemphigus vulgaris and may be obscured by eosinophilic spongiosis, as in this field.

Paraneoplastic Pemphigus

Criteria for diagnosis

- Painful mucosal erosions and ulcers with or without skin lesions (blisters, plaques, and erosions)
- An underlying neoplasm
- Varying degrees and combinations of keratinocyte necrosis, intraepidermal acantholysis and interface inflammation (Fig. 4.17)
- Indirect immunofluorescence that demonstrates circulating antibodies to other epithelia in addition to the skin and oral mucosa
- Direct immunofluorescence demonstrating intercellular and basement membrane zone deposition of IgG and sometimes C3 in a linear or granular pattern.

Differential diagnosis

- Other forms of pemphigus
- Erythema multiforme and toxic epidermal necrolysis
- Interface drug eruptions.

Pitfalls

- Histopathologic features vary considerably, in part due to the site of the biopsy and the age of the lesion
- Often the finding is interface dermatitis without appreciable acantholysis or blister formation, leading to confusion with EM and other interface diseases
- False-negative indirect immunofluorescence results occur.
- Without identification of characteristic immunopathologic features, EM and other disorders can be difficult to exclude.

Pearls

- Common associated neoplasms are lymphomas (particularly chronic lymphocytic leukemia/small lymphocytic lymphoma), thymomas and Castleman's disease
- Necrotizing tracheobronchitis and/or bronchiolitis obliterans commonly develop
- Survival is poor overall and many patients die as a result of complications from the airway involvement
- Treatment of the underlying neoplasm is sometimes (but not always) curative
- Hemorrhagic mucositis with painful oral and perioral erosions and conjunctival erosions are characteristic
- Demonstration of antibodies that recognize bladder epithelium, if positive, is by itself virtually diagnostic if the remainder of the clinical and histopathologic features are characteristic of paraneoplastic pemphigus
- Otherwise, confirmation of the diagnosis requires one of the following:
    - Direct immunofluorescence showing intercellular and linear basement membrane zone deposition of IgG and/or C3
    - Indirect immunofluorescence demonstrating serum antibodies that bind to the cell surface of stratified squamous mucosa and nonstratified squamous mucosa (monkey esophagus or urinary bladder are commonly used substrates)
    - Immunoprecipitation assays demonstrating serum antibodies that recognize the following antigens:
        - 250 kd desmoplakin I
        - 230 kd bullous pemphigoid antigen I
        - 210 kd desmoplakin II
        - 190 kd periplakin
        - 170 kd unidentified antigen.

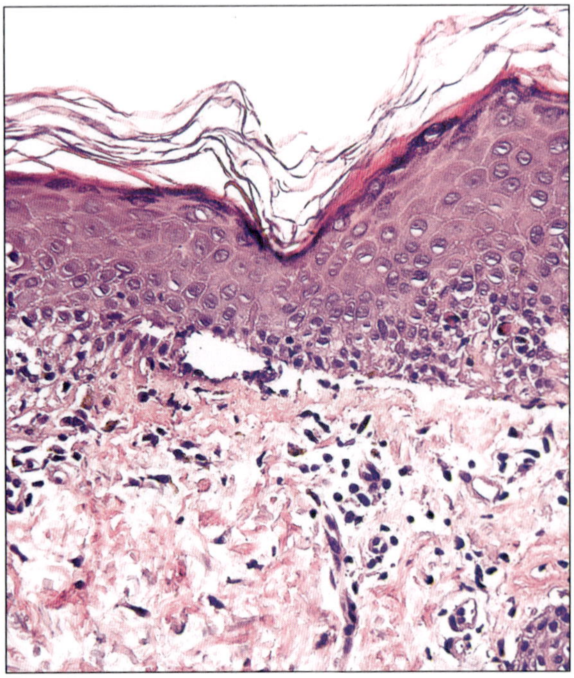

Fig. 4.17: Paraneoplastic pemphigus. This patient had a systemic B-cell lymphoma. The biopsy demonstrates a mixed interface inflammatory infiltrate in addition to keratinocyte necrosis and subtle acantholysis. Some of the clefting appears subepidermal while other areas seem to be intraepidermal. (Please see Figs 3.20A and B for additional images of paraneoplastic pemphigus presenting as interface dermatitis).

Bullous Pemphigoid (Figs 4.18A to F)

■ *Criteria for diagnosis*

- Tense blisters with or without an erythematous base
- Subepidermal blister
- *Direct immunofluorescence*: Linear deposition of IgG and C3 along basement membrane zone
- Salt-split skin DIF; linear IgG along blister "roof".

■ *Differential diagnosis*

- Epidermolysis bullosa acquisita
- Linear IgA bullous dermatosis
- Cicatricial pemphigoid
- Other subepidermal blistering diseases.

■ *Pitfalls*

- Pemphigoid may present with an urticarial phase characterized by nonspecific eosinophilic spongiosis that overlaps with urticaria and the urticarial phase of other autoimmune blistering disorders, such as pemphigus vulgaris
- Bullous pemphigoid cannot be reliably distinguished from EBA without examination of salt-split skin DIF.

■ *Pearls*

- The vast majority of cases present in the elderly
- Blisters are often preceded by an early urticarial phase characterized by pruritic, persistent urticarial plaques
- Trunk and proximal extremities are the most affected but acral and mucosal sites are occasionally involved.

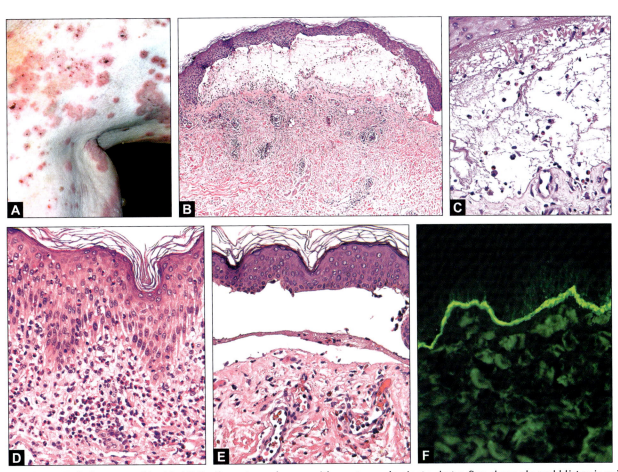

Figs 4.18A to F: Bullous pemphigoid. (A) Erythematous plaques with crusts predominate, but a firm dome-shaped blister is evident at the angle of the axilla; (B) The stereotypical histopathologic finding is a unilocular subepidermal blister; (C) Most blisters contain numerous eosinophils in addition to fibrin; (D) Prebullous or urticarial phase pemphigoid may show eosinophilic spongiosis without any evidence of a blister; (E) Occasionally the blisters contain few if any inflammatory cells (so-called cell poor pemphigoid). Usually, however, at least one or two eosinophils are evident within the blister, underlying dermis or adjacent epidermis; (F) Direct immunofluorescence demonstrates linear deposition of IgG and C3 within the basement membrane zone.

Pemphigoid (Herpes) Gestationis

■ *Criteria for diagnosis*

- Pruritic urticarial papules, plaques, and blisters beginning on the abdomen in the second or third trimester of pregnancy (Fig. 4.19A)
- Subepidermal blister with eosinophils and papillary dermal edema (Fig. 4.19B)
- *Direct immunofluorescence*: Linear C3 at dermoepidermal junction, sometimes accompanied by IgG.

■ *Differential diagnosis*

- Bullous arthropod bite reaction
- Bullous drug eruption
- Pruritic urticarial papules and plaques of pregnancy (PUPPP)/ polymorphous eruption of pregnancy (PEP).

■ *Pitfalls*

- Scattered necrotic keratinocytes may be present and cause confusion with a bullous drug eruption or bullous arthropod bite reaction
- Occasionally a well-formed subepidermal blister is absent and without DIF, definitive distinction from PUPPP/PEP is impossible.

■ *Pearls*

- Lesions characteristically begin around umbilicus and spread to trunk and proximal extremities
- Face and mucosa are typically spared
- Recurs with subsequent pregnancies
- Bullous pemphigoid is extremely uncommon in women of child-bearing age and can usually be eliminated
- The other conditions in the differential diagnosis do not have linear C3 deposition on DIF
- May also be triggered by oral contraceptives, hormone replacement therapy or menses in women who have developed the condition during pregnancy
- Uncommonly, the newborn may have small blisters that resolve spontaneously
- Uncommonly, there is an exacerbation immediately postpartum.

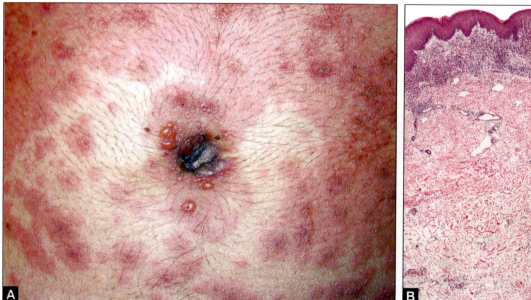
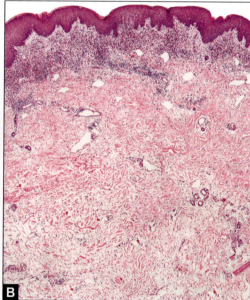

Figs 4.19A and B: Pemphigoid gestationis. (A) Erythematous plaques and blisters around the umbilical region is the classic presentation, but lesions may involve other sites; (B) The histopathologic features are identical to those of bullous pemphigoid. Early lesions may show the same prebullous finding of eosinophilic spongiosis.

Cicatricial Pemphigoid (Figs 4.20A to D)

■ *Criteria for diagnosis*

- Blisters and erosions on mucosal surfaces and (less commonly) the skin that produce dermal granulation tissue and scarring
- Subepidermal/subepithelial blister
- Skin lesions without involvement of mucosa is exceptionally rare and is referred to as the Brunsting-Perry variant or localized variant of cicatricial pemphigoid.

■ *Differential diagnosis*

- Epidermolysis bullosa acquisita
- Bullous pemphigoid
- Linear IgA
- Sweet's syndrome.

■ *Pitfalls*

- In mucosal lesions, lymphocytes and plasma cells may be the predominant inflammatory cell type
- In some cases, neutrophils may predominate; eosinophils are usually fewer in number.

■ *Pearls*

- Conventional cicatricial pemphigoid has a female to male ratio of 2:1
- Only 25% of cases involve the skin
- Eighty-five percent of cases involve oral mucosa
- Sixty-five percent involve the eye and can result in blindness
- Lesions on the scalp may produce scarring alopecia
- Extension of clefts and blistering along adnexal epithelium is a clue to cicatricial pemphigoid (but is not entirely specific)
- Dermal granulation tissue and scarring are helpful clue but do not exclude EBA
- Localized/Brunsting-Perry variant is more common in men.

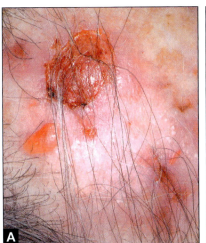
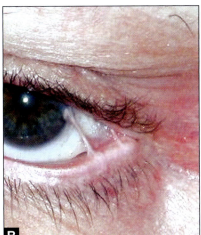
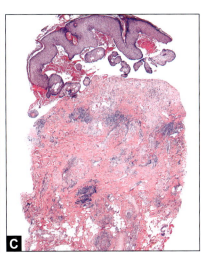
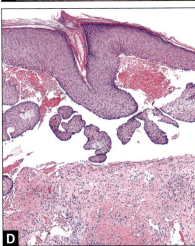

Figs 4.20A to D: Cicatricial pemphigoid. (A) Blisters, erosions and milia are present on the sun-damaged skin of this man's scalp; (B) Conjunctival scarring has resulted in fibrous adhesions (symblepharon); (C) A subepidermal blister cavity is present and contains dislodged sebaceous glands, indicating that the cleavage plane extends along adnexal epithelium; (D) There is granulation tissue and scarring of the dermis.

Epidermolysis Bullosa Acquisita
(Figs 4.21A to C)

Criteria for diagnosis

- Blisters on nonerythematous skin that resolve with atrophic scars and milia
- Subepidermal blister without keratinocyte necrosis
- *Direct immunofluorescence* : Linear basement membrane zone C3 and IgG deposition
- Immunoreactants localize to floor of blister on salt-split skin.

Differential diagnosis

- Porphyria cutanea tarda/pseudoporphyria
- Cell-poor bullous pemphigoid
- Bullous lupus erythematosus
- Congenital epidermolysis bullosa.

Pitfalls

- Bullous pemphigoid cannot be reliably distinguished from EBA without examination of salt-split skin DIF.

Pearls

- Predilection for middle-aged and elderly adults (which helps to exclude congenital epidermolysis bullosa)
- Lesions favor trauma-prone skin, particularly the dorsa of the hands and feet
- Nail dystrophy may be present
- Dermal fibrosis (scarring) and milia are common and are a clue to the diagnosis
- Most cases exhibit little inflammation
- Antibodies to type VII collagen appear to be the most common cause.

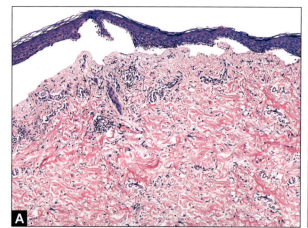
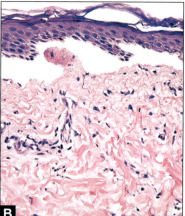
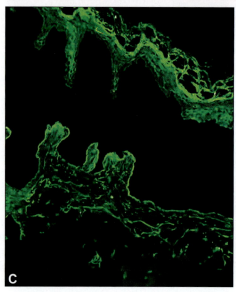

Figs 4.21A to C: Epidermolysis bullosa acquisita. (A) The usual histopathologic features are a subepidermal blister with little or no inflammation; (B) The dermal papilla are often preserved; (C) On salt-split skin examination by direct immunofluorescence, the immunoreactants (IgG and C3) localize to floor of blister.

Porphyria/Pseudoporphyria (Figs 4.22A to E)

■ Criteria for diagnosis

- Blisters, erosions, scars and milia (particularly on dorsum of hands, face and ears)
- Pseudoporphyria is clinically indistinguishable from porphyria cutanea tarda.

■ Differential diagnosis

- Epidermolysis bullosa acquisita.

■ Pitfalls

- Porphyria, many of its variants and pseudoporphyria cannot be distinguished histopathologically.

■ Pearls

- Predilection for dorsum of the hands, face and ears (sun-exposed areas)
- Hypertrichosis and scleroderma-like thickening of the skin can also occur
- Hepatic disease (viral hepatitis, alcoholic liver damage, etc.) commonly associated.

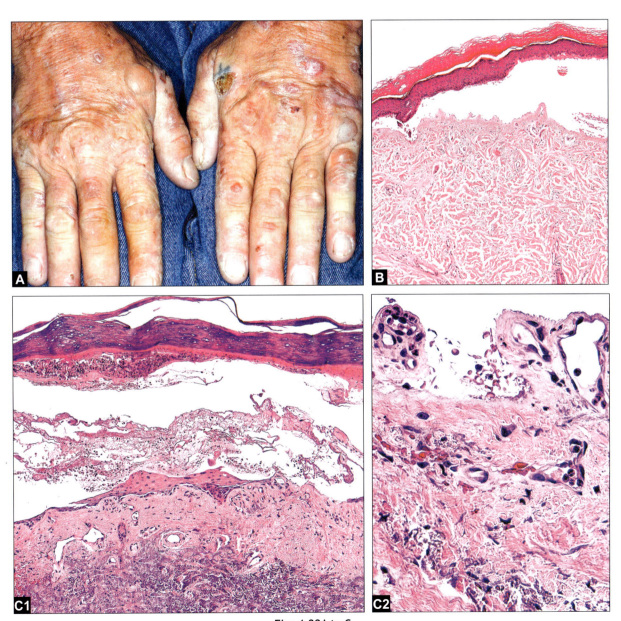

Figs 4.22A to C

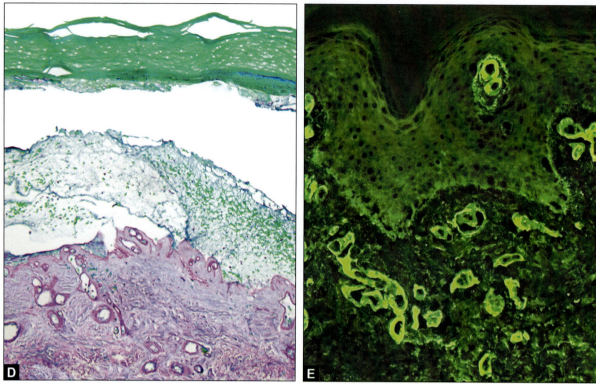

Figs 4.22A to E: Porphyria cutanea tarda. (A) Tense blisters, erosions, and scars cover the dorsum of the hands; (B) The classic histopathologic finding is a subepidermal paucicellular blister with retention of the dermal papilla (festooning); (C) The blisters are often impetiginized, however, and may contain red blood cells, serum and various inflammatory cells. There is also re-epithelialization (epidermal regrowth) in some cases, as seen in the center of this field; (D) Porphyria. Staining with periodic acid-Schiff stain highlights the characteristic thickening of vessel walls; (E) Direct immunofluorescence demonstrates thick perivascular deposits of IgG.

Bullous Lupus Erythematosus

▪ Criteria for diagnosis

- Widespread blisters with a predilection for sun-exposed skin
- Subepidermal blister with numerous neutrophils within the blister cavity or the underlying papillary dermis (Fig. 4.23A)
- Clinical and laboratory findings indicative of lupus erythematosus.

▪ Differential diagnosis

- Dermatitis herpetiformis (Fig. 4.23B)
- Linear IgA bullous dermatosis
- Cicatricial pemphigoid
- Epidermolysis bullosa acquisita
- Sweet's syndrome
- Bullous leukocytoclastic vasculitis (LCV).

▪ Pitfalls

- Clinically and histopathologically, there is often little or no resemblance to the typical lesions of lupus erythematosus (i.e. basal vacuolar change, epidermal atrophy and basement membrane zone thickening are uncommon)

- Leukocytoclastic vasculitis may be present, causing confusion with bullous LCV.

▪ Pearls

- Sun-exposed skin is favored but lesions may occur anywhere
- Predilection for trunk and flexural surfaces
- Most common in young black females
- Blisters are commonly preceded by erythematous plaques
- Occasional cases are accompanied by marked dermal edema (Fig. 4.23C)
- If performed, DIF often reveals granular or linear deposition of IgG, IgA, IgM and C3 along the dermoepidermal junction in both lesional and clinically normal-appearing skin (and if positive, can differentiate bullous lupus from the other entities in the differential diagnosis).

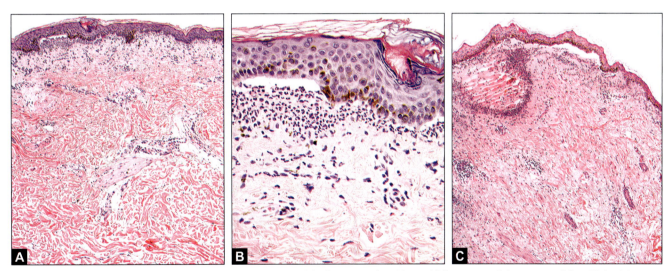

Figs 4.23A to C: Bullous lupus erythematosus. (A) The usual finding is a subepidermal blister containing neutrophils; (B) In this case, the neutrophils within the papillary dermis impart an appearance very similar to dermatitis herpetiformis; (C) In some examples there is edema and cellular debris.

Dermatitis Herpetiformis

■ *Criteria for diagnosis*

- Crops of recurrent intensely pruritic papules, erosions and blisters (Fig. 4.24A)
- Subepidermal blister with dermal neutrophils within upper dermis/dermal papilla (Figs 4.24B and C)
- *Direct immunofluorescence*: Granular deposition of IgA along basement membrane zone in perilesional skin (Fig. 4.24D).

■ *Differential diagnosis*

- Clinical differential considerations often include nonspecific dermatitis, folliculitis and other inflammatory processes
- Histopathologically dermatitis herpetiformis may closely simulate linear IgA dermatosis.

■ *Pitfalls*

- Intact blisters are seldom seen since the severe pruritus causes excoriation

- Excoriated papules are therefore the most common clinical finding
- Clinical impression is often that of nonspecific eczematous dermatitis, folliculitis or insect bite reaction and DH may not be included.

■ *Pearls*

- Extensor surfaces of the extremities (especially knees and elbows) are favored sites
- Lesions are usually bilateral and symmetrically distributed
- Most patients have a gluten-sensitive enteropathy (celiac sprue)
- Linear IgA bullous dermatosis is differentiated by its linear pattern of IgA deposition and the clinical scenario.

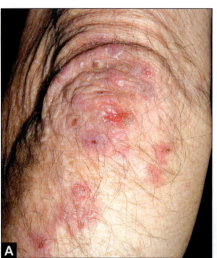
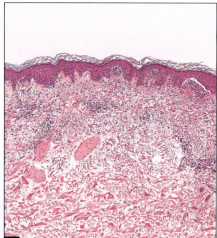
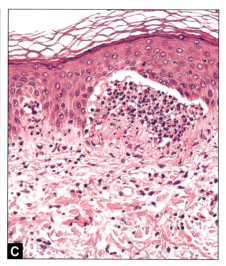
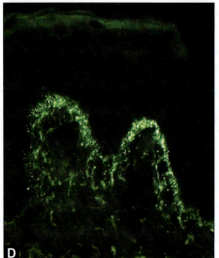

Figs 4.24A to D: Dermatitis herpetiformis. (A) Intact blisters are rarely seen due to the intense pruritus. Excoriations, such as these on the elbow are a more common presentation; (B) At low power, dermal papilla are occupied by small microabscesses; (C) High magnification shows that neutrophils predominate, particularly within early lesions; (D) Direct immunofluorescence examination reveals granular IgA deposition at the basement membrane.

Linear IgA Bullous Dermatosis
(Figs 4.25A to C)

■ Criteria for diagnosis

- Crops of clear or hemorrhagic blisters, either discrete or closely grouped
- Subepidermal blister with dermal neutrophils and eosinophils
- Direct immunofluorescence: Linear deposition of IgA along basement membrane zone in perilesional skin.

■ Differential diagnosis

- Histopathologically may simulate dermatitis herpetiformis, "chronic bullous disease of childhood" (see below), bullous pemphigoid, EBA and bullous lupus erythematosus.

■ Pitfalls

- In addition to IgA deposition, there may also be linear deposition of C3 and other immunoreactants.

■ Pearls

- So-called "chronic bullous disease of childhood" is likely the same entity
- Linear IgA bullous dermatosis is best differentiated by its linear pattern of IgA deposition (not granular, as in dermatitis herpetiformis) and the clinical scenario
- May be idiopathic or drug induced
- Vancomycin accounts for approximately half of the drug induced cases
- Oral lesions are common.

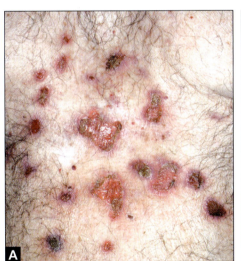
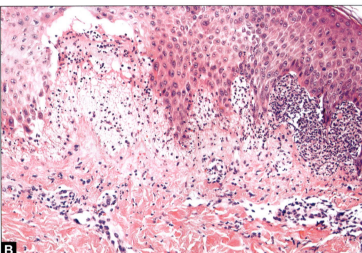
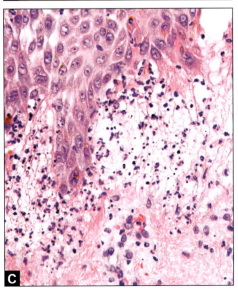

Figs 4.25A to C: Linear IgA bullous dermatosis. (A) Erythematous crusted erosions resulting from excoriated blisters; (B) Many cases closely resemble dermatitis herpetiformis with dermal papillae occupied by an inflammatory infiltrate rich in neutrophils; (C) Neutrophils often predominate, but it is important to remember that eosinophils may be equally or even more numerous in some cases.

Bullous Arthropod Bite Reaction
(Figs 4.26A to C)

■ *Criteria for diagnosis*

- Edematous papules, vesicles or blisters
- Solitary or grouped in clusters of several lesions
- Intraepidermal or subepidermal vesicles with spongiosis and a superficial and deep perivascular inflammatory infiltrate with eosinophils.

■ *Differential diagnosis*

- Autoimmune blistering diseases
- Bullous light eruption.

■ *Pitfalls*

- Nonspecific histopathologic features make definitive diagnosis difficult.

■ *Pearls*

- Multiloculated blisters, especially with epidermal necrosis, are more common in bullous arthropod bite than in autoimmune blistering disorders

- A large central vesicle with adjacent vesicles of progressively diminishing size is particularly characteristic of a bite reaction.
- Epidermal necrosis and/or pustule formation may accompany the blister
- A dense superficial and deep perivascular infiltrate containing eosinophils is almost always present, a finding that would be unusual in autoimmune blistering diseases
- Focal degeneration or necrosis of dermal collagen is a helpful clue
- Predilection for children, particularly the lower extremities
- Fleas, chiggers and bed bugs are among the most common causes.

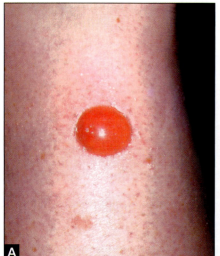 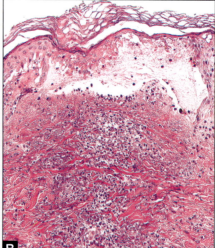 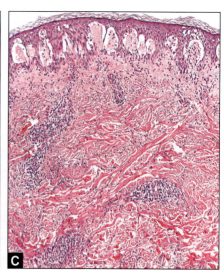

Figs 4.26A to C: Bullous arthropod bite reaction. (A) There is a tense blister very similar to the type often seen in bullous pemphigoid; (B) In this example, there is a subepidermal blister and mixed inflammation. A clue to the fact that this is a bite reaction is the necrotic/degenerating collagen beneath the blister, a finding more typical of a bite reaction than of most autoimmune blistering diseases; (C) In other cases, the epidermis is occupied by a multiloculated blister or a series of vesicles.

Bullous Light Eruption

■ *Criteria for diagnosis*

- Macules, papules, plaques and less commonly, vesicles
- Onset within hours or days after sun exposure (Fig. 4.27)
- Subepidermal edema, mixed inflammation and blister formation.

■ *Differential diagnosis*

- Bullous arthropod bite reaction
- Other bullous diseases, particularly those with deep dermal inflammation (rather than only superficial inflammation).

■ *Pitfalls*

- Rare cases of lupus erythematosus may have papillary dermal edema and even neutrophils, closely simulating bullous light eruption and other blistering diseases.

■ *Pearls*

- Bullous light eruption is an exaggerated presentation of polymorphous light eruption
- Onset typically after first prolonged exposure to sunlight (ultraviolet A and sometimes ultraviolet B) after prolonged period of low sun exposure
- Usually seen in early spring or summer, but onset after a sunny winter vacation is also a common history
- Photo distribution of lesions is supportive of the diagnosis
- Forearms and other intermittently exposed skin are common sites, while chronically sun-exposed skin is often spared due to "hardening" of these sites.

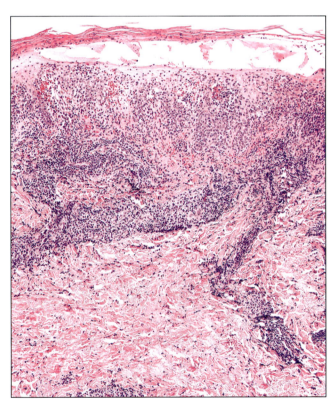

Fig. 4.27: Occasionally severe reactions to light exposure may result in blisters. The epidermis is thinned, there is marked edema and the inflammatory infiltrate involves the deeper dermis in addition to the superficial region.

Bullous Erythema Multiforme

■ *Criteria for diagnosis*

- Vacuolar type interface lymphocytic infiltrate with keratinocyte necrosis and variable papillary dermal edema in bullous EM.

■ *Differential diagnosis*

- Paraneoplastic pemphigus
- Toxic epidermal necrolysis
- Other interface vacuolar dermatoses that have developed blistering (e.g. bullous drug eruption, bullous lichen planus, etc.).

■ *Pitfalls*

- Eosinophils may be numerous, especially in cases caused by drugs, and may closely simulate bullous pemphigoid (Fig. 4.28).

■ *Pearls*

- Clues to the etiology may be found at the edge of the blister (e.g. wedge-shaped hypergranulosis of bullous lichen planus would not be seen in bullous EM)

- Extensive keratinocyte necrosis favors bullous EM over bullous pemphigoid and many other bullous disorders.

Blisters Due to Dermolysis

A number of other diseases may result in blistering. All appear to cause blistering by destruction of the basement membrane zone and therefore the blisters are subepidermal (Fig. 4.29).

Examples of other causes of blisters that are not true blistering disorders are:

- Blister overlying scars
- Suction blisters
- Bullous lichen sclerosus
- Bullous amyloidosis.

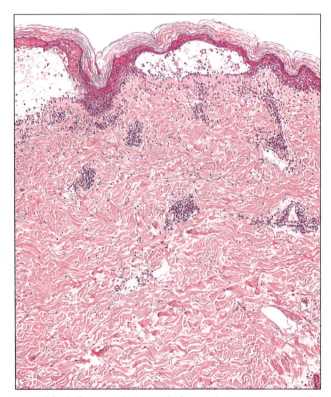

Fig. 4.28: Bullous erythema multiforme. In some cases, erythema multiforme may contain numerous eosinophils and blisters may form closely simulating bullous pemphigoid.

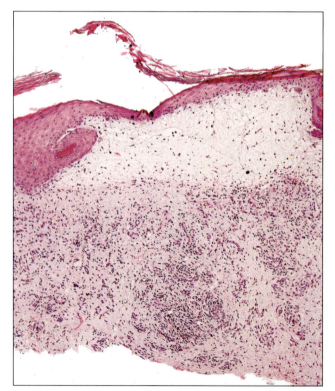

Fig. 4.29: Bullous edema. Severe edema such as this can cause a subepidermal blister that can be mistaken for a "genuine" blistering disease.

BIBLIOGRAPHY

1. Caux F. Diagnosis and clinical features of epidermolysis bullosa acquisita. Dermatol Clin. 2011;29(3):485-91.
2. Frew JW, Murrell DF. Paraneoplastic pemphigus (paraneoplastic autoimmune multiorgan syndrome): clinical presentations and pathogenesis. Dermatol Clin. 2011;29(3):419-25.
3. Intong LR, Murrell DF. Pemphigoid gestationis: pathogenesis and clinical features.Dermatol Clin. 2011;29(3):447-52.
4. James KA, Culton DA, Diaz LA. Diagnosis and clinical features of pemphigus foliaceus.Dermatol Clin. 2011;29(3):405-12.
5. Lara-Corrales I, Pope E. Autoimmune blistering diseases in children. Semin Cutan Med Surg. 2010;29(2):85-91.
6. Schmidt E, della Torre R, Borradori L. Clinical features and practical diagnosis of bullous pemphigoid. Dermatol Clin. 2011;29(3):427-38.
7. Schmidt E, Zillikens D. Modern diagnosis of autoimmune blistering skin diseases.Autoimmun Rev. 2010;10(2):84-9.
8. Venning VA. Linear IgA disease: clinical presentation, diagnosis, and pathogenesis. Dermatol Clin. 2011;29(3):453-8.

CHAPTER 5

Follicular Processes

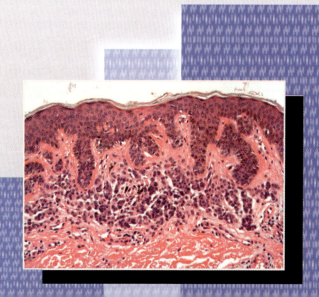

INTRODUCTION

Follicular processes can be subdivided into diseases that involve three different portions of the hair follicle:

1. The follicular epithelium itself—folliculitis (Box 5.1)
2. Diseases that are folliculocentric and involve the perifollicular epithelium—perifolliculitis (Box 5.2)
3. Diseases which are associated with a decrease in the number of hair follicles—alopecia (Boxes 5.3 and 5.4)

Folliculitis can be classified as either infectious or noninfectious. Infectious folliculitis is often due to Staphylococcus but can also be due to Pseudomonas, fungi (Majocchi's granuloma), Pityrosporum organisms, herpes virus, Demodex organisms, or other kinds of infectious agents. Causes of noninfectious folliculitis include acne and other acneiform diseases.

INFECTIOUS BACTERIAL FOLLICULITIS

▪ *Criteria for diagnosis (Figs 5.1A to C)*

Presence of Bacteria Associated with Neutrophils
- Clues for diagnosis
  - Neutrophils within the follicular infundibulum and isthmus
  - Occasional disruption of follicular epithelium
  - Neutrophils in the interstitium between collagen bundles
  - Subcorneal pustule formation (Fig 5.1A).

▪ *Differential diagnosis*

- Fungal or viral folliculitis versus noninfectious causes of folliculitis (Box 5.1).

▪ *Pitfalls*

- Propionibacterium acnes is associated with acne vulgaris and could be confused with Staphylococcal folliculitis
- Early lesions of pyoderma gangrenosum can present as folliculitis.

▪ *Pearls*

- Neutrophils predominate in bacterial folliculitis
- Histiocytes are prominent in fungal folliculitis
- Lymphocytes predominate in herpes folliculitis.

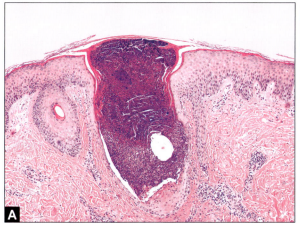
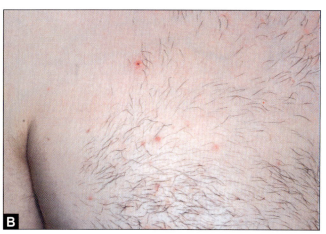
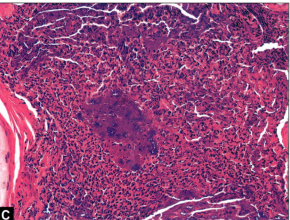

Figs 5.1A to C: Folliculitis. (A) Follicular based pustule; (B) Follicular based papules and pustules; (C) Bacteria in the center of the pustule.

MAJOCCHI'S GRANULOMA

■ *Criteria for diagnosis*

Fungi within or Surrounding Hair Shafts (Figs 5.2A and B)
- Clue for diagnosis
  - Granulomatous inflammation
  - Occasional eosinophils.

■ *Differential diagnosis*

Other infectious and noninfectious folliculitis (Boxes 5.1 and 5.2).

■ *Pitfalls*

- Pityrosporum organisms are normally found within follicular infundibuli and unless hyphal forms are noted or organisms present within the dermis caution should be made in diagnosing Pityrosporum or fungal folliculitis.

■ *Pearls*

- Deep folliculitis containing giant cells is a clue to Majocchi's granuloma.

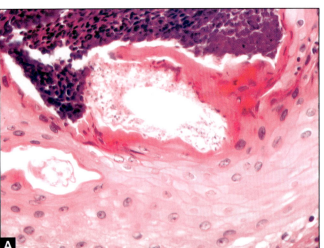 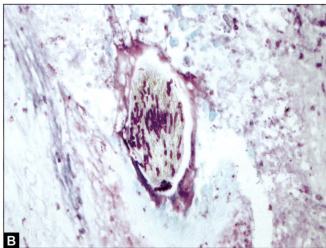

Figs 5.2A and B: Majocchi's granuloma. (A) Fungi surrounding a hair follicle; (B) Periodic acid-Schiff stain highlights the fungi around.

HERPES ZOSTER

■ *Criteria for diagnosis*

Multinucleated Keratinocytes with Nuclear Molding

- Clues for dlagnosis
  - Ballooning necrosis of follicular epithelium (Fig. 5.3A)
  - Follicular keratinocytes with steel gray nuclei (Fig. 5.3B)
  - Dense superficial and deep lymphocytic infiltrate
  - Occasional eosinophils.

■ *Differential diagnosis*

Herpes Simplex Viral infection

- Trichodysplasia Spinulosa due to polyoma virus (see also Boxes 5.1 and 5.2)

■ *Pitfalls*

- A dense lymphocytic infiltrate with atypical lymphocytes can be seen in vicinity of herpes folliculitis (Resnik KS, DiLeonardo M). The atypical infiltrate can mimic lymphoma cutis. Some early herpetic lesions can also mimic eythema multiforme before the characteristic follicular involvment becomes evident.

■ *Pearls*

- Granulomatous vasculitis can be a sequela of herpes zoster infection.

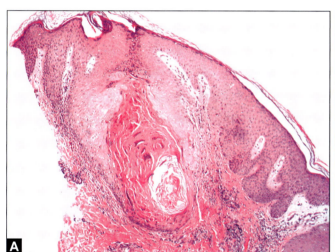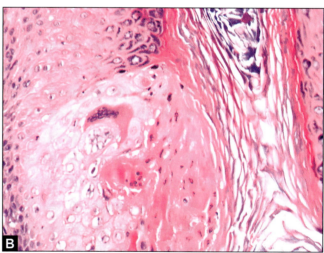

Figs 5.3A and B: Herpes zoster. (A) Ballooning necrosis of follicular epithelium; (B) Multinucleated giant cell and nuclei with steely grey nuclei.

NONINFECTIOUS CAUSES OF FOLLICULITIS (BOX 5.1)

Acne Vulgaris and Variants

Acne vulgaris and its variants are typically best diagnosed because of characteristic clinical features and usually do not require biopsy (Figs 5.4A and B). An important clue to the diagnosis is the presence of comedones (Fig. 5.4C).

Rosacea (Figs 5.5A to C)

Rosacea is an inflammatory disease of the pilosebaceous unit exacerbated by sun damage in genetically predisposed individuals. The sun damage eliminates the structural support in the dermis around blood vessels causing the blood vessels to dilate, and the lack of support around hair follicles causes the follicular infundibulum to dilate allowing *Demodex* organisms to proliferate along with debris. The accumulation of keratinaceous debris, bacteria and *Demodex* organisms is associated with perifollicular inflammation (Figs 5.5A and B).

■ *Differential diagnosis*

Box 5.1: Noninfectious causes for folliculitis

- Acne vulgaris and variants
  - Acne conglobata, nodular acne, acne mechanica, acne cosmetica, pomade acne, acne fulminans
- Acne necrotica
- Acne rosacea
- Acne keloidalis
- Behcet's disease
- Eosinophilic folliculitis of HIV
- Eosinophilic folliculitis (Ofuji's disease)
- Erythema toxicum neonatorum
- Folliculitis of pregnancy
- Medication induced acne
  - Steroid
  - Epidermal growth factor inhibitors
  - Lithium
  - Halogenoderma
- Pseudofolliculitis
- Pyoderma gangrenosum

■ *Criteria for diagnosis*

- Dilated follicular infundibulum containing *Demodex* organisms
- Perifollicular lymphohistiocytic infiltrate
- Occasional granulomas
- Solar elastosis
- Telangiectasias
- Occasional eosinophils.

■ *Pitfalls*

- Perifollicular sarcoidal granulomas resembling sarcoidosis can be seen in granulomatous rosacea (Fig. 5.5B)
- Granulomas with caseating necrosis resembling tuberculosis can be seen in the lupus miliaris disseminatus faciei variant of Rosacea.

■ *Pearls*

- Rosacea invariably occurs in sun damaged skin (Fig. 5.5C).

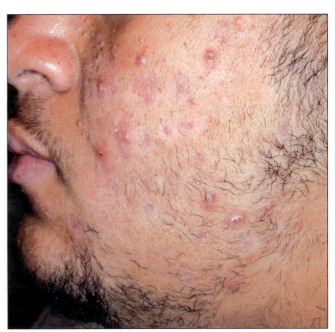

Fig. 5.4A

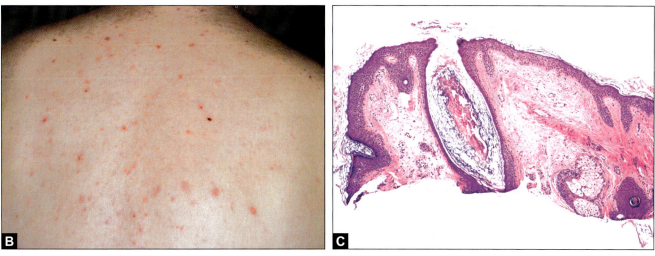

Figs 5.4A to C: (A) Acne with scarring on face; (B) Acne also commonly involves the black and chest; (C) Comedone—dilated follicular orifice containing debris and bacteria.
Note: Unlike infectious folliculitis, the inflammatory infiltrate is usually very sparse in comedones

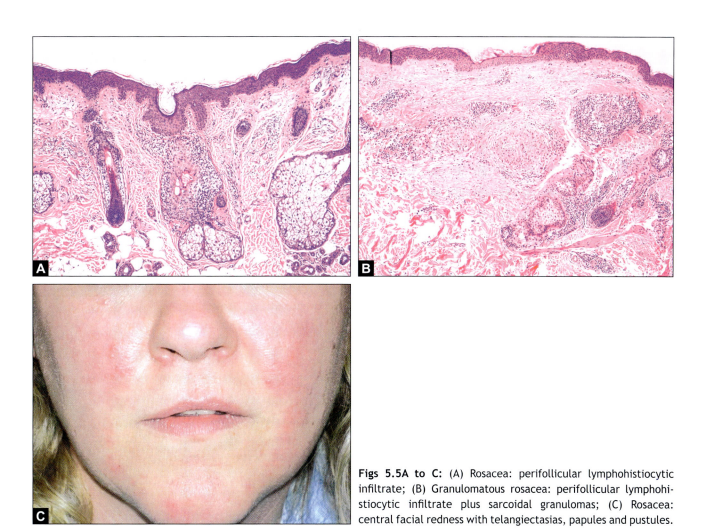

Figs 5.5A to C: (A) Rosacea: perifollicular lymphohistiocytic infiltrate; (B) Granulomatous rosacea: perifollicular lymphohistiocytic infiltrate plus sarcoidal granulomas; (C) Rosacea: central facial redness with telangiectasias, papules and pustules.

Eosinophilic Folliculitis (Ofuji's Disease) and Eosinophilic Folliculitis of HIV Disease (Fig. 5.6)

■ *Criteria for diagnosis*
- Pustule composed of eosinophils within follicular infundibula.

■ *Differential diagnosis*
- Erythema toxicum neonatorum
- Folliculocentric insect bite reaction
- Fungal eosinophilic folliculitis.

■ *Pitfalls*
- Insect bite reactions can often be folliculocentric.

■ *Pearls*
- Eosinophils predominate in Ofuji's disease.

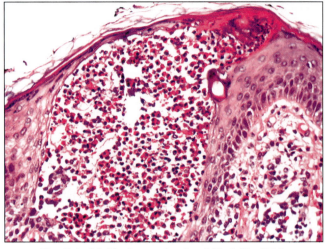

Fig. 5.6: Ofuji's disease (eosinophilic folliculitis).

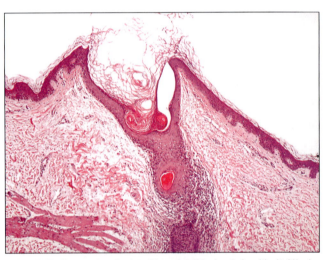

Fig. 5.7: Keratosis pilaris—dilated follicular infundibuli filled with keratin and overlying hyperkeratosis.

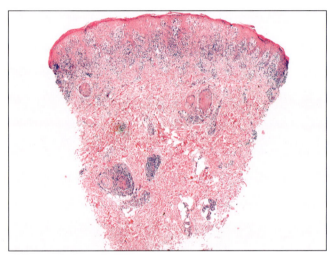

Fig. 5.8: Lichen striatus—psoriasiform lichenoid pattern with periadnexal inflammation.

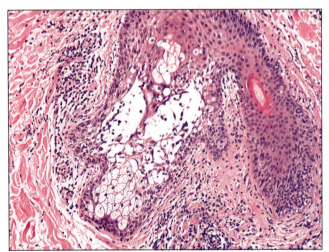

Fig. 5.9: Follicular mucinosis—mucin deposition within follicular epithelium.

Box 5.2: Causes for perifolliculitis

- Lymphocytic inflammation
  - Lupus erythematosus/dermatomyositis
  - Lichen planopilaris
  - Keratosis pilaris and variants (Fig. 5.7).
  - Lichen striatus (Fig. 5.8).
  - Follicular mycosis fungoides
  - Follicular mucinosis (Fig. 5.9).
  - Drug reaction (epidermal growth factor inhibitors)
- Lymphohistiocytic inflammation
  - Rosacea (also see folliculitis)

ALOPECIA

The alopecias can be divided into two main categories: scarring and nonscarring alopecia (Boxes 5.3 and 5.4). There may be overlapping features because some types of alopecia, classically classified as nonscarring, may develop scarring over time. Diagnosis of nonscarring alopecia can often be made by clinical examination of the scalp, although biopsies must sometimes be performed.

Nonscarring Alopecia

■ *Criteria for diagnosis*

- *Alopecia areata*: Lymphocytes and occasional eosinophils surrounding anagen hair follicles (Figs 5.10A to C)
- *Androgenetic alopecia*: Miniaturization of hair follicles (Figs 5.11A and B)
- *Trichotillomania or Traction alopecia*: Empty hair shafts and trichomalacia (degenerating hair shafts) and increased number of catagen hair follicle (Figs 5.12A and B)
- *Telogen effluvium*: Increased number of telogen hair follicles without hair miniaturization (Fig. 5.14).

■ *Differential diagnosis*

- Scarring Alopecia (see box 5.4)
- Syphilis

■ *Pitfalls*

- The "moth eaten" clinical pattern of alopecia encountered in secondary syphilis can mimic alopecia areata on biopsy, but plasma cells are usually more conspicuous.

■ *Pearls*

- Dilated follicular infundibuli resembling Swiss cheese on horizontal sections is clue to alopecia areata (Muller et al.).

Box 5.3: Nonscarring alopecia
• Alopecia areata (Figs 5.10A to C).
• Androgenetic alopecia (Figs 5.11A and B).
• Trichotillomania (Figs 5.12A to C).
• Traction alopecia (Fig. 5.13).
• Telogen effluvium (Figs 5.14 A and B).
• Disorders of hair shaft

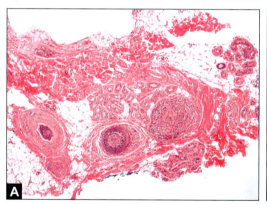
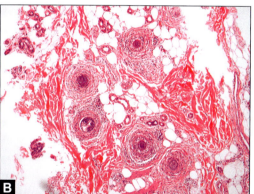
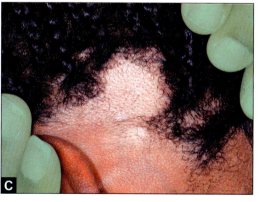

Figs 5.10A to C: Alopecia areata. (A) Lymphocytic inflammation around anagen hair follicle and a catagen hair on left; (B) Perifollicular lymphocytic infiltrate; (C) Round circular foci of nonscarring alopecia.

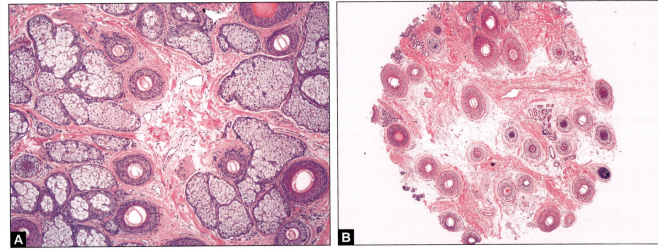

Figs 5.11A and B: Androgenetic alopecia. (A) Non-inflammatory alopecia with miniaturization of hair follicles; (B) Non-inflammatory alopecia with hair shafts of different sizes/miniaturization.

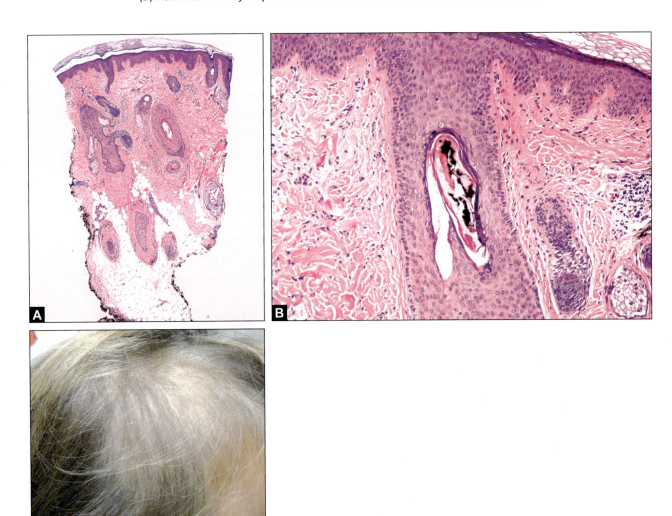

Figs 5.12A to C: Trichotillomania. (A) Noninflammatory alopecia with catagen hair follicle; (B) Trichomalacia; (C) Thinning of hair due to trichotillomania. *Courtesy:* Dr Renee Straub.

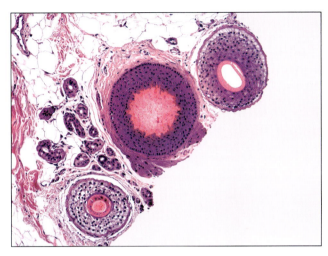

Fig. 5.13: Traction alopecia—reduced number of hair follicles with preserved vellus hairs.

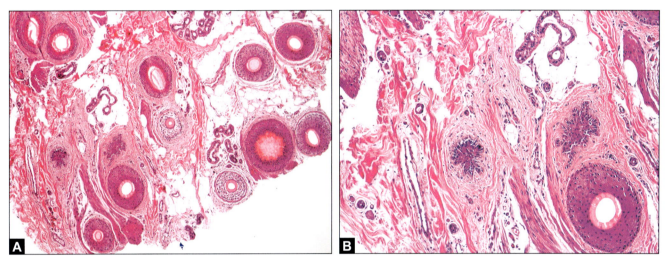

Figs 5.14A and B: Telogen effluvium—increased number of telogen follicles and catagen follicle.

Scarring Alopecia

■ *Criteria for diagnosis*

- Decreased number of hair follicles
- Hair follicles replaced by fibrous tracks
- Lymphocytes predominate in lupus erythematosus, lichen planopilaris and central centrifugal scarring alopecia
    - Lymphocytes around follicular infundibula—lichen planopilaris (Figs 5.16A to C).
    - Interface dermatitis plus mucin—cutaneous lupus erythematosus (Fig. 5.15).
    - Central centrifugal scarring alopecia—Epithelial thinning with surrounding perifollicular fibrosis (Figs 5.17A and B)
- Neutrophils predominate
    - Folliculitis decalvans—predominately folliculocentric inflammation (Fig. 5.18).
    - Disecting cellulitis (Fig. 5.18).

■ *Pitfalls*

- Chronic nonscarring alopecia such as androgenetic alopecia can lead to permanent scarring.

■ *Pearls*

- Compound follicles (tufted folliculitis), i.e. more than one hair shaft within follicular epithelium is a clue to an old lesion of neutrophilic scarring alopecia (Elston DM, Pincus LB, et al.).

Box 5.4: Differential of scarring alopecia

- Lupus erythematosus (Fig. 5.15).
- Lichen planopilaris (Figs 5.16A to C).
    - Variant: Frontal fibrosing alopecia
- Central centrifugal cicatricial alopecia (Figs 5.17A and C).
    - Synonym's/variants: Follicular degeneration syndrome, Pseudopelade of Brocq
- Folliculitis decalvans (Fig. 5.18).
- Dissecting cellulitis (Figs 5.19A and B).
- Acne keloidalis (Figs 5.20 A to C).

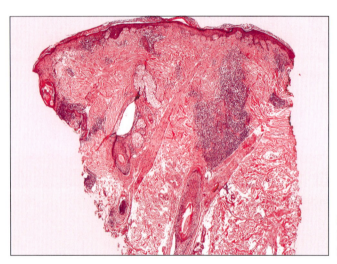

Fig. 5.15: Cutaneous lupus erythematosus—dense perifollicular lymphocytic infiltrate associated with interface changes along the dermal epidermal junction.

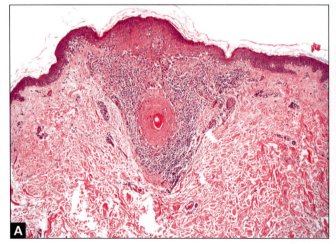

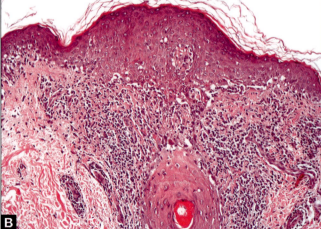

Figs 5.16A and B

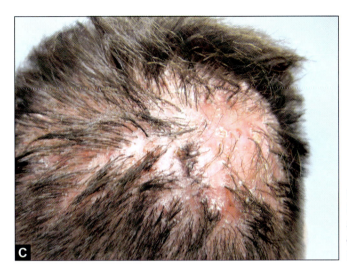

Figs 5.16A to C: Lichen planopilaris. (A) Folliculocentric lichenoid inflammation; (B) Higher power (Note hypergranulosis and saw toothing); (C) Scarring alopecia with perifollicular erythema.
Courtesy: Dr Renee Straub

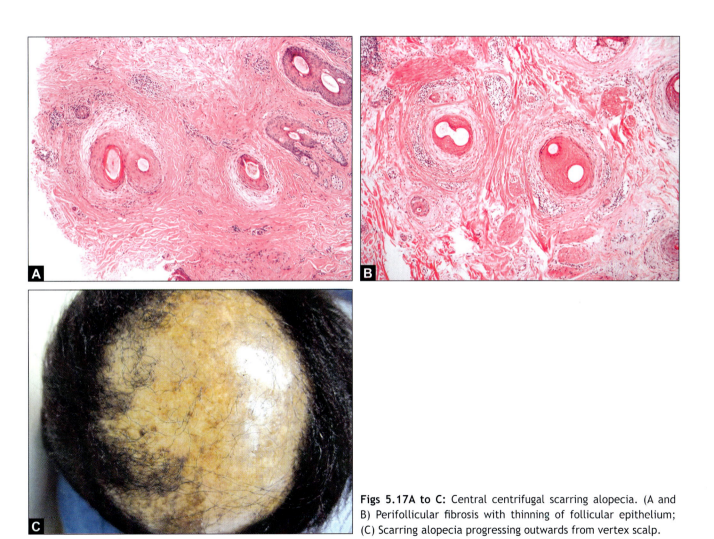

Figs 5.17A to C: Central centrifugal scarring alopecia. (A and B) Perifollicular fibrosis with thinning of follicular epithelium; (C) Scarring alopecia progressing outwards from vertex scalp.

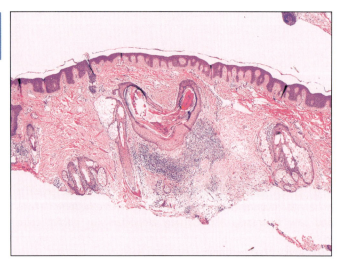

Fig. 5.18: Folliculitis decalvans—acute and chronic deep folliculitis with fibrosis.

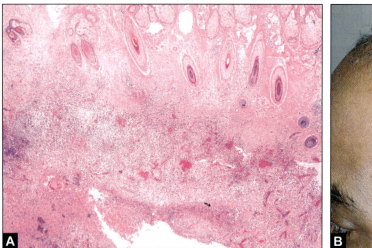

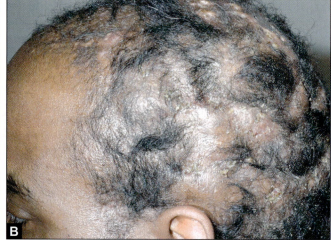

Figs 5.19A and B: (A) Dissecting cellulitis—hair shaft with surrounding granulomatous inflammation and mixed inflammatory infiltrate and fibrosis in periphery; (B) Disecting cellulitis with patches of scarring alopecia.

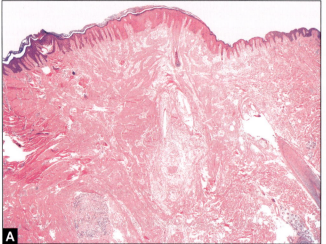

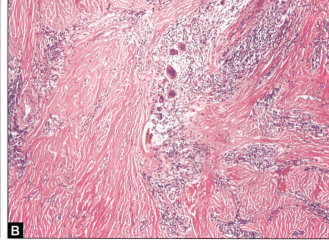

Figs 5.20A and B

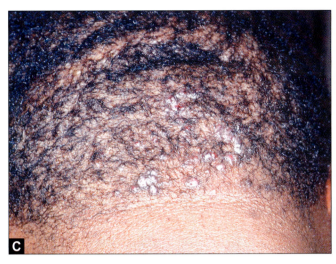

Figs 5.20A to C: Acne keloidalis. (A) Scarring alopecia with perifollicular granulomatous inflammation; (B) Sclerotic collagen bundles visible in higher magnification; (C) Papules and nodules associated with alopecia nape of neck and occipital scalp.

BIBLIOGRAPHY

1. Boer A, Herder N, Winter K, et al.. Herpes folliculitis: clinical, histopathological, and molecular pathologic observations. Br J Dermatol. 2006;154(4):743-6.
2. Elston DM. Tufted folliculitis. J Cutan Pathol. 2011.
3. Eudy G, Solomon AR. The histopathology of noncicatricial alopecia. Semin Cutan Med Surg. 2006;25(1):35-40.
4. Helm KF, Menz J, Gibson LE, et al. A clinical and histopathologic study of granulomatous rosacea. J Am Acad Dermatol. 1991;25(6 Pt 1):1038-43.
5. Muller CS, L. El Shabrawi-Caelen L. 'Follicular Swiss cheese' pattern—another histopathologic clue to alopecia areata. J Cutan Pathol. 2011;38(2):185-9.
6. Nervi SJ, Schwartz RA, Dmochowski M. Eosinophilic pustular folliculitis: a 40 year retrospect. J Am Acad Dermatol. 2006;55(2):285-9.
7. Osio A, Mateus C, Soria JC, et al. Cutaneous side-effects in patients on long-term treatment with epidermal growth factor receptor inhibitors. Br J Dermatol. 2009;161(3):515-21.
8. Pincus LB, Price VH, McCalmont TH. The amount counts: distinguishing neutrophil-mediated and lymphocyte-mediated cicatricial alopecia by compound follicles. J Cutan Pathol. 2011;38(1):1-4.
9. Resnik KS, DiLeonardo M. Herpes incognito. Am J Dermatopathol. 2000;22(2):144-50.
10. Somani N, Bergfeld WS. Cicatricial alopecia: classification and histopathology. Dermatol Ther. 2008;21(4):221-37.
11. Sperling LC, Cowper SE. The histopathology of primary cicatricial alopecia. Semin Cutan Med Surg. 2006;25(1):41-50.
12. Sperling LC, Homoky C, Pratt L, et al. Acne keloidalis is a form of primary scarring alopecia. Arch Dermatol. 2000;136(4):479-84.
13. Sperling LC, Solomon AR, Whiting DA. A new look at scarring alopecia. Arch Dermatol. 2000;136(2):235-42.
14. Sperling LC. Scarring alopecia and the dermatopathologist. J Cutan Pathol. 2001;28(7):333-42.
15. Stefanato CM. Histopathology of alopecia: a clinicopathological approach to diagnosis. Histopathology. 2010;56(1):24-38.

CHAPTER 6

The Nodular and Diffuse Dermal Infiltrative Patterns

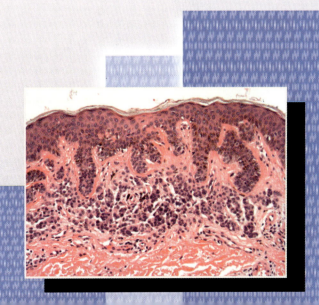

INTRODUCTION

Nodular and/or diffuse inflammatory infiltrates of the dermis are produced by a wide variety of diseases. They can be divided into general categories based on the presence of granulomas, the type as a rule, careful search for microorganisms (usually including histochemical stains) is warranted whenever a granulomatous or suppurative dermatitis is encountered. The clinical and etiological details of the many infections that may cause this pattern are beyond the scope of this book, but the common patterns that they produce and the histochemical stains that aid in their detection are important for every histopathologist to know (Tables 6.1 to 6.9).

The differential diagnosis of palisading granulomas can include one of the most disastrous pitfalls in pathology—the tendency for epithelioid sarcoma to mimic a palisading granulomatous disease. Although rare, this is a well-documented differential diagnostic dilemma with very serious implications. As a result, great care is necessary to exclude this possibility both clinically and histopathologically.

THE GRANULOMATOUS PATTERN (TABLE 6.1)

Sarcoidosis

■ *Criteria for diagnosis*

- Smooth flesh-colored brown papules, nodules or plaques; often violaceous nodules on cheeks, nose and earlobes (lupus pernio) (Fig. 6.1A)
- Sarcoidal granulomas within dermis and/or subcutis (Figs 6.1B and C)
- Absence of microorganisms (confirmed by histochemical stains or cultures)
- Clinical evidence of sarcoidosis (e.g. lung, eye, lymph node involvement).

■ *Differential diagnosis*

- Foreign body reaction (especially to silicates, zirconium, beryllium and tattoo pigments)
- Infections (tuberculoid leprosy, tuberculosis, leishmaniasis, etc.)
- Granulomatous rosacea, cutaneous Crohn's disease, cheilitis granulomatosa (Melkersson-Rosenthal syndrome)
- Granulomas associated with lymphoproliferative disorders.

■ *Pitfalls*

- In addition to the classic "naked granulomas" (granulomas without significant additional inflammation), sarcoidosis may also present with central fibrinoid necrosis that simulates the caseation necrosis of a tuberculoid granuloma; occasionally lymphocytes are present
- Sarcoid granulomas occasionally contain polarizable crystals, making distinction from foreign body granulomas difficult; the presence of polarizable material does not exclude sarcoidosis
- Lesions of sarcoidosis commonly develop at sites of trauma, including in tattoos and scars, making it difficult to determine whether granulomas are a reaction to a pigment or a foreign material or are a manifestation of sarcoidosis.

■ *Pearls*

- Sarcoidal granulomas are nonspecific and clinical evidence of sarcoidosis is necessary to confirm the diagnosis (lung, eye, lymph node involvement, etc.)
- Serum angiotensin converting enzyme (ACE) levels are often elevated
- So-called "asteroid bodies" are sometimes seen in sarcoidosis but are not specific and are seen in many granulomatous reactions, particularly foreign body reactions (Fig. 6.1D).

Table 6.1: The sarcoidal/foreign body type granulomatous pattern			
Disease	Histopathologic Findings	Histochemical Stains	Clinical
Sarcoidosis	Granulomas (rare caseation)	Negative GMS, PAS, AFB, and Gram stains	Cutaneous nodules, ulcers, fistulas in patients with Crohn's disease
Foreign body reaction	Sarcoidal granulomas (rare caseation)	Negative GMS, PAS, AFB, and Gram stains	History of exposure to certain materials
Cutaneous Crohn's disease	Noncaseating granulomas within dermis and subcutis	Negative GMS, PAS, AFB, and Gram stains	Cutaneous nodules, ulcers, fistulas in patients with Crohn's disease
			Usually perianal, genital, or facial
Melkersson-Rosenthal syndrome	Small noncaseating granulomas within dermis and subcutis that impinge on lymphatics	Negative GMS, PAS, AFB, and Gram stains	Lip swelling
			Unilateral facial paralysis
			Furrowed tongue

Contd...

Disease	Histopathologic Findings	Histochemical Stains	Clinical
Primary cutaneous tuberculosis *M. tuberculosis*	Granulomas (+/- caseation) Suppurative dermatitis Sometimes ulceration	Fite or Ziehl-Neelsen type AFB stains may reveal organisms	Exogenous inoculation Indurated plaque, eventually with regional lymphadenopathy
Lupus vulgaris *M. tuberculosis*	Granulomas (+/- caseation) Suppurative dermatitis with necrosis	Fite or Ziehl-Neelsen type AFB stains Organisms rarely identified	Most common cutaneous form Infiltrated plaques with crusts Favors head and neck
Scrofuloderma *M. tuberculosis*	Necrotic sinus tract (connecting to underlying lymph node or joint)	Fite or Ziehl-Neelsen type AFB stains Organisms rarely identified	Rare Subcutaneous nodule that may form connection to overlying skin Favors head and neck
Tuberculids *M. tuberculosis* *hypersensitivity reaction*	Necrosis, mixed inflammation, sometimes vasculitis, sometimes palisading granulomas	No organisms present on stains	Erythema induratum Papulonecrotic tuberculid Lichen scrofulosorum
Tuberculoid leprosy *M. leprae*	Elongated oval granulomas, sometimes extending along nerves	Fite stain	Asymmetric plaques on trunk or limbs Enlarged nerve entering and exiting plaque
Candidiasis *C. albicans*	Usually confined to stratum corneum; nodular and diffuse pattern seen when hair follicle epithelium is involved or in systemic disease Yeasts and pseudohyphae	PAS GMS	Vesicles, pustules, and crusted erosions Skin folds
Aspergillosis *A. flavus* *A. fumigatus* *A. niger*	Thin septate hyphae 45° angle branching No yeast	PAS GMS	Cutaneous involvement rare Usually part of systemic infection Plaques rapidly evolve to eschar
Zygomycosis *Rhizopus* *Mucor* *Absidia*	Thick nonseptate hyphae 90° angle branching No yeast	PAS GMS	Immunocompromised patients, especially leukemia Indurated lesion that becomes necrotic with an erythematous halo No specific site
Dermatophytosis	Thin septate hyphae	PAS GMS	Blisters Hands and feet
Blastomycosis *Blastomyces dermatitidis*	Thick-walled round cell with multiple nuclei Broad-based buds on surface	PAS GMS	Many cases secondary to pulmonary disease but primary cutaneous inoculation also occurs Papules, nodules, verrucous plaques, or fungating tumors
Cryptococcosis	Yeast Often short chains of yeast Sieve-like appearance (in 'gelatinous' form)	PAS GMS Mucicarmine – red capsule Alcian blue – blue capsule	Immunocompromised Variable appearance including nodules, ecchymoses, and cellulitis Favors face, neck, and forearm

Contd...

Disease	Histopathologic Findings	Histochemical Stains	Clinical
Lobomycosis *Lacazia loboi* *(aka Loboa loboi)*	Yeast Often short 'chains' of yeast Sieve-like appearance	PAS GMS Negative for mucicarmine and Alcian blue	Dermal nodules with varying pigmentation, epidermis not involved Traumatic inoculation Favors extremities and external ear
Syphilis (secondary and tertiary forms) *Treponema pallidum*	Secondary - superficial and deep dermal lymphocytic infiltrate with variable number of plasma cells Tertiary - gummatous necrosis with peripheral inflammation	Warthin-Starry Steiner stain	Secondary - macules or papules with a guttate psoriatic appearance, palmoplantar predilection, moth-eaten alopecia Tertiary - chronic gummatous ulcer
Leishmaniasis *Leishmaina sp.*	Round to oval basophilic structures without a capsule Often localized to periphery of macrophage (marquee sign)	Giesma	Acute, chronic, recidivous (lupoid), disseminated, tardive, and leishmanid forms
Protothecosis *p. wikerhamii*	Multinucleated giant cells and macrophages containing morula-like sporangia	PAS GMS	Traumatic inoculation in an immunocompromised host

(GMS: Gomori methenamine silver; PAS: Periodic acid-Schiff; AFB: Acid-fast bacillus).

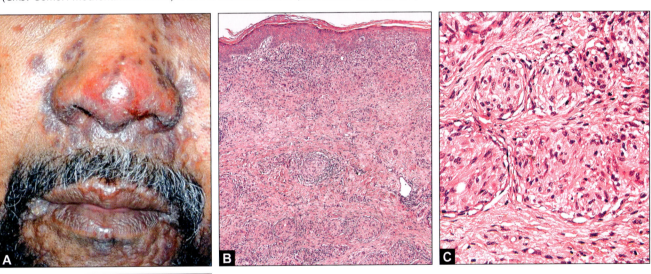

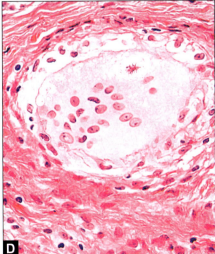

Figs 6.1A to D: Sarcoidosis. Smooth violet-brown dermal papules and nodules on the face representative of the lupus pernio subtype of cutaneous sarcoidosis. Lupus pernio is frequently associated with respiratory tract sarcoidosis; (B) Discrete granulomas are present throughout the entire dermis; (C) The granulomas are compact, rounded aggregates of macrophages; (D) Occasionally, multinucleated giant cells contain so called "asteroid bodies", which are small, brightly eosinophilic stellate structures. They are not specific for sarcoidosis, however.

Foreign Body Granulomatous Reactions (Table 6.2)

■ *Criteria for diagnosis*

- Granulomas containing foreign material (or cornified cells/keratin fragments) (Fig. 6.2A)
- No clinical evidence of sarcoidosis
- Absence of microorganisms (confirmed by histochemical stains).

■ *Differential diagnosis*

- Sarcoidosis and other causes of sarcoidal granuloma
- Chalazion.

■ *Pitfalls*

- Refractile and/or polarizable crystals alone are not sufficient for diagnosis since they may be encountered in sarcoidosis as well (Fig. 6.2B)

- Cornified cells and keratin fragments cause "foreign body" reactions that may be indistinguishable from genuine foreign body granulomas; ruptured cysts, glands or follicles must be excluded carefully; keratin fragments are occasionally sparse or altogether absent in resolving lesions.

■ *Pearls*

- Careful search for microorganisms is always warranted to exclude infectious causes
- The most common polarizable foreign materials are suture, starch, silica and talc (Fig. 6.2C) (Table 6.2)
- Clinical assessment of possible exposure to granuloma-inducing foreign materials may be helpful in confirming diagnosis.

Table 6.2: Granulomatous reactions to foreign materials		
Material	*Histopathologic Features*	*Common Causes and/or Clinical Scenario*
Keratin	Keratin fragments Rarely intact hair shafts	Ruptured cyst or follicles Barbers and dog groomers
Suture	Refractile fibers or fragments Polarizable round cords or fragments	Prior biopsy or surgery
Collagen	Granuloma formation Sarcoidal and/or palisading	Bovine collagen injections
Gout (Sodium urate)	Amorphous aggregates of pale eosinophilic or amphophilic material Negatively birefringent Angular clefts Palisading granulomatous inflammation Preserved crystals may be evident if fixed in alcohol rather than formalin	Nodules on digits (especially big toe) or ear
Tattoo	Pigment granules Black in carbon tattoos Any color in decorative tattoos	Carbon Graphite Cinnabar Cobalt blue Chrome green
Oils	Round and oval clear spaces vaguely resembling adipocytes Lipid droplets stainable for oil red-O stain and Sudan IV on frozen sections	Mineral oil Paraffin (especially in penis) Cottenseed oil Sesame oil Camphor
Injected steroids	Clear ovoid spaces or clefts Sometimes filled with amorphous, granular material	History of steroid injection
Aluminum	Basophilic granular material Nonpolarizable	Vaccination sites (aluminum sometimes an adjuvant in vaccines)

Contd...

Material	Histopathologic Features	Common Causes and/or Clinical Scenario
Beryllium	Sarcoidal granulomas Central necrosis or hyalinization sometimes Nonpolarizable	Fluorescent light bulb particles
Mercury	Black or dark brown globules Free within dermis and / or contained in macrophages	Broken thermometers Mercury-containing topicals
Starch	Foreign body-type granulomas PAS and GMS positive particles Polarizable white 'maltese cross' shaped particles	Surgical glove powder IV drug injection sites
Silica (silicon dioxide)	Foreign body-type granulomas Polarizable white granules or crystals	Wounds contaminated by glass fragments or soil
Talc (magnesium silicate)	Foreign body-type granulomas Polarizable white granules or crystals	
Zirconium	Foreign body-type granulomas Nonpolarizable	Deodarants

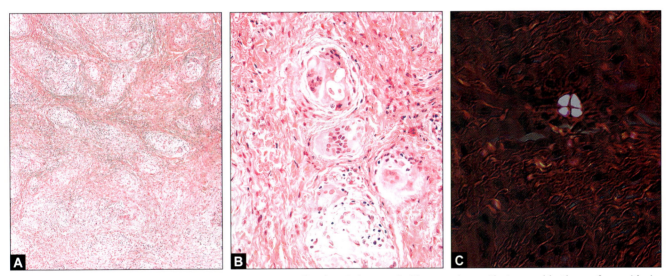

Figs 6.2A to C: Foreign body granulomatous reaction. (A) The dermis is occupied by granulomas that resemble those of sarcoidosis; (B) In some cases, relatively large foreign bodies may be seen within multinucleated giant cells. The granuloma at the top of the field contains refractile foreign material; (C) Examination with polarized light demonstrates refractile particles with a "Maltese cross" appearance.

Granulomatous Rosacea

▪ *Criteria for diagnosis*

- Clinical features or history of rosacea, especially advanced form with yellow-brown facial nodules (Lewandowsky's rosacea) (Fig. 6.3A)
- Granulomas with central caseation along with a perivascular and/or perifollicular lymphoplasmacytic infiltrate centered on follicles (Figs 6.3B and C)
- Absence of microorganisms (confirmed by histochemical stains).

▪ *Differential diagnosis*

- Cheilitis granulomatosa
- Sarcoidosis
- Cutaneous Crohn's disease
- Lupus miliaris disseminatus faciei
- Cutaneous tuberculosis (lupus vulgaris form in particular)
- Chronic granulomatous disease.

▪ *Pitfalls*

- Caseating necrosis is not uncommon and the appearance may closely simulate an infection (e.g. mycobacterial granulomas).

▪ *Pearls*

- Granulomas in acne rosacea likely result from rupture of markedly inflamed follicles
- Lupus miliaris disseminatus faciei is most likely an exaggerated form of granulomatous rosacea (see below)
- In cheilitis granulomatosa, the granulomas are characteristically directly adjacent to lymphatics (not centered on follicles) and localized to the deep dermis and subcutis
- Sarcoidosis lacks the abundant lymphoplasmacytic infiltrate typical of granulomatous rosacea
- The granulomas of cutaneous Crohn's disease are not centered on follicles and tend to involve the deep dermis and subcutis.

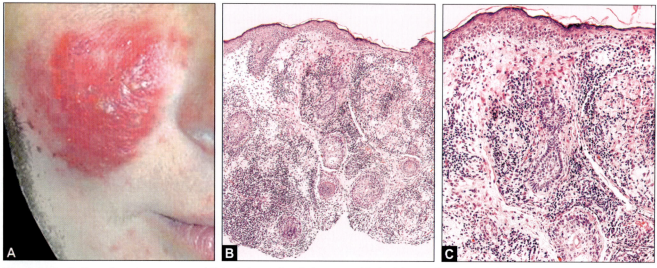

Figs 6.3A to C: Granulomatous rosacea. (A) An indurated red plaque studded with pustules on the cheek; (B) Noncaseating granulomas fill the dermis. A lymphoplasmacytic infiltrate is also present; (C) The granulomas are located around follicles.

Lupus Miliaris Disseminatus Faciei (Acne Agminata)

■ Criteria for diagnosis

- Yellow-brown papules on the central face, particularly the periorbital region, forehead and cheeks (Fig. 6.4A)
- Macrophages surrounding areas of caseation (sometimes with multinucleated giant cells) (Figs 6.4B and C)
- Absence of microorganisms (confirmed by histochemical stains if necessary).

■ Differential diagnosis

- Granulomatous infections (especially mycobacterium)
- Granulomatous rosacea.

■ Pitfalls

- Caseating granulomas may be identical to infectious granulomas, particularly mycobacteria.
- Some granulomas may be centered on follicles, suggesting suppurative folliculitis.

■ Pearls

- Considered an exaggerated form of granulomatous rosacea by some, but clinical presentation is distinct and many patients do not have other features typical of rosacea.

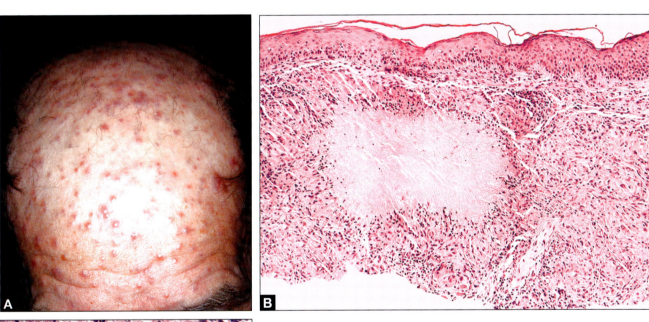

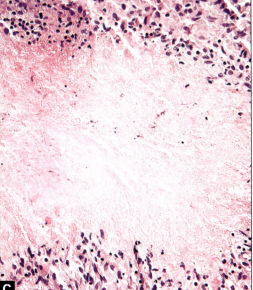

Figs 6.4A to C: Lupus miliaris disseminatus faciei. (A) Smooth violet-pink papules and nodules on the face and scalp; (B) The dermis contains a well-defined area of caseation; (C) The caseation is surrounded by macrophages. In many instances, histochemical stains for microorganisms must be performed to exclude an infectious etiology.

Chalazion

■ *Criteria for diagnosis*

- Painless nodule on eyelid
- Granulomas surrounding round, clear spaces adjacent to inflamed sebaceous (meibomian) glands (Fig. 6.5A)
- Absence of microorganisms (confirmed by histochemical stains if necessary).

■ *Differential diagnosis*

- Granulomatous rosacea/lupus miliaris disseminates faciei
- Ruptured cyst or hair follicle
- Infections.

■ *Pitfalls*

- Small samples may not include the characteristic granulomas with clear vacuoles at their centers.

■ *Pearls*

- Caused by rupture of sebaceous glands around eyelid (meibomian glands) (Fig. 6.5B).
- Clinical presentation is usually characteristic.
- Vacuoles within granulomatous inflammatory infiltrate along with characteristic clinical presentation are essentially diagnostic (Fig. 6.5C).

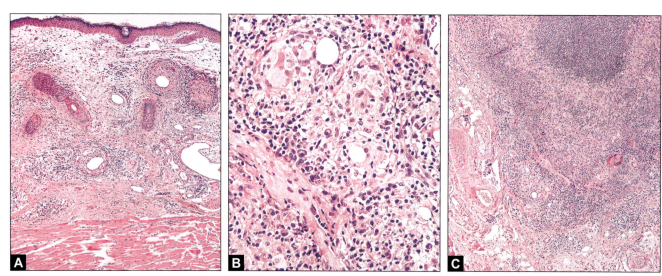

Figs 6.5A to C: Chalazion. Granulomas containing round, clear spaces on the eyelid are virtually diagnostic of a chalazion; (B) The clear vacuoles are formed by collections of sebum resulting from a ruptured sebaceous (Meibomian) gland; (C) In many cases there is mixed inflammation and abscess formation in addition to granulomas.

Cheilitis Granulomatosa
(Melkersson-Rosenthal Syndrome)

■ *Criteria for diagnosis*
- Localized swelling of the lip and face.
- Granulomas adjacent to or impinging on lymphatics.

■ *Differential diagnosis*
- Granulomatous rosacea.

■ *Pitfalls*
- A deep biopsy is necessary as in many cases the granulomas are only seen around the lymphatics of the subcutis or deep dermis (Figs 6.6A and B).

■ *Pearls*
- Cheilitis granulomatosa is usually an isolated disorder, but it may be seen in the setting of Melkersson-Rosenthal syndrome, a triad which includes:
  - Lip swelling
  - Unilateral facial paralysis
  - Furrowed tongue

- The complete triad is encountered only in very rare instances.
- In some cases, the swelling involves the face and eyelids (biopsies have shown features identical to cheilitis granulomatosa)
- Some consider cheilitis granulomatosa as a variant of granulomatous rosacea; others argue that it is distinct since the granulomas are deep and not centered on follicles.

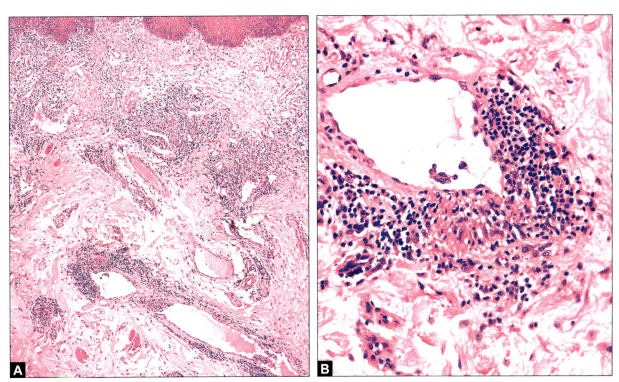

Figs 6.6A and B: Cheilitis granulomatosa. (A) Lymphocytes, plasma cells and macrophages are present in a dermis that contains markedly dilated lymphatics; (B) The inflammatory infiltrate and a small granuloma impinge on dilated lymphatics.

Cutaneous Crohn's Disease

■ *Criteria for diagnosis*

- Clinical history of Crohn's disease
- One of the following cutaneous presentations:
  - Nodules or plaques (with or without ulceration) in genital, perianal or flexural skin
  - Perianal ulcers, fistulas or sinus tracts
  - Swelling in or around the lips
  - Small confluent nodules (cobblestoning) of the mucosa
- Noncaseating granulomas accompanied by mixed inflammation within the dermis and subcutis; vasculitis is sometimes present (Figs 6.7A and B).

■ *Differential diagnosis*

- Hidradenitis suppurativa (for perianal lesions)
- Cheilitis granulomatosa (for perioral lesions)
- Interstitial granulomatous dermatitis (IGD)
- Granulomatous infections
- Hermansky-Pudlak disease.

■ *Pitfalls*

- Occasionally, cutaneous lesions may precede gastrointestinal involvement by years, but a definitive diagnosis of cutaneous Crohn's disease is difficult to establish in this circumstance
- Rarely, the lesions may arise within skin distant from the anus or mouth (so-called "metastatic Crohn's disease")
- In some cases, vasculitis and diffuse dermal inflammation may predominate and granulomas may be few or difficult to discern.

■ *Pearls*

- Erythema nodosum and pyoderma gangrenosum are the most common cutaneous manifestations of Crohn's disease; granulomatous lesions are comparably rare
- Cutaneous lesions often (but not always) respond to treatment of the gastrointestinal symptoms
- Granulomatous panniculitis is particularly common in cutaneous Crohn's disease.

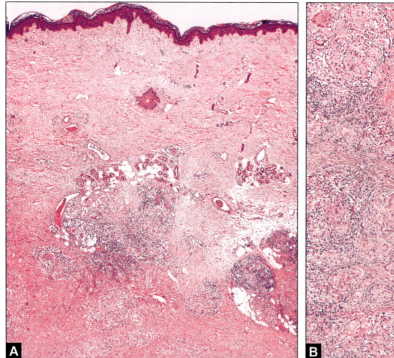
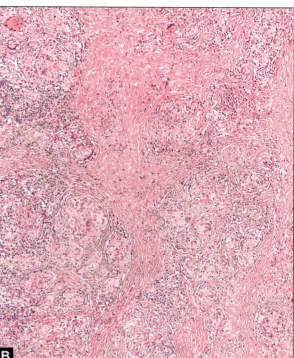

Figs 6.7A and B: Cutaneous Crohn's disease. (A) Noncaseating granulomas occupy the mid and lower reticular dermis; (B) The granulomas contain numerous multinucleated giant cells.

Ruptured Cysts and Hair Follicles/Acneiform Papules

■ *Criteria for diagnosis*

- Clinical history of a cutaneous nodule or inflamed follicle/acneiform papule
- A mixed inflammatory infiltrate with histiocytes and granulomatous inflammation surrounding keratin fragments ± fragments of cytologically banal epithelium (Fig. 6.8A).

■ *Differential diagnosis*

- Granulomatous rosacea
- Various other causes of granulomatous inflammation.

■ *Pitfalls*

- Occasionally, the inflammatory reaction and resulting fibrosis or granulation tissue completely obliterates the cyst or follicle; keratin fragments may be present but sometimes even these are absent (Fig. 6.8B).
- If the clinical history is not straightforward, histochemical stains for microorganisms may be warranted.

■ *Pearls*

- In cases in which there is only inflammation and fibrosis with no residual evidence of the destroyed cyst or follicle, a descriptive diagnosis may be used with the comment that the findings are consistent with the site of an obliterated ruptured cyst or follicle.

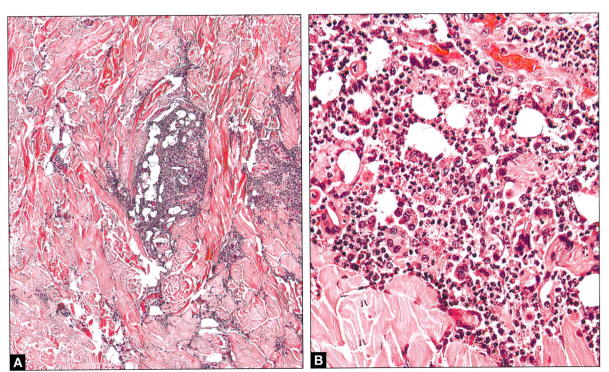

Figs 6.8A and B: Ruptured cyst. (A) In this case there is no evidence of cyst epithelium, but there is granulomatous inflammation with clear vacuoles in some areas; (B) Close inspection reveals keratin fragments within the vacuoles, suggesting that the inflammation is within the vicinity of a ruptured cyst or follicle, or is at the site of a resolving rupture.

Granulomatous Reactions to Deep Fungal Infections (and Filamentous Bacteria) (Figs 6.9A to C)

■ *Criteria for diagnosis*

- Granulomatous and suppurative inflammatory infiltrate
- Identification of fungal elements with corroborating culture results and/or an established history of a specific fungal infection.

■ *Differential diagnosis*

- Virtually all other causes of granulomatous inflammation.

■ *Pitfalls*

- Recent data have demonstrated that morphology alone is unreliable in the definitive diagnosis of many infections, particularly fungal infections, even in the hands of experienced pathologists (Sangoi et al. 2009)
- Since, treatment regimens have become increasingly specific for certain organisms, overly definitive diagnoses may lead to inappropriate therapy
- Misinterpretation of septate versus nonseptate hyphae has particular potential for adverse consequences, e.g. a diagnosis of a *Zygomycetes* species (often mistakenly assumed to be *Mucorales genera*) when the organism is actually *Aspergillus* and may result in unnecessary treatment with amphotericin, a drug with potentially severe side effects
- Tangentially sectioned bulbous hyphae may simulate an empty *Coccidioides spherule*
- *Coccidioides* endospores in clusters or overlapping empty spherules may simulate a budding yeast that could be misinterpreted as *Blastomyces, Paracoccidioides* or Cryptococcus
- Rarely, *Histoplasma capsulatum* organisms may not be intracellular and may simulate *Candida species*
- Some filamentous bacteria (higher bacteria) may resemble fungal elements and stain with periodic acid-Schiff (PAS) and Gomori methenamine silver (GMS).

■ *Pearls*

- Clues to a deep fungal infection are:
  - Pseudoepitheliomatous hyperplasia
  - Neutrophilic microabscesses within the epidermis
  - Abscesses and suppurative granulomas
  - Multinucleated giant cells within the dermis or subcutis
  - Round "empty" spaces within multinucleated dermal giant cells
  - Necrosis
  - Vascular occlusion
- Unless the histopathologic features are unmistakable (e.g. the fruiting heads of *Aspergillus* species are seen (rare) or an unequivocal intact endospore-filled spherule of *Coccidioides*), correlation with the results of prior or concurrent culture results should be recommended in the diagnosis of many infections
- Cultures of *Dermatophytes*, *Histoplasma* and *Paracoccidioides* require up to 7–10 days
- Most other fungal cultures (including hyphal fungi) have a rapid turn around time of 3 days or less
- When dermal fungal elements are identified, classification into one of the five basic categories may be attempted: (1) Septated hyphae; (2) Nonseptated hyphae; (3) Granules composed of hyphae or filaments; (4) Yeast forms with pseudohyphae; (5) Yeast forms without pseudohyphae
- Attempting more precise classification on tissue biopsy alone is not recommended in the absence of cultures.

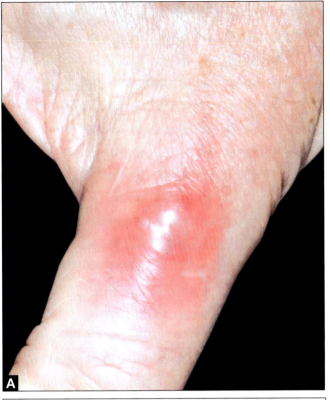

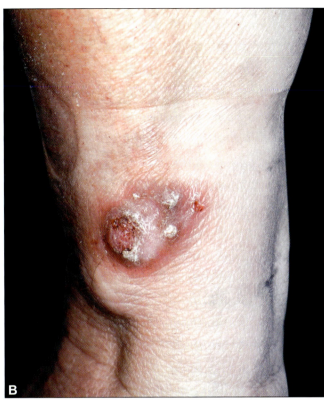

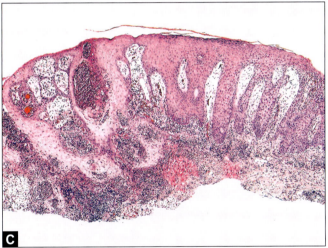

Figs 6.9A to C: Deep fungal infection. (A) A red tender nodule on the finger that did not resolve after treatment with oral antibiotics for presumed bacterial infection. Tissue culture revealed *Alternaria* species (phaeohyphomycosis); (B) Persistent crusted, keratotic plaque on the forearm of an immunosuppressed renal transplant recipient. Clinical diagnosis was squamous cell carcinoma or keratoacanthoma; (C) Deep fungal infection. Common to many deep fungal infections is pseudoepitheliomatous hyperplasia of the epidermis and neutrophilic abscesses within the epithelium. Granulomas and mixed inflammation are present in the underlying dermis.

Septated Hyphal Fungal Organisms

Nodular Granulomatous Perifolliculitis (Majocchi's Granuloma)

- Caused by dermatophyte infection of hair shafts (most often *Trichophyton rubrum*) that leads to follicular rupture with fungi and keratinous debris resulting in a mixed dermal inflammation that includes granulomas (simulating other deep fungal infections) (Figs 6.10A to C)
- Septated hyphae and arthrospores are usually seen, but occasionally a mycetoma may form.

Aspergillosis

Figures 6.11A to C show aspergillosis.

- *A. flavus, A. niger* and *A. fumigatus* are primary causes
- Predisposing conditions are neutropenia, hematologic malignancies, immunosuppression for organ transplantation and chronic granulomatous disease
- Relatively thin (compared to Zygomyces) septated hyphae that branch at 45° angles
- Variable granulomatous infiltrate with mixed inflammation
- Disseminated disease is a rapidly progressive, usually widespread infection that involves multiple organs in addition to skin
- Skin lesions often contain intravascular hyphae that penetrate vessel walls (Fig. 6.11A)
- Primary cutaneous lesions are most often necrotic ecthyma-like papules usually develop within burns, catheter sites and beneath adhesive tape.

Hyalohyphomycosis

Fusarium

- Frequent cause of corneal and nail infections
- Primary cutaneous infections most commonly occur within burns, surgical sites or traumatic injury with retained foreign body
- Disseminated disease usually follows primary pulmonary infection, especially in those with hematolymphoid malignancies, neutropenia, graft-versus-host disease or prolonged corticosteroid therapy
- Histopathologic features are identical to aspergillosis (Figs 6.12A to C).

Penicillium:

- Most commonly seen in South China and Thailand
- Papular eruption that progresses to cutaneous ulcers and abscesses with generalized lymphadenopathy
- Organisms are small yeast (resembling *H. capsulatum*) that multiply by binary fission (rather than the budding of *Histoplasma*).

Chromomycosis (Chromoblastomycosis)

- Caused by organisms that inhabit soil, vegetation and wood (Figs 6.13A and B)
- Common in farmers and others who work outdoors
- Traumatic inoculation is the most common source of infection.

Phaeohyphomycosis

Figures 6.14A to D show phaeohyphomycosis.

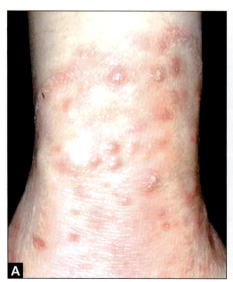
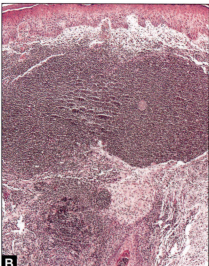
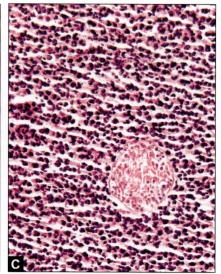

Figs 6.10A to C: Nodular granulmatous perifolliculitis (Majocchi's granuloma). (A) This patient presented with a slowly expanding scaly annular plaque with follicular papules and pustules that did not improve with topical corticosteroids; (B) Inflammation due to the fungal infection has led to follicular rupture with massive abscess formation and a granulomatous response; (C) A fragmented hair shaft contains fungi.

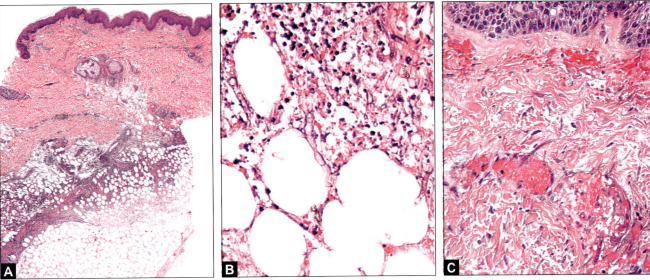

Figs 6.11A to C: (A) The subcutis is occupied by a dense inflammatory infiltrate surrounding zones of necrosis; (B) Septated hyphae are evident even without the aid of fungal stains. (C) Hyphae are penetrating vessel walls within the upper dermis.

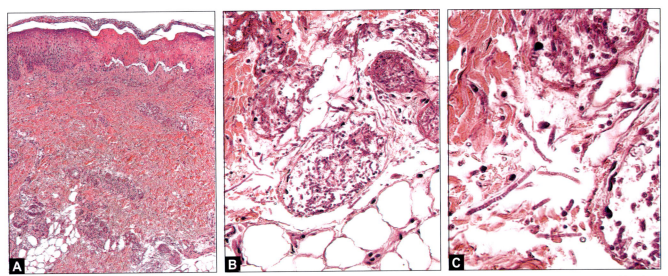

Figs 6.12A to C: Fusarium. (A) The dermis contains congested vessels and hemorrhage; (B) At higher magnification, the fungal hyphae are seen within and around the dilated vessels of the dermis and subcutis; (C) The septated fungi are virtually identical to aspergillus species by light microscopy.

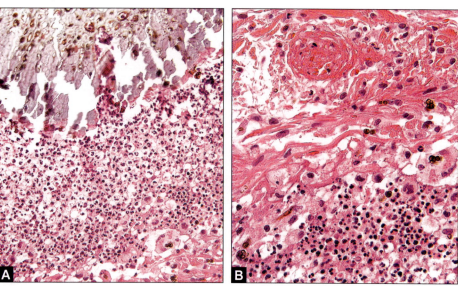

Figs 6.13A and B: Chromomycosis. (A) The infection is caused by organisms that inhabit soil, vegetation and wood, and may follow trauma, such as that induced by the splinter seen here. Note the brown, rounded pigmented bodies at the lower right; (B) The brown sclerotic (Medlar) bodies are evident within giant cells and surrounded by inflammation within the dermis.

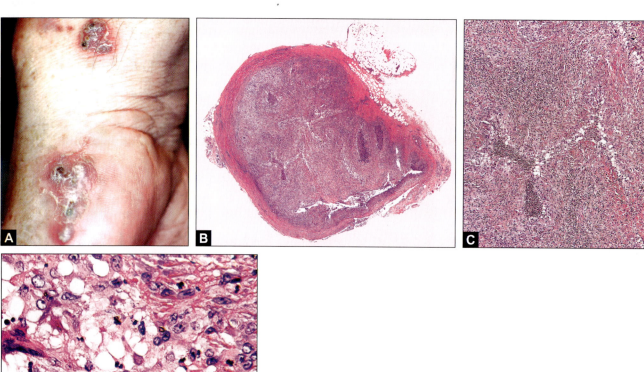

Figs 6.14A to D: Phaeohyphomycosis. (A) Crusted plaques on the forearm of an immunosuppressed patient. Tissue culture revealed *Exophiala werneckii* and the patient later presented with sporotrichoid spread with multiple lesions on the arm. The lesions lacked the draining sinuses that would be expected in a mycetoma; (B) A circumscribed nodule is present within the deep dermis and subcutis; (C) A mixed granulomatous and suppurative infiltrate are evident; (D) Pigmented hyphae and yeast forms are present but the sclerotic (Medlar) bodies of chormomycosis are absent.

Exophiala and phialophora species:
- Direct inoculation of skin, usually producing a solitary nodule
- Usually involves extremities, especially fingers and hands, knees, ankles
- Circumscribed cyst-like abscess cavity with suppurative granulomatous inflammation (resembling mycetomas)
- Organisms often (but not always) pigmented
- Budding yeast, pseudohyphae (resembling Candida) or septated hyphae.

Alternariosis

Figures 6.15A and B show alternariosis.
- Caused by *Alternaria*, a pigmented fungus of the phaeohyphomycete group
- Ubiquitous in soil and plant material and most lesions occur by direct. Inoculation (trauma) in outdoor workers, especially those who work in logging or are exposed to splinters or wood dust
- Occasionally causes onychomycosis
- Primary form (direct skin inoculation) results in ulcerating nodules, sometimes with a warty appearance
- Endogeneous form with secondary dissemination to skin can occur in immunocompromised patients with primary lung infection
- Suppurative granulomatous dermatitis and/or panniculitis are typical of skin lesions
- Brown, broad, branching septate hyphae with round or oval spores, usually in clusters
- Difficult to differentiate from other phaeohyphomycoses.

Nonseptated Fungal Organisms

Zygomycetes

Figures 6.16A and B show *Zygomycosis* (mucormycosis).

Mucorales (Mucor, Rhizopus and Absidia)

- Cutaneous infection simulates cellulitis and often has an ecthyma-like necrotic crust
- Diabetes, leukemia and neutropenia are predisposing conditions
- Necrosis, thrombosis and infarction are common.
- Large, hollow-appearing, broad nonseptated hyphae that branch at 90° angles
- Hyphae may be present in vessel walls
- Rapidly progressive disease is common in immunocompromised patients and sinonasal infection can lead to brain invasion and death within days

- Aspergillosis is the major differential diagnostic consideration and distinction based on morphology in skin biopsies is unreliable.

Entomophthorales

- Unlike the *Mucorales*, *Entomophthorales* may infect immunocompetent and immunocompromised patients
- Subcutaneous swelling is the most common clinical presentation
- Conidiobolus occurs primarily in agricultural workers and commonly involves the nasal mucosa before spreading to the skin of the head and neck
- Basdiobolus is primarily a disease of children.

Granule-Forming Filaments (Mycetoma)

- Chronic infection of skin or subcutis
- May be caused by filamentous bacteria (actinomycotic mycetoma) or fungi (eumycotic mycetoma)
- Both forms produce nodules with sinuses that drain purulent material containing grains; aggregates of microorganisms surrounded by eosinophilic hyaline material representing immunoglobulins
- Most common in tropical and subtropical regions
- Occurs after traumatic inoculation of skin, most commonly on the foot
- Presents as nodules that drain through sinus tracts
- New nodules may form even after initial lesion heals
- Abscesses containing organisms, often surrounded by granulation tissue, granulomas, and/or fibrosis.

Actinomycotic Mycetoma (Bacteria)

Figures 6.17A and B show *Actinic (bacterial) Mycetoma*.

Nocardiosis

- Acid-fast filamentous bacteria
- Thin branching filaments that tend to break into small fragments resembling bacilli.

Actinomyces, Streptomyces

- Nonacid fast filamentous bacteria.

Eumycotic Mycetoma (Fungi)

Figures 6.17C and D show *Eumycotic mycetoma*.

Brown Hyphae

- Dematiaceous fungi.

Clear Hyphae

- Other fungi.

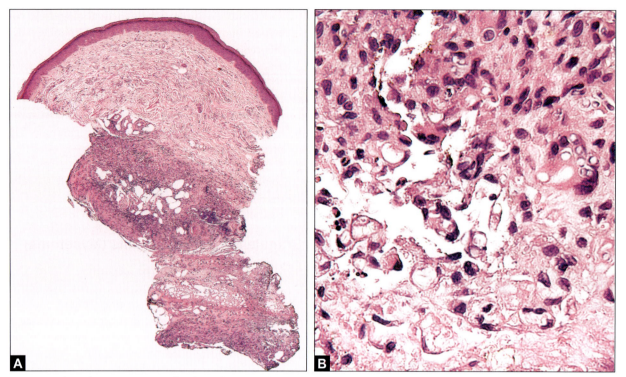

Figs 6.15A and B: Alternariosis. (A) The deep dermis and subcutis contain granulomatous and suppurative inflammation; (B) Open, rounded yeast forms are present within multinucleated giant cells and free within the tissue.

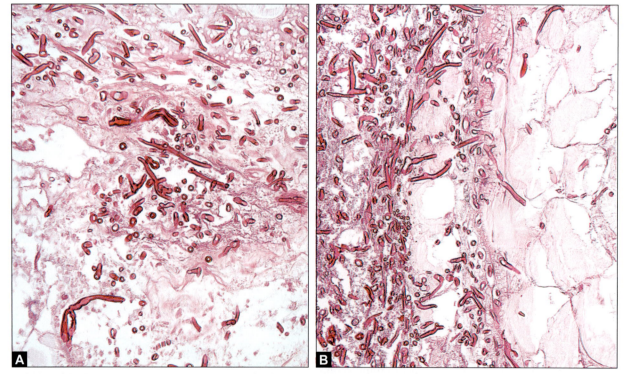

Figs 6.16A and B: Zygomycosis (mucormycosis). (A) The fungi are wide and often easily visualized on H and E stains alone; (B) It is often said that *Zygomyces* can be reliably differentiated from aspergillosis based on their right-angle branching and absence of septa. As this image shows, not all branching is at 90°, and due to folding of the organisms within the plane of section, some hyphae actually appear septated. Thus, cultures are recommended for definitive diagnosis.

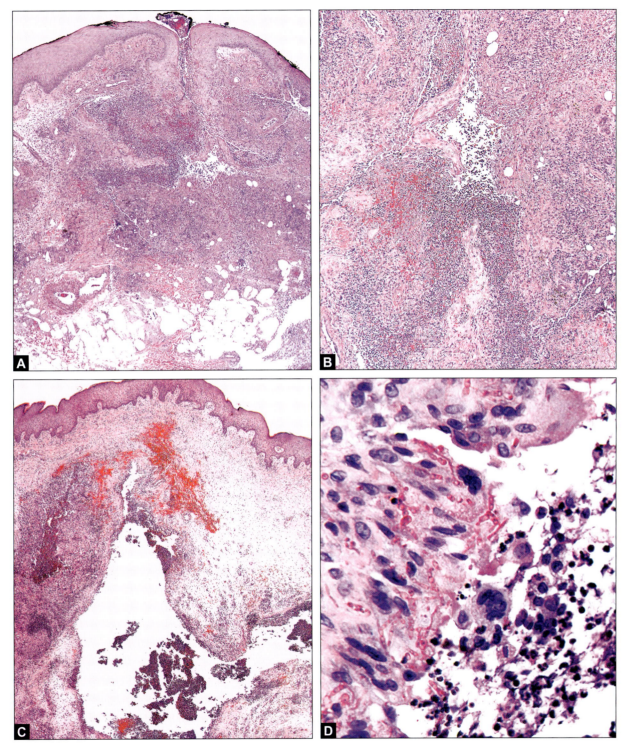

Figs 6.17A to D: Actinic (bacterial) mycetoma. (A) The deep dermis contains a mixed inflammatory infiltrate that connects to the skin surface by a fistula tract. *Madurella mycetomatis*, *Nocardia*, *Streptomyces* and *Actinomyces* are among the most common causes of bacterial mycetoma; (B) There is mixed granulomatous and suppurative inflammation at the base of the fistula; (C) Eumycotic mycetoma. The dermis contains a large cystic cavity lined by macrophages and neutrophils; (D) A periodic acid-Schiff stain highlights fungi within the inflammatory infiltrate.

Yeast-Like Fungal Organisms with Pseudohyphae

Disseminated Candidiasis

Figure 6.18 shows disseminated candidiasis.
- Occurs in patients who are immunocompromised, have central venous catheters or are on broad spectrum antibiotics
- Hematogenous spread from urinary tract or gastrointestinal tract infection
- Macules, papules, petechiae or ecthyma gangrenosum-like lesions
- Mixed dermal infiltrate with yeast and pseudohyphae
- Often accompanied by vasculitis
- Poor prognosis.

Other Molds (with Septated or Nonseptated Hyphae)

- Other molds may be indistinguishable from candida species since pseudohyphae may not always be reliably identified, and even distinction between septated and nonseptated hyphae may not be possible.

Yeast without Pseudohyphae (Table 6.3)

Disseminated Candidiasis

- See above
- Occurs in patients who are immunocompromised, have central venous catheters or are on broad spectrum antibiotics
- Hematogenous spread from urinary tract or gastrointestinal tract infection
- Macules, papules, petechiae or ecthyma gangrenosum-like lesions.

Coccidiomycosis

- Is caused by *Coccidioides immitis*
- Is found in soil in desert regions of South-western region of North America and parts of Mexico, Central America and South America
- Is acquired by inhalation of arthrospores in dust
- May develop in healthy patients or those who are immunocompromised
- Primary cutaneous lesions occur due to traumatic inoculation, most often in farmers or healthcare workers (nurses, morticians)
- Dissemination from lung infection is rare; lesions are verrucous plaques or nodules with ulceration and crusting.
- Fully evolved lesions have pseudoepitheliomatous epidermal hyperplasia and a mixed inflammatory infiltrate including giant cells; organisms (spherules containing

endospores) may be contained in giant cells or free within the dermal collagen
- Gomori methanamine silver stain is the best since PAS stains the endospores but not the spherules
- Myospherulosis—aggregates of degenerating erythrocytes-may simulate the organisms, an important pitfall.

Cryptococcosis

Figure 6.19A to E show cryptococcosis.
- Caused by *Cryptococcus neoformans*
- Found in soil, pigeon droppings and fruit
- Usually acquired by inhalation, with primary infection in the lung
- Skin lesions occur in approximately 10% of patients with disseminated infection and the clinical appearance varies markedly
- Histopathologic features also vary and include a "gelatinous pattern" in which numerous organisms are contained within a mucoid dermal infiltrate with minimal inflammation (Fig. 6.19B)
- In other cases, there is suppurative granulomatous inflammation
- The organisms usually have a polysaccharide (mucoid) capsule and produce small, narrow-based buds
- The capsule is bright pink on mucicarmine stain; GMS and PAS stains highlight the central spherical yeast (Fig. 6.19D).

Histoplasmosis

Figures 6.20A to E show histoplasmosis
- Is caused by two related fungi; *H. capsulatum* var. *capsulatum* and *H. capsulatum* var. *duboisii*
- *H. capsulatum* var. *capsulatum* is found in soil, bat droppings and poultry
- Is most common in North America's Ohio and Mississippi. river valleys but is encountered worldwide
- Spore inhalation is the usual mode of infection
- Disseminated disease is uncommon but is seen in immunocompromised patients, especially those with HIV/AIDS
- Cutaneous lesions are rare (fewer than 10% of cases) and their clinical appearance varies markedly
- The most common histopathologic pattern is diffuse aggregates of macrophages, some multinucleated containing small basophilic yeast surrounded by a clear halo, but granulomas may also be seen
- *H. capsulatum* var. *duboisii* is most frequently encountered in equatorial Africa
- The appearance is similar to *capsulatum* but the yeasts are much larger and are often contained primarily within multinucleated giant cells.

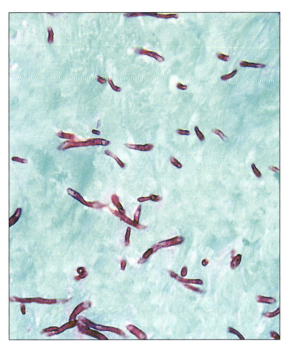

Fig. 6.18: Disseminated candidiasis. The organisms, easily visualized on this PAS stain, consist of a mixture of budding yeast and pseudohyphae.

Table 6.3: Pseudoepitheliomatous hyperplasia with suppurative granulomas			
Disease	*Histopathologic Clues*	*Histochemical Stains*	*Clinical*
Blastomycosis	Pseudoepitheliomatous hyperplasia	GMS	Endemic in wooded areas of South Central and Southeastern United States
("North American Blastomycosis")	Intraepidermal microabscesses	PAS	
Blastomyces dermatitidis			Most common in adult males who work outdoors
			Verrucous plaques with pus-tules at their periphery; ulcers occasionally
			Skin lesions develop in more than half of those with dis-seminated disease
			Erythema nodosum is associ-ated with pulmonary blasto-mycosis
Pyoderma Vegetans	Pseudoepitheliomatous hyperplasia	Gram stain	Verrucous or vegetating plaques with pustules, sinus tracts, or ulcer
('Blastomycosis-like pyoderma')	Intraepidermal microabscesses		
S. aureus	Sinus tracts		Intertriginous areas, face, legs are favored sites
Pseudomonas aeruginosa			May overlap with pyoderma gangrenosum (i.e. some patients have inflammatory bowel disease and other conditions often associated with PG)
Beta-hemolytic Streptococcus			

Contd...

Disease	Histopathologic Clues	Histochemical Stains	Clinical
Chromomycosis *Fonsecaea pedrosi* *Phialophora sp.* *Cladosporium sp.*	Pseudoepitheliomatous hyperplasia Intraepidermal microabscesses	GMS PAS	Scaly papule that evolves into verrucous plaque or nodule Develops at site of minor trauma with contact with plants or soil
Sporotrichosis *Sporothrix schenckii*	Sporothrix "asteroids"—yeast like form surrounded by eosinophilic hyaline projections Organisms may be few but are usually found in suppurative foci if multiple serial sections are examined	GMS PAS	Multiple nodules distributed along lymphatics, usually on the arm
Chromomycosis *Fonsecaea pedrosi* *Phialophora sp.* *Cladosporium sp.*	Brown clustered yeast like bodies ('medlar bodies'; 'copper penny sign') No hyphae (unlike pheaohyphomycosis)		Scaly papule that evolves into verrucous plaque or nodule developing at site of minor trauma with contact with plants or soil
Coccidiomycosis *Coccidioides immitis*	Pseudoepitheliomatous epidermal hyperplasia and a mixed inflammatory infiltrate including giant cells; organisms (spherules containing endospores) may be contained in giant cells or free within the dermal collagen Myospherulosis—aggregates of degenerating erythrocytes—may simulate the organisms, an important pitfall	GMS (methanamine silver stain) is best since PAS stains the endospores but not the spherules	Verrucous plaques or nodules with ulceration and crusting Primary cutaneous lesions occur due to traumatic inoculation, most often in farmers or health care workers (nurses, morticians); dissemination to skin from lung infection is rare Organisms found in desert regions of Southwestern region of North America, and parts of Mexico, Central America, and South America Acquired by inhalation of arthrospores in dust and soil May affect healthy or immuno-compromised patients
Paracoccidiomycosis ("South American Blastomycosis") *Paracoccidioides brasiliensis*	Pseudoepitheliomatous hyperplasia with mixed dermal inflammation and granulomas in most cases Granulomas vary from compact and well-formed to loose collections of macrophages	GMS	Oral and mucosal lesions are is often present, but skin lesions are rare; both are usually arise from disseminated systemic infection occurred through respiratory infection Endemic areas include parts of Brazil, Argentina, Colombia, and Venezuela Most cases (more than 90%) occur in males

Contd...

Disease	Histopathologic Clues	Histochemical Stains	Clinical

Halogenodermas
  Iododerma
  Bromoderma
  Fluroderma
	Pseudoepitheliomatous hyperplasia
	Intraepidermal microabscesses within or around follicular infundibula and dermal abscesses with a mixture of eosinophils and neutrophils
	Granulomatous forms have scattered multinucleated cells but fewer than those usually seen in chromomycosis, sporotrichosis, and other deep fungal infections
		None	Acneiform papules (that may ulcerate), granulomatous dermatitis, or vegetative plaques
			Iododerma usually caused by potassium salts in expectorants; rare causes are radiocontrast media and amiodarone
			Bromoderma and fluoroderma are exceedingly rare

Hidradenitis suppurativa	Squamous-lined sinus tracts and pseudoepitheliomatous hyperplasia Neutrophils, often abscess formation		Clinical history of chronic relapsing suppurative inflammation of axilla, inguinal folds, and genitals (areas containing apocrine glands)

(GMS: Gomori methenamine silver; PAS: Periodic acid-Schiff).

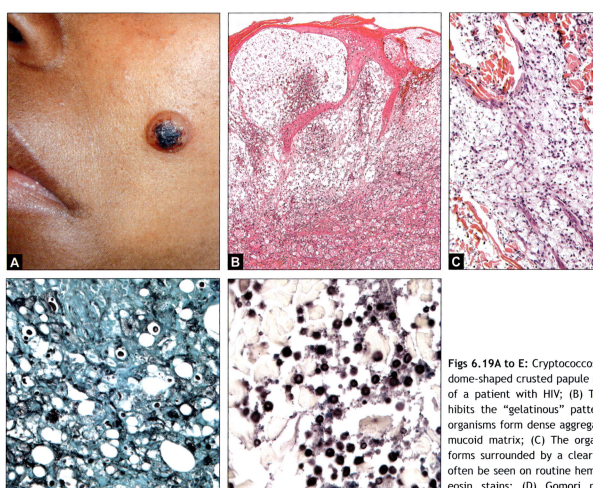

Figs 6.19A to E: Cryptococcosis. (A) Large dome-shaped crusted papule on the cheek of a patient with HIV; (B) This case exhibits the "gelatinous" pattern in which organisms form dense aggregates within a mucoid matrix; (C) The organisms—yeast forms surrounded by a clear "halo", can often be seen on routine hematoxylin and eosin stains; (D) Gomori methenamine silver stains highlight the organisms (except for their capsules); (E) Mucicarmine stains the capsule a dark red color.

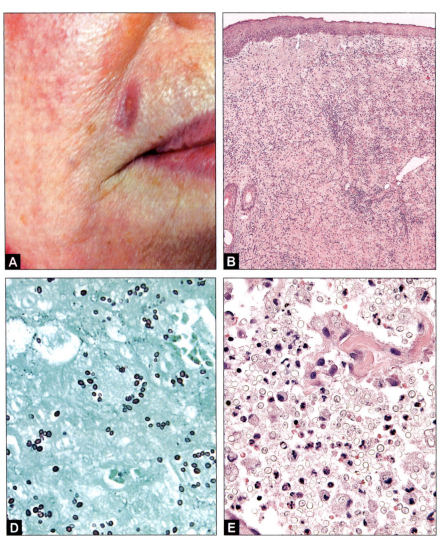

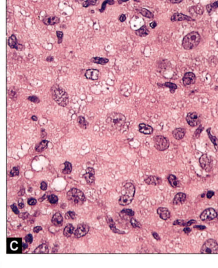

Figs 6.20A to E: Histoplasmosis. *Histoplasma capsulatum*. (A) Pink plaque on the cheek; (B) The dermis is occupied by diffuse sheets of macrophages; (C) Close inspection shows that the macrophages contain clear spaces that impart a vacuolated appearance; (D) Gomori methenamine silver stains the organisms strongly; (E) Histoplasmosis *Histoplasma capsulatum* var. *duboisii*. This variant is larger than *capsulatum* and is often easily visualized without the aid of fungal stains.

Blastomycosis

Figures 6.21A to C show blastomycosis.
- Is caused by *Blastomyces dermatitidis*
- Is found in wood, soil and bird droppings
- Often occurs in healthy (not immunocompromised) patients, as opposed to many other deep fungal infections
- Skin lesions may be primary cutaneous (direct inoculation) or disseminated from pulmonary infection
- *Primary cutaneous form*: Ulcerating pustules that appear 1 or 2 weeks after inoculation; may produce lymphadenopathy and spread in a lymphangitic pattern (similar to sporotrichosis)
- *Disseminated form*: Skin lesions are common; may be solitary or multiple; begin as papules but evolve into crusted verrucous nodules or ulcerated plaques with raised serpiginous borders
- Early lesions contain mostly neutrophils and numerous organisms; fully evolved lesion has pseudoepitheliomatous epidermal hyperplasia with granuloma formation; organisms may be contained in giant cells or free within the dermal collagen (Figs 6.21A and B).

Paracoccidioides

- Is caused by *Paracoccidioides brasiliensis*
- Is found in contaminated soil
- Most cases are acquired from inhalation of conidia within soil
- Primary cutaneous lesions (direct inoculation of skin) are very rare
- Lesions commonly involve the mucocutaneous junction of the nose and mouth, or less often, other regions of the face
- Ulcerated nodules with verrucous hyperplasia are typical.
- Eosinophils are sometimes prominent
- Classic appearance is multiple narrow buds arising from a central yeast form (the so-called "mariner's wheel" form) often within giant cells.

Sporothrix

Figures 6.22A to C show sporotrichosis.

- Is caused by *Sporothrix schenkii*
- Organisms are ubiquitous in decaying plant material and wood
- Infection results from skin inoculation by wood splinters, thorns or moss
- An ulcerating nodule at site of inoculation followed by the appearance of additional nodules in a linear (lymphocutaneous) array (sporotrichoid spread)
- Suppurative and granulomatous dermal inflammation is with rare organisms, sometimes within multinucleated giant cells
- Splendore-Hoeppli phenomenon is occasionally seen
- Most infections remain skin-limited.

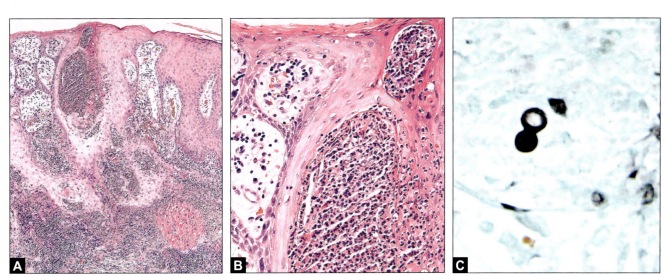

Figs 6.21A to C: Blastomycosis. (A) Pseudoepitheliomatous epidermal hyperplasia is characteristic; (B) The epithelial "tongues" often contain neutrophilic abscesses; (C) Broad-based budding can be seen with fungal stains, such as Gomori methenamine silver.

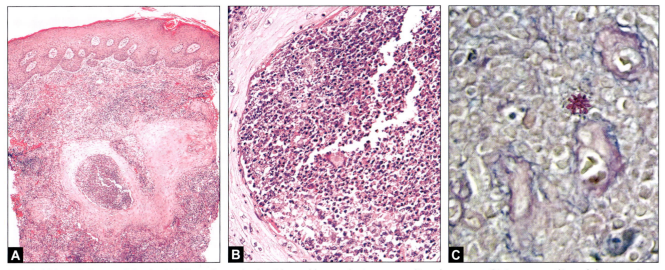

Figs 6.22A to C: Sporotrichosis. (Λ) There is marked epidermal hyperplasia surrounding abscesses; (B) A vague outline of the organisms may be seen with careful inspection of hematoxylin and eosin stained slides; (C) A periodic acid-Schiff stain highlights a yeast form surrounded by radiating "spokes", a finding that is often associated with sporotrichosis (but is not specific for it).

Other Molds (Septate/Nonseptate Hyphae)

While aspergillosis is the most commonly encountered mold in most regions, it must be remembered that Hyalohyphomycoses such as Fusarium, Scedosporium, and Penicillium, as well as other hyaline septate molds (including dermatophytes) may closely resemble Aspergillus species and may require different therapies. Again, overly specific diagnosis based on morphology alone is not recommended."

Granulomatous Reactions to Other Infections

■ *Criteria for diagnosis*
- Granulomatous and suppurative dermal and/or subcutaneous inflammation
- Identification of organisms with corroborating culture results and/or an established history of a specific infection.

■ *Differential diagnosis*
- Other causes of suppurative granulomatous inflammation.

■ *Pitfalls*
- Many organisms are difficult to visualize, even with histochemical stains
- Well-formed granulomas are not always encountered, and a more diffuse mixed inflammatory infiltrate may predominate.

■ *Pearls*
- Clinical features and correlation with cultures usually establish the diagnosis

- Immunohistochemical methods are available for the detection of some pathogens (*Treponema pallidum*).

Tuberculosis (Table 6.4)

Figures 6.23A to C show tuberculosis mycobacterial infection.
- Caused by *Mycobacterium tuberculosis*
- Granulomas (± caseation) with suppurative dermatitis and sometimes ulceration
- Organisms, when present, are usually only identifiable with histochemical stains for acid-fast bacilli
- Several cutaneous variants exist (see Table 6.1).

Nontuberculous Mycobacterial Infections ("Atypical" Mycobacteria) (Table 6.5)

Figures 6.23D to G show nontuberculous mycobacterial infection.
- Caused by:
  - *M. marinum*
  - *M. kansasii*
  - *M. fortuitum*
  - *M. chelonei*
  - *M. avium intracellulare*
  - *M. ulcerans*
- Necrosis and abscess formation in early lesions, with progression to granulomatous inflammation
- Organisms are often easily seen in early phases but may be scant in some situations (see Table 6.1).

Table 6.4: Cutaneous tuberculosis variants (Mycobacterium tuberculosis infection)			
Variant	Histopathologic Findings	Organisms	Clinical Features
Tuberculous chancre	Granulomas, usually caseating Suppurative dermatitis Sometimes ulceration	Usually seen in caseating areas	Exogenous inoculation Indurated plaque, eventually with regional lymphadenopathy
Lupus vulgaris	Granulomas (+/- caseation) Suppurative dermatitis with necrosis	Occasionally seen in deep suppurative areas	Most common cutaneous form Infiltrated plaques with crusts Favors head and neck
Scrofuloderma	Necrotic sinus tract (connecting to underlying infected lymph node or joint space)	Occasionally seen in deep suppurative areas	Rare Underlying infection that extends upward into skin Favors head and neck
Orificial tuberculosis	Mixed inflammation with rare granulomas	Usually numerous	Ulcerative lesions around mouth, nose, anus, genitalia
Miliary tuberculosis	Abscess surrounded by histiocytic infiltrate	Absent in indolent form; present in aggressive form	Rare form presenting with disseminated lesions

Table 6.5: Nontuberculous mycobacterial infections			
Organism	*Histopathologic Features*	*Density of Organisms*	*Clinical Features*
M. marinum	Abscess formation followed by granulomas; epidermal hyperplasia common; Long, broad bacilli	Usually scant (except in immunocompromise)	80% acquired after injury from fish tanks, or fishing equipment; most common on arms, often with 'sporotrichoid' lymphatic spread
M. kansasii	Abscess formation followed by granulomas; large, broad bacilli with 'coarse' appearance	Numerous	Skin lesions are rare except in disseminated infection in immunocompromised patients Nodules, ulcers, or cellulitis
M. fortuitum chelonei	Abscess formation followed by granulomas	Numerous; often in clusters	Contamination of wounds or surgical sites; disseminated lesions in immunocompromise
M. avium intracelluare	Abscess or diffuse lymphohistiocytic infiltrate that may resemble lepromatous leprosy	Numerous; usually intracellular ('pseudo-gaucher cells')	Subcutaneous nodules that eventually ulcerate
M. ulcerans	Coagulative necrosis and ulceration but minimal inflammation ('anergic')	Numerous; often clustered on collagen bundles or adipocytes	Slow growing erythematous nodule that evolves in ulcer with 'undermined' border (Buruli ulcer)

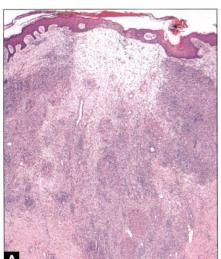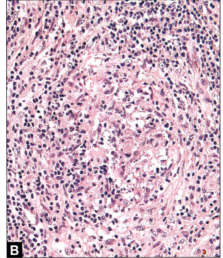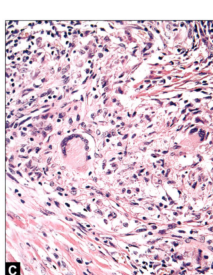

Figs 6.23A to C

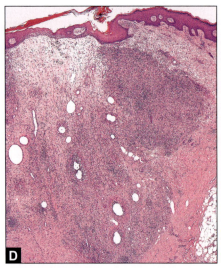

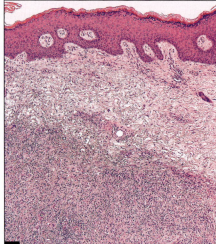

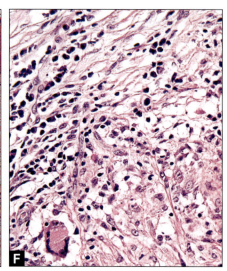

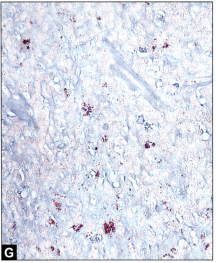

Figs 6.23A to G: Tuberculosis mycobacterial infection. (A) The dermis is occupied by a nodular and diffuse infiltrate; (B) The nodular component is made up of granulomas surrounded by lymphocytes (tuberculoid granulomas); (C) The granulomas often include multinucleated cells of the "Langhans" type, meaning that the nuclei are distributed at the periphery of the cell in a horseshoe-like pattern; (D) Nontuberculous mycobacterial infection. This case was caused by infection with *Mycobacterium chelonei*; (E) A large nodular collection of macrophages and other inflammatory cells occupies the dermis; (F) Granulomas with multinucleated giant cells flanked by lymphocytes are usually present; (G) Stains for acid-fast bacteria highlight numerous organisms, many in clusters, in this case.

Leprosy, Tuberculoid Type

Figures 6.24A to C show tuberculoid leprosy.
- Is caused by *Mycobacterium leprae*
- Granulomas are present with numerous multinucleated giant cells (especially Langhans type) and lymphocytes
- Is distributed along nerves but also extend into adjacent dermis
- The causative bacilli are rarely found in this form of leprosy; Fite stain (or Wade-Fite stain, a modified Ziehl-Neelsen stain) may on occasion reveal an organism or two.

Secondary or Tertiary Syphilis
- Is caused by the spirochete *Tertiary pallidum*.
- Granulomatous inflammation is typically only seen in nodular lesions
- Granulomas may be sarcoidal, tuberculoid or (rarely) palisading
- Mixed inflammation is common and plasma cells may be numerous
- Organisms vary in number and may be few; Warthin-Starry stains or an immunohistochemical stain specific for *T. pallidum* is the most reliable method of identifying them.

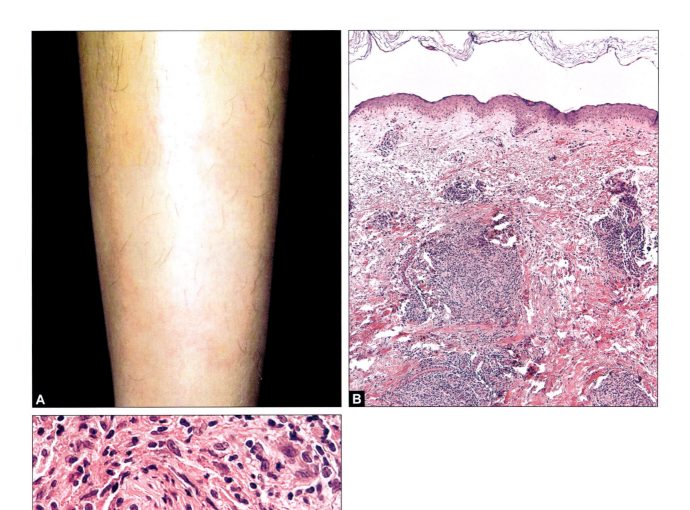

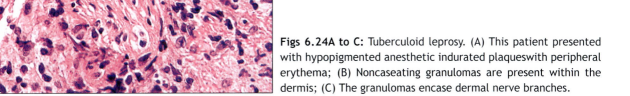

Figs 6.24A to C: Tuberculoid leprosy. (A) This patient presented with hypopigmented anesthetic indurated plaqueswith peripheral erythema; (B) Noncaseating granulomas are present within the dermis; (C) The granulomas encase dermal nerve branches.

Leishmaniasis (Chronic form)

Figures 6.25A to C show leishmaniasis.

- Caused by various species of the *Leishmania* protozoas (unicellular parasites)
- Granulomas composed of epithelioid histiocytes are sometimes seen, but an infiltrate of dermal histiocytes is common to all forms
- The organisms (amastigotes referred to Donovan bodies) are within histiocytes and have round basophilic nuclei and small basophilic rodlike kinteoplast
- See "infectious causes of diffuse histiocytic infiltrate" for additional details.

Protothecosis

- Infection by the *Achlorophyllic algae, Prototheca widerhamii* or *P. zopfii*, which are ubiquitous in water, soil and vegetation
- Occurs in tropical and temperate zones
- Three forms: (1) localized infection of the olecranon bursa in immunocompetent persons; (2) cutaneous lesions or; (3) disseminated disease in immunocompromised patients
- Olecranon bursa protothecosis develops weeks after elbow injury and presents as swollen bursa with draining sinuses surrounded by epithelial hyperplasia;-

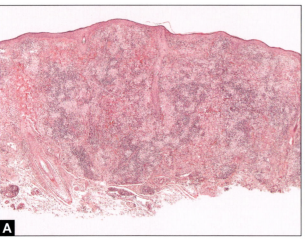

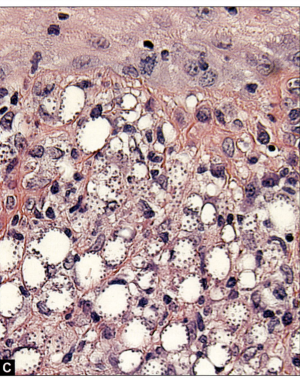

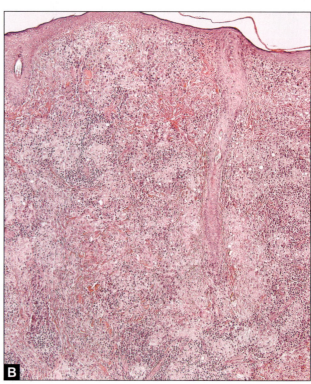

Figs 6.25A to C: Leishmaniasis. (A) A nodular infiltrate occupies large sections of the dermis; (B) Even at medium magnification, cells that appear to contain clear cytoplasmic vacuoles can be seen; (C) At high power, macrophages occupied by amastigotes are evident. The microorganisms are often distributed as a "ring" around the periphery of a central clearing.

suppurative granulomatous infection with caseation necrosis containing the prototheca organisms is evident histopathologically (Fig. 6.26)

- Cutaneous forms produce multiple indistinct indurated macules, sometimes with ulceration, histopathologic features are more variable but granulomas are usually seen at least focally
- Organisms are typically pleomorphic, but classically large morula forms are evident; spheres with internal septate (conferring the "soccer ball" appearance)
- The primary differential diagnostic consideration is chromomycosis.

Cat-Scratch Disease

- Caused by *Bartonella henselae*

- A palisading granulomatous appearance is the most common presentation (see palisading granulomas) (Fig. 6.27A)
- Warthin-Starry or other silver stains highlight microorganisms in some cases but not all (Fig. 6.27B)

Pyoderma Vegetans (Blastomycosis-like Pyoderma)

- Most common causes are Staphylococcus aureus, Pseudomonas aeruginosa, and Beta-hemolytic Streptococcus
- Pseudoepitheliomatous hyperplasia with intraepidermal microabscesses is the most common histopathologic finding

Figures 6.28A and B show blastomycosis-like pyoderma.

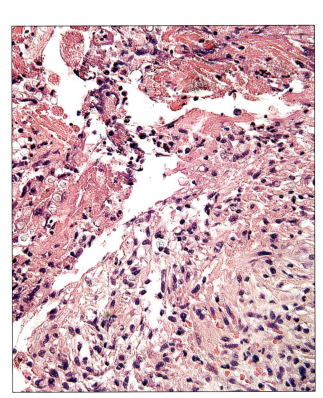

Fig. 6.26: Protothecosis. There is granulomatous inflammation and close inspection may reveal the outlines of the organisms. Some have prominent septations.

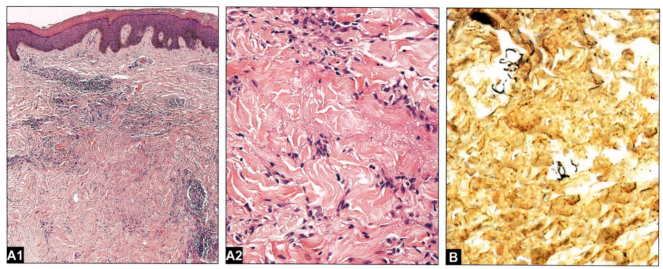

Figs 6.27A and B: Cat-scratch disease. (A) Within the skin, the most common presentation is poorly formed palisading granulomas that resemble those of early granuloma annulare; (B) Occasionally silver stains (such as, Warthin-Starry pictured here) will demonstrate organisms.

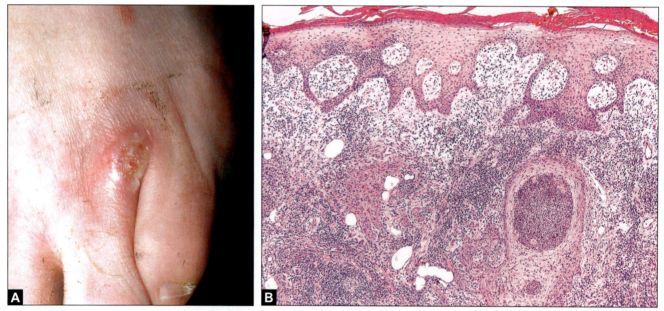

Figs 6.28A and B: Blastomycosis-like pyoderma. (A) Pink eroded plaque on the dorsal foot that drained purulent material. Tissue culture revealed *Staphylococcus aureus*; (B) As the name implies, the histopahthologic features are very similar to those of deep fungal infections, such as blastomycosis, including pseudoepitheliomatous hyperplasia with intraepidermal and dermal abscess formation.

Granuloma Annulare (Figs 6.29A to F)

■ *Criteria for diagnosis*

- Flesh colored erythematous or violaceous papules that often coalesce into annular, arcuate or polycyclic configurations
- Palisading granulomas formed by macrophages surrounding degenerating collagen (Fig. 6.29C)
- Granulomas are relatively discrete and separated by areas of normal-appearing dermis.

■ *Differential diagnosis*

- Other palisading granulomas, especially necrobiosis lipoidica
- Epithelioid sarcoma.

■ *Pitfalls*

- Epithelioid sarcoma is a well-known simulator of granuloma annulare since it may form palisading tumor cells around central areas of necrotic tumor

- Early lesions ("interstitial" or "incomplete" granuloma annulare) lack well-formed palisading granulomas and may simulate other histiocytic infiltrates (see below) (Fig. 6.29E).

■ *Pearls*

- The presence of normal dermis between the granulomas ("islands") is the most reliable feature differentiating granuloma annulare from necrobiosis lipoidica.

Table 6.6: Causes of palisading granulomas		
Disease	*Histopathologic Clues*	*Clinical*
Granuloma annulare	Palisades of macrophages around degenerating collagen	Papules that coalesce into annular plaques
	Round or ovoid	
	Focal; intervening normal dermis between granulomas	
Necrobiosis lipoidica	Horizontal palisades of macrophages admixed with plasma cells	Plaques on shins
		Most common in diabetics
	Diffuse; involves entire dermis and superficial subcutis	
Rheumatoid nodule	Usually subcutaneous	Adults with rheumatoid arthritis
	Palisades of macrophages around eosinophilic 'fibrinoid' necrosis	Subcutaneous nodules on elbows, knuckles, and Achilles tendon area
Rheumatic fever nodule	Similar to rheumatoid nodule	Most common in children with acute rheumatic fever
		Skin over bony prominences and occiput are most common sites
Necrobiotic xanthogranuloma	Palisades usually poorly formed	Indurated papules and plaques with predilection for periorbital area (rare at other sites)
	Cholesterol clefts and foamy macrophages	
	Large foreign body type and Touton giant cells	IgG paraproteinemia in 80%
Epithelioid sarcoma	Palisades of tumor cells (not macrophages) surrounding central necrosis; IHC can be useful in determining that the cells are tumor cells (i.e. they are CD34+, cytokeratin +, etc.) rather than macrophages (the latter would express CD68).	Plaque or nodule, sometimes ulcerated
		Distal extremities of young adults is characteristic site
	Cytologic atypia may be minimal in superficial areas	

Contd...

Color Atlas of Differential Diagnosis of Dermatopathology

Disease	Histopathologic Clues	Clinical
Cat-scratch disease *Bartonella henselae*	Palisades of macrophages and lymphocytes around central abscess and necrotic debris	Crusted papule or nodule develops at site of a cat's scratch; lymphadenopathy/adenitis develops approximately two weeks later
	Rod shaped bacteria may be identified with Warthin-Starry stain	
	May be within macrophages and free within the abscess cavity	Systemic symptoms occur in only about 1%
Lymphogranuloma venereum *Chlamydia trachomatis*	Epidermis normal or ulcerated	Multiple herpetiform genital ulcers
	Diffuse mixed suppurative granulomatous infiltrate	Marked regional lymphadenopathy
	Intracellular microorganisms are Giemsa positive coccoid bodies	
Deep fungal infections	See Table 6.3	See Table 6.3

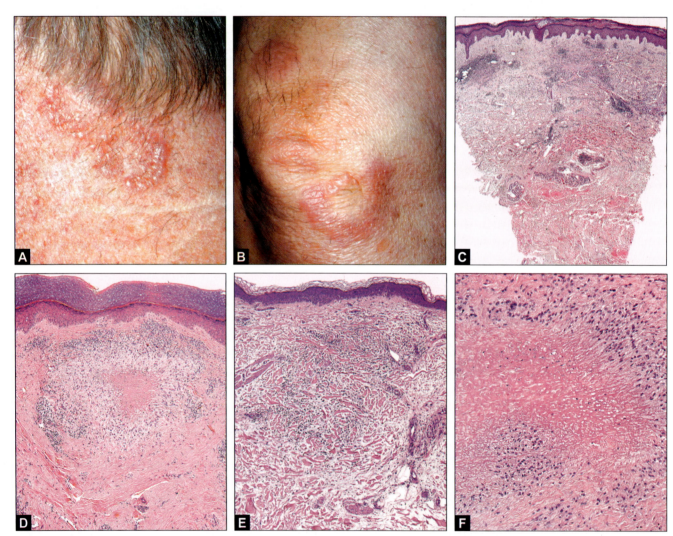

Figs 6.29A to F: Granuloma annulare. (A) Smooth, pink, dermal papule coalescing into annular plaques on the neck; (B) Smooth, red annular plaques on the elbows; (C) The dermis contains discrete granulomas with palisades of macrophages surrounding a central zone of degenerating collagen. Note that the dermis between the granulomas appears normal (in contrast to necrobiosis lipoidica); (D) In established lesions, the palisading architecture is distinctive; (E) In early lesions, the lesions are much less discrete and the primary finding is infiltration of the dermis by macrophages, often accompanied by some mucin. Some refer to this as the "incomplete" or "interstitial" form of granuloma annulare; (F) The deep form of granuloma annulare tends to have larger palisading granulomas within the deep dermis and subcutis. The differential diagnosis often includes rheumatoid nodules, deep infections and in some cases, epithelioid sarcoma.

Interstitial/Incomplete Granuloma Annulare

- Early lesions (often referred to as the "interstitial" or "incomplete" form of granuloma annulare) lack well-formed palisading granulomas and instead appear as macrophages distributed in a more haphazard distribution accompanied by small collections of extracellular mucinous material

Necrobiosis Lipoidica

■ *Criteria for diagnosis*

- Yellowish plaques, most often on the shins (Fig. 6.30A)
- Granulomatous inflammation throughout the entire dermis (and often extending into the subcutis) (Fig. 6.30B)
- Palisades of macrophages, lymphocytes and plasma cells with zones of degenerating collagen oriented in parallel to the epidermis (Fig. 6.30C).

■ *Differential diagnosis*

- Granuloma annulare
- Other palisading granulomas.

- The differential for this form may include IGD (see below).

Deep Granuloma Annulare

- "Deep" granuloma annulare occurs in the subcutis and has a predilection for children, often on the extremities, buttocks and scalp; granulomas are usually well-formed and may closely simulate rheumatoid nodule.

■ *Pitfalls*

- Some lesions have vasculitis and can be mistaken for various forms of vasculitis.

■ *Pearls*

- At least two-thirds of patients with necrobiosis lipoidica have diabetes mellitus.
- The diffuse involvement of the entire dermis (without 'islands' of normal dermis) helps exclude granuloma annulare in many cases.

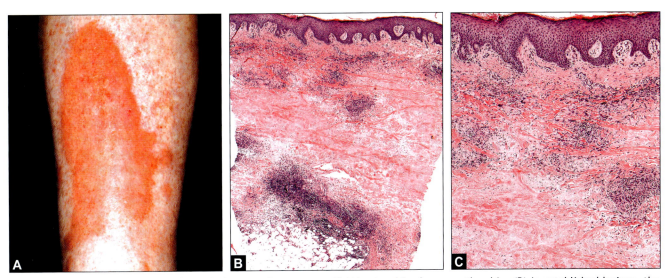

Figs 6.30A to C: Necrobiosis lipoidica. (A) Large yellow-orange slightly atrophic plaque on the shin; (B) In established lesions, the entire dermis is altered (either sclerotic, inflamed or both) and the changes extend into the subcutis. Unlike granuloma annulare, none of the dermis appears normal; (C) The palisading architecture of necrobiosis lipoidica is usually less apparent than in granuloma annulare. Instead, the dermis is occupied by horizontal layers of mixed granulomatous inflammation and degenerating or sclerotic collagen, imparting the "layer cake" appearance.

Necrobiotic Xanthogranuloma (Figs 6.31A to C)

■ Criteria for diagnosis

- Indurated papules, nodules or plaques developing in a patient with IgG paraproteinemia
- Broad zones of granulomatous inflammation with lipid filled "foam cells", multinucleated giant cells and cholesterol clefts.

■ Differential diagnosis

- Necrobiosis lipoidica
- Infectious causes of suppurative granulomatous inflammation.

■ Pitfalls

- The characteristic foam cells and cholesterol clefts may be few in some cases.

■ Pearls

- Periorbital region is the most common site; lesions may also occur on the trunk and extremities, however
- Lipid-filled foam cells, multinucleated giant cells with foamy cytoplasm (Touton giant cells) and foreign body-type giant cells associated with cholesterol clefts are fairly specific for necrobiotic xanthogranuloma and are rarely seen in the other differential diagnostic considerations
- Almost all patients have an IgG paraproteinemia and some may contain plasma cell aggregates within the bone marrow, very few actually have a plasma cell malignancy (myeloma)
- Plane xanthomas may have some overlapping features and may be a closely related condition.

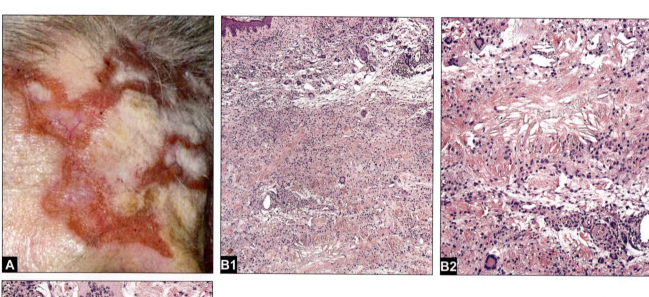

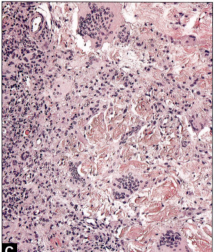

Figs 6.31A to C: Necrobiotic xanthogranuloma. (A) Expanding plaques with orange-red leading borders and atrophic depigmented centers on the forehead; (B) The dermis contains a mixed granulomatous infiltrate. A characteristic finding is clefts that are formed by extracellular lipid (the lipid itself dissolves during tissue processing, leaving only the cleft-like spaces); (C) The giant cells are often much larger than those seen in most other granulomatous infiltrates. Their nuclei are usually more numerous, and the cytoplasm may have irregular elongated or angular contours.

Rheumatoid Nodule (Figs 6.32A to D)

Criteria for diagnosis

- Nodules around joints or on the feet
- Deep dermal or subcutaneous palisading granulomas with central zones of eosinophilic fibrinoid material.

Differential diagnosis

- Deep granuloma annulare
- Rheumatic fever nodules
- Infectious causes of suppurative granulomatous inflammation
- Epithelioid sarcoma.

Pitfalls

- Epithelioid sarcoma may simulate rheumatoid nodules in both anatomic location and histopathologic appearance
- The deep form of granuloma annulare may contain more eosinophilic than basophilic material and therefore may appear similar or identical to rheumatoid nodules.

Pearls

- Clinical presentation is often helpful in distinguishing rheumatoid nodule from deep granuloma annulare.

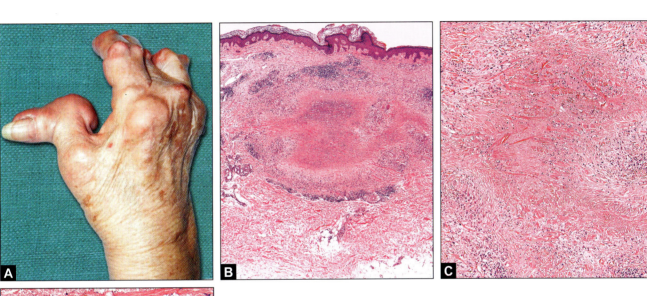

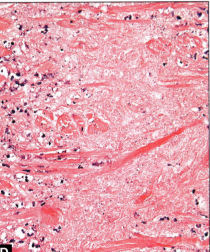

Figs 6.32A to D: Rheumatoid nodule. (A) Large, nontender, subcutaneous nodules and on the hand of a patient with arthritis mutilans caused by rheumatoid arthritis; (B) The granulomas of rheumatoid nodules tend to be well-formed with a distinct palisading architecture and broad central zones of degenerating collagen; (C) The centers of the granulomas are often occupied by brightly eosinophilic degenerating collagen; (D) Often, partially intact collagen bundles are found within some of the granulomas.

Arthropod and Arachnid Bite Reactions

■ *Criteria for diagnosis*

- Erythematous papule or nodule, often excoriated (arthropod bite) or ulcerated (arachnid bite)
- Mixed dermal inflammation with eosinophils, usually both superficial and deep, often with a wedge-shaped distribution (Figs 6.33A and B)
- Epidermal spongiosis often, ulceration (at bite site) sometimes
- Degenerating collagen
- Marked dermal edema, secondary vasculitis and necrosis may occur in arachnid bites.

■ *Differential diagnosis*

Arthropod bites
- Other causes of a hypersensitivity reaction (drug reactions, viral exanthems, etc.)
- Lymphomatoid papulosis

Arachnid bites
- Pyoderma gangrenosum
- Cellulitis
- Primary vasculitis

■ *Pitfalls*

- Definitive diagnosis is not possible unless insect parts are retained in the biopsied skin
- Bite reactions may contain numerous large CD30+ cells; this must not be overinterpreted as evidence of lymphomatoid papulosis.

■ *Pearls*

- Large CD30+ lymphocytes are common in bite reactions, even in small clusters or aggregates
- Degenerated collagen (collagen bundles with "fuzzy" indistinct edges surrounded by amorphous fibrinoid or basophilic material) is a helpful clue to a bite reaction (Fig. 6.33B)
- Other clues include the wedge shaped dermal inflammatory infiltrate and spongiotic vesicles within the epidermis.

Table 6.7: The neutrophilic/suppurative dermatitis pattern		
Disease	*Histopathologic Clues*	*Clinical*
Sweet's syndrome	Diffuse dermal neutrophilic infiltrate with leukocytoclasis and variable subepidermal edema Absence of microorganisms The density of the neutrophilic infiltrate in Sweet's syndrome is usually greater than that of cellulitis Ulceration is typical of pyoderma gangrenosum but rare in Sweet's syndrome	Clinical history of an infection, malignancy (usually leukemia or lymphoma), a chronic disease (e.g. inflammatory bowel disease), or use of certain medications (e.g. minocycline, sulfas, GCSF) Constitutional symptoms—fever, arthralgias, myalgias, headache, and malaise—are common, in contrast to pyoderma gangrenosum Tender erythematous to violaceous plaques, nodules, or bulla Elevated peripheral blood neutrophil count and elevated erythrocyte sedimentation rate support the diagnosis
Leukemia cutis	Atypical cells infiltrate the dermis diffusely, characteristically encircling individual collagen bundles with only minimal collagen degenerative change Atypical or immature-appearing myeloid cells or blastic lymphocytes	Many patients have a known history of underlying leukemia Certain medications (particularly immune modulating drugs) can produce a nearly identical reaction
Pyoderma gangrenosum	Epidermal ulcer overlying a dermis occupied by a diffuse neutrophilic infiltrate that extends under the adjacent intact epidermis ('undermining' inflammation) May resemble other neutrophilic dermatoses leukocytoclastic vasculitis, suppurative folliculitis before the characteristic ulcer develops	Ulcerated painful erythematous papules or nodules that develop raised violaceous borders Pathergy is characteristic (but not specific) Less likely to have constitutional symptoms by comparison to Sweet's syndrome

Contd...

Disease	Histopathologic Clues	Clinical
Behcet's Disease	Suppurative folliculitis, vasculitis, subcorneal pustules, ulcers, and diffuse dermal neutrophilic infiltrates	Recurrent oral ulcers
		Recurrent genital ulcers
		Uveitis
		Erythema nodusm, papulopustular lesions or acneiform (suppurative folliculitis) lesions
		Positive pathergy test
Rheumatoid neutrophilic dermatitis	Diffuse dermal neutrophilic infiltrate	Clinical history of rheumatoid arthritis
		Papules, nodules, and plaques with a predilection for extensor surfaces and neck
		Infections must be carefully excluded since many patients are on corticosteroids; mycobacterial infections particularly common
		Patients with rheumatoid arthritis may develop pyoderma gangrenosum as well
Bowel-associated neutrophilic dermatitis	The infiltrate (neutrophils) is primarily localized to the superficial dermis	Clinical history of a gastrointestinal disease (e.g. ulcerative colitis), liver disease, jejunoileal bypass, or Billroth II surgery
	As in Sweet's syndrome, there is papillary dermal edema	Occurs in up to 20% of patients with a jejunoileal bypass
	Usually does not ulcerate like pyoderma gangrenosum, but the conditions share many other features	
Cellulitis/Erysipelas	Cellulitis: Dermal edema and abscess formation	*Cellulitis:*
Group A Streptococci	Erysipelas: Marked dermal edema and lymphatic dilatation, sometimes with subepidermal blister formation	Tender edematous and erythematous plaques
Streptococcus pyogenes		*Erysipelas:*
S. aureus		Usually caused by S. pyogenes (beta hemolytic streptococcus) in adults;
H. influenzae		In children: *Group A Streptococci, S. aureus, H. influenzae*
		Erythematous plaques that become edematous and often have scalloped borders
		Blisters may develop, and some become hemorrhagic
Ecthyma	Ulceration, sometimes with identifiable organisms, overlying a diffuse neutrophilic dermal infiltrate	Isolated or solitary crusted ulcers, often on the extremities
Staphylococcus aureus		
Streptococcus pyogenes		
Ecthyma Gangrenosum	Extensive epidermal necrosis with dermal infarction; inflammatory infiltrate is sparse, composed of lyphocytes and neutrophils around blood vessels	Usually presents with disseminated bullae and necrotic ulcers
Pseudomonas (sepsis)		Caused by pseudomonas sepsis in critically ill patients; often fatal
	Gram-negative bacilli may be visible witin the dermis (light blue rods on H&E, bright red on Gram stain)	

Contd...

Disease	Histopathologic Clues	Clinical
Suppurative folliculitis	Neutrophils and necroinflammatory debris centered on follicle	Follicular-centered pustules and nodules
S. aureus	Gram positive cocci within follicles	
	Expansion of follicles by bacteria and necro-inflammatory debris, eventually leading to rupture and diffuse dermal inflammation, often with keratin debris	
Atypical mycobacterial infection	See Table 6.5	
Pheaohyphomycosis	Cyst-like cavity or abscess in lower dermis or subcutis	Crusted plaques and nodules, sometimes with sporotrichoid spread
Exophiala jeanselmei	Mixed granulomatous and suppurative infiltrate in some cases	Lacks the draining sinuses that would be expected in a mycetoma
Wangiella dermatitidis	Splinter or foreign body often evident	
Phialophora sp.	Brown pigmented septate hyphae and yeasts (but NOT the sclerotic 'Medlar bodies' of chormomycosis)	
Bacillary angiomatosis	Resemble pyogenic granuloma or edematous granulation tissue	Papules and nodules resembling pyogenic granulomas, often in groups
Bartonella henselae	Psuedoepitheliomatous hyperplasia	May become pedunculated
Bartonella quintana	Amorphous basophilic or amphophilic material (contains the organisms, which are gram-negative bacilli)	Most cases arise in immunocompromised patients
	Organisms often numerous and may be visualized on H & E	HIV is most common setting
		Occasional cases in patients with leukemia or organ transplant-related immunosuppression

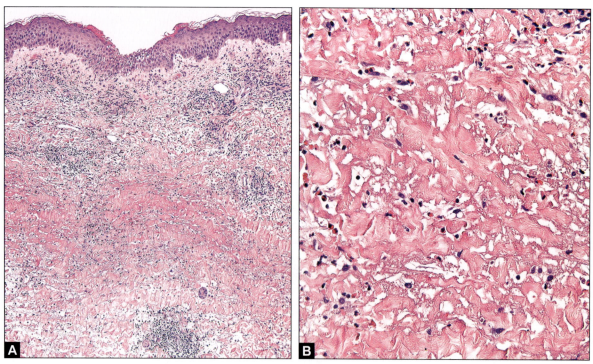

Figs 6.33A and B: Arthropod bite reaction. (A) In addition to mixed inflammation, a feature common to many arthropod/arachnid bite reaction is strands of basophilic degenerative material; (B) The numerous eosinophils are a clue to an arthropod bite.

Sweet's Syndrome (Acute Febrile Neutrophilic Dermatosis) (Figs 6.34A to D)

■ *Criteria for diagnosis*

- Clinical history of an infection, malignancy (usually leukemia or lymphoma), a chronic disease (e.g. inflammatory bowel disease) or use of certain medications (see below)
- Tender erythematous to violaceous plaques, nodules or bulla
- Elevated peripheral blood neutrophil count and elevated erythrocyte sedimentation rate
- Diffuse dermal neutrophilic infiltrate with leukocytoclasis and variable subepidermal edema
- Absence of microorganisms.

■ *Differential diagnosis*

- Leukocytoclastic vasculitis
- Bacterial cellulitis
- Leukemia cutis
- Interstitial granulomatous dermatitis
- Blistering diseases (when bulla are present)
- Cellulitis and other infections
- Pyoderma gangrenosum, bowel bypass syndrome and rheumatoid neutrophilic dermatitis.

■ *Pitfalls*

- In some cases, the neutrophils are most numerous around blood vessels and may simulate leukocytoclastic vasculitis

- Leukemia cutis may be difficult to exclude, especially since Sweet's syndrome may occur in patients with leukemia
- Occasionally, the neutrophilic infiltrate extends into the epidermis and ulceration or blistering (bullous Sweet's syndrome) can occur simulating a blistering disease or pyoderma gangrenosum.

■ *Pearls*

- The density of the neutrophilic infiltrate in Sweet's syndrome is usually greater than that of cellulitis
- Constitutional symptoms like fever, arthralgias, myalgias, headache and malaise are common in contrast to pyoderma gangrenosum
- Ulceration is typical of pyoderma gangrenosum and rare in Sweet's syndrome
- Up to 40% of cases may be associated with a hematolymphoid malignancy
- An elevated peripheral blood neutrophil count and elevated erythrocyte sedimentation rate are usually present and are strong support for the diagnosis
- Drugs that have been associated with Sweet's syndrome include minocycline, trimethoprim-sulfamethoxazoe, all-trans retinoic acid and granulocyte colony stimulating factor.

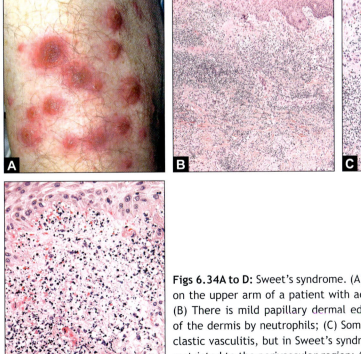

Figs 6.34A to D: Sweet's syndrome. (A) Boggy, red, crusted plaques on the upper arm of a patient with acute myelogenous leukemia; (B) There is mild papillary dermal edema and diffuse infiltration of the dermis by neutrophils; (C) Some areas resemble leukocytoclastic vasculitis, but in Sweet's syndrome the neutrophils are not restricted to the perivascular region; (D) Leukocytoclastic debris is marked in many areas.

Pyoderma Gangrenosum (Figs 6.35A to C)

■ *Criteria for diagnosis*

- Ulcerated painful erythematous papules or nodules that develop raised violaceous borders
- Epidermal ulcer overlying a dermis occupied by a diffuse neutrophilic infiltrate that extends under the adjacent intact epidermis (undermining inflammation).

■ *Differential diagnosis*

- Sweet's syndrome
- Suppurative folliculitis and cellulitis
- Bechet's disease
- Leukocytoclastic vasculitis.

■ *Pitfalls*

- In many cases, pyoderma gangrenosum cannot be distinguished histopathologically from other neutrophilic dermatoses
- In early lesions, the inflammation may be centered on follicles, simulating ecthyma or suppurative folliculitis

- Before ulceration occurs, the features may be difficult to differentiate from Sweet's syndrome or leukocytoclastic vasculitis.

■ *Pearls*

- The diagnosis is best made clinically, but histopathology assists in excluding other causes of neutrophilic infiltrates, such as infections
- Pathergy—flaring or enlargement of the lesions in response to trauma (e.g. biopsy) is characteristic (but not specific) of pyoderma gangrenosum
- Although like Sweet's syndrome it is often associated with underlying diseases, such as leukemia/lymphoma, inflammatory bowel disease or rheumatoid arthritis, pyoderma gangrenosum usually lacks constitutional symptoms (arthralgias, malaise, etc.).

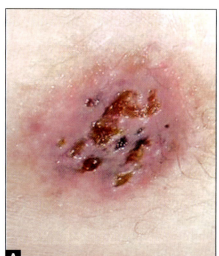
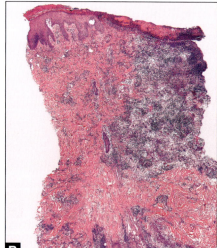
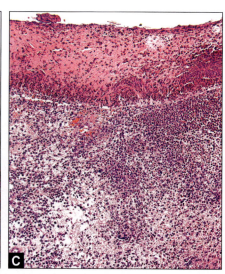

Figs 6.35A to C: Pyoderma gangrenosum. (A) Cribriform ulcer with undermined violet border on the leg of a patient with inflammatory bowel disease; (B) This biopsy from the edge of an ulcer demonstrates the diffuse inflammation of the dermis; (C) As in Sweet's syndrome, neutrophils usually predominate.

Behcet's Disease

Criteria for diagnosis

- Diagnosis is clinical and requires:
  - Recurrent oral ulcers
  - Two or more of the following:
    - Recurrent genital ulcers
    - Uveitis
    - Erythema nodosum, papulopustular lesions or acneiform (suppurative folliculitis) lesions
    - Positive pathergy test
- Histopathologic findings are nonspecific and include suppurative folliculitis, vasculitis, subcorneal pustules, ulcers and diffuse dermal neutrophilic infiltrates.

Differential diagnosis

- Folliculitis
- Infections of many types
- Leukocytoclastic vasculitis of other causes
- Other neutrophilic/suppurative dermatoses (e.g. Sweet's syndrome, pyoderma gangrenosum).

Pitfalls

- Histopathologic features are not specific
- Secondary infection of an ulcer or other lesion of Bechet's may lead to erroneous diagnosis of an infectious disease.

Pearls

- Clinical features provide the only means of definitive diagnosis
- Other than oral and genital ulcers, papulopustular lesions are the most common skin manifestation
- Pathergy-sterile pustules that develop at the site of mild trauma (e.g. injections) are an important but nonspecific diagnostic clue.

Rheumatoid Neutrophilic Dermatosis

Criteria for diagnosis

- Clinical history of rheumatoid arthritis
- Papules, nodules and plaques with a predilection for extensor surfaces and neck
- Dermal neutrophilic infiltrate
- Absence of microorganisms (may require tissue culture).

Differential diagnosis

- Folliculitis
- Infections (especially mycobacterial)
- Other neutrophilic/suppurative dermatoses (e.g. Sweet's syndrome, pyoderma gangrenosum).

Pitfalls

- Histopathologic features are not specific
- Infections must be carefully excluded since many patients are on corticosteroids; mycobacterial infections may be particularly common
- Patients with rheumatoid arthritis may develop pyoderma gangrenosum.

Pearls

- Clinical features are necessary for definitive diagnosis
- Patients with both pyoderma gangrenosum and rheumatoid neutrophilic dermatosis have been documented, suggesting that these neutrophilic dermatoses may form a continuum.

Interstitial Granulomatous Dermatitis and Palisaded Neutrophilic Granulomatous Dermatitis

Criteria for diagnosis

- Interstitial granulomatous dermatitis and palisaded neutrophilic granulmatous dermatitis (PNGD) likely represent a continuum of related reactions to immune complex deposition
- Both have been associated with a multitude of disorders including numerous autoimmune diseases (particularly rheumatoid arthritis but virtually all others as well), malignancies and infection
- Both have heterogeneous clinical presentations, including linear cords (the so-called rope sign), plaques or papules
- The histopathologic features are similarly heterogeneous accounting for the various designations; IGD and/or PNGD are probably sufficient descriptors for the majority of histopathologic features
- Interstitial granulomatous dermatitis: Individual collagen bundles are surrounded by an infiltrate of macrophages sometimes admixed with other inflammatory cell types including eosinophils and neutrophils; collagen degeneration is relatively inconspicuous (Figs 6.36A and B)
- Palisaded neutrophilic granulomatous dermatitis: Variably formed "palisades" of macrophages and other inflammatory cells surround zones of basophilic degenerating collagen (Fig. 6.37A)
- Either may have a component of leukocytoclastic vasculitis in some cases (Fig. 6.37B).

Differential diagnosis

- Interstital granuloma annulare
- Interstitial granulomatous drug eruption
- Pyoderma gangrenosum
- Sweet's syndrome
- Rheumatoid neutrophilic dermatosis.

■ Pitfalls

- In some cases vasculitis may dominate the histopathologic picture
- Some cases of IGD are virtually identical to the interstitial/incomplete form of granuloma annulare
- Interstitial granulomatous dermatitis may be difficult or impossible to differentiate from interstitial granulomatous drug eruption, particularly since the latter may occur in response to drugs used in the treatment of the many disorders associated with IGD.

■ Pearls

- The clinical history is indispensible in most instances, since the histopathologic spectrum is so broad
- Since IGD and PNGD have been associated with virtually the same list of underlying diseases, their distinction is usually not of great clinical importance.

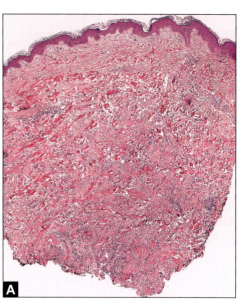
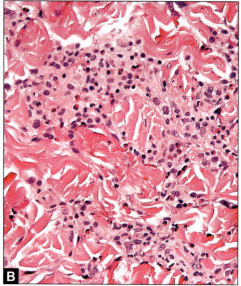

Figs 6.36A and B: Interstitial granulomatous dermatitis. (A) An infiltrate of macrophages occupies the dermis; (B) The macrophages surround relatively intact collagen bundles. In some cases, they are accompanied by neutrophils or in this case, eosinophils.

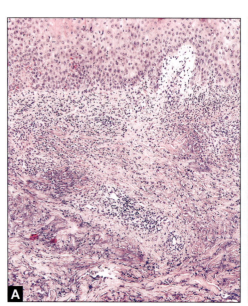
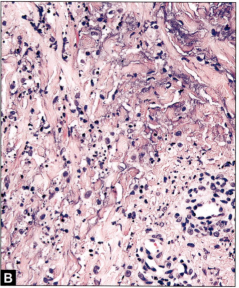

Figs 6.37A and B: Palisaded neutrophilic granulomatous dermatitis. (A) There is basophilic degeneration of the dermal collagen along with leukocytoclastic debris; (B) Some areas resemble a leukocytolastic vasculitis, but the cell debris and the basophilic degenerative collagen are distributed throughout the entire dermis. Unlike interstitial granulomatous dermatitis which usually spares the papillary dermis, palisaded neutrophilic granulomatous dermatitis often involves the full thickness of the dermis and may extend into the subcutis.

Gastrointestinal Associated Neutrophilic Dermatosis (Bowel-Bypass Syndrome) (Figs 6.38A to C)

■ *Criteria for diagnosis*

- Clinical history of a gastrointestinal disease (e.g. ulcerative colitis), liver disease, jejunoileal bypass, or Billroth II surgery
- Neutrophilic dermatosis.

■ *Differential diagnosis*

- Pyoderma gangrenosum
- Sweet's syndrome
- Rheumatoid neutrophilic dermatosis.

■ *Pitfalls*

- In some cases vasculitis is prominent

- Differentiation from pyoderma gangrenosum may be impossible (and arbitrary) when ulceration is present.

■ *Pearls*

- Most lesions do not exhibit the progressive ulceration of pyoderma gangrenosum
- Pyoderma gangrenosum and gastrointestinal associated neutrophilic dermatosis may represent part of a continuum and in cases with extensive overlap the distinction is arbitrary
- Up to 20% of patients with a jejunoileal bypass develop the disease.

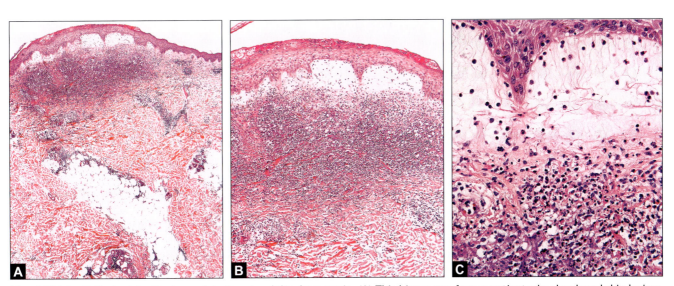

Figs 6.38A to C: Gastrointestinal associated neutrophilic dermatosis. (A) This biopsy was from a patient who developed skin lesions after gastrointestinal bypass surgery; (B) The infiltrate is primarily localized to the superficial dermis; (C) As in Sweet's syndrome, there is papillary dermal edema and a primarily neutrophilic infiltrate.

Hidradenitis Suppurativa (see Table 6.3)

■ *Criteria for diagnosis*

- Clinical history of chronic relapsing suppurative inflammation of axilla, inguinal folds and genitals (areas containing apocrine glands)
- Squamous lined sinus tracts extending from follicular epithelium (Figs 6.39A and B)
- Suppurative inflammation/abscess formation and fibrosis.

■ *Differential diagnosis*

- Folliculitis
- Deep fungal infections or bacterial infections.

■ *Pitfalls*

- Almost all lesions are secondarily infected, often by multiple types of microorganisms making distinction from a primary infectious disease difficult in the absence of typical history of a chronic relapsing condition.

■ *Pearls*

- The pathogenesis remains ill-defined; primary inflammation of the apocrine glands has been postulated but others believe the disease results from follicular occlusion
- The clinical presentation is often diagnostic in and of itself; biopsies are uncommonly performed but surgical excision of the affected skin remains a common treatment.

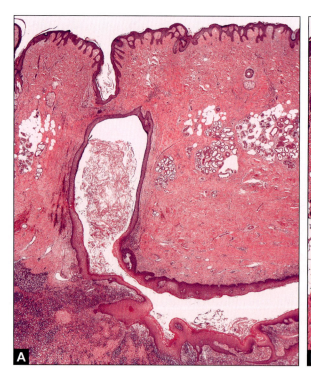
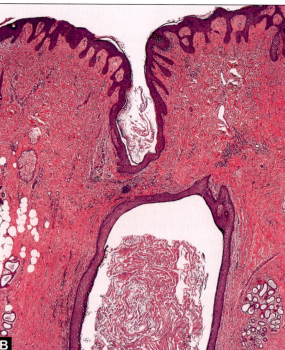

Figs 6.39A and B: Hidradenitis suppurativa. (A) The development of large sinus tracts is characteristic; (B) The sinus tracts are lined by squamous epithelium and are often surrounded by granulation tissue as well.

Infectious Causes of Diffuse Suppurative/Neutrophilic Dermatitis

Bacillary Angiomatosis

- Bartonella henselae or Bartonella quintana
- Angioma-like papules
- Histopathologic resemblance to lobular capillary hemangioma (pyogenic granuloma), sometimes with purple clumps of bacteria visible on hematoxylin and eosin (H&E)
- Warthin-Starry stain may highlight rods.

Bartonellosis (Verruga Peruana)

- Bartonella bacilliformis
- Angioma-like papules
- Warthin-Starry and/or Giemsa positive rods
- Rocha-Lima bodies within endothelial cells
- Resemblance to lobular capillary hemangioma (pyogenic granuloma).

Botryomycosis (Bacterial Pseudomycosis)

- A deep bacterial infection that may be caused by various bacteria, most commonly *Staphylococcus aureus,* but also *Pseudomonas, E. coli, Proteus* and *Streptococci* (Fig. 6.40A)

- Like mycetoma, it presents as nodules with draining sinuses containing granules that often exhibit the Splendore-Hoeppli phenomenon; basophilic bacteria surrounded by an eosinophilic hyaline matrix containing IgG and C3 (Fig. 6.40B).

Toxic Shock Syndrome

- *S. aureus*
- Erythroderma, accentuated in flexures, desquamation within a febrile septic patient
- Clusters of necrotic keratinocytes and underlying dermal neutrophilic infiltrate
- Organisms not seen
- Unlike Staphylococcal scalded skin syndrome, toxic shock affects adults, as well as children and may occur in immunocompetent adults.

Suppurative Folliculitis/Furunculosis

- *S. aureus*
- Follicular-centered pustules and nodules
- Gram positive cocci within follicles
- Expansion of follicles by bacteria and necroinflammatory debris, eventually leading to rupture and diffuse dermal inflammation (Figs 6.40C and D).

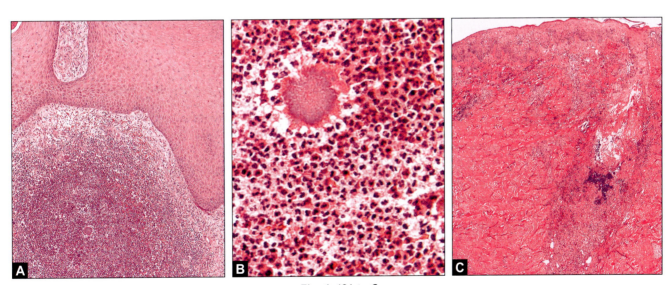

Figs 6.40A to C

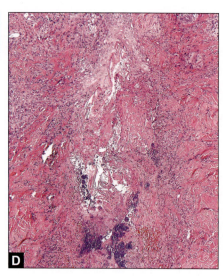

Figs 6.40A to D: Botryomycosis. (A) The low-power appearance is similar to deep fungal infections, with pseudoepitheliomatous hyperplasia and dermal abscesses; (B) Granules exhibiting the Splendore-Hoeppli phenomenon, basophilic bacteria surrounded by an eosinophilic hyaline matrix containing immunoglobulins are a common feature (similar to those of a mycetoma); (C) Suppurative folliculitis. The dermis contains a mixed inflammatory infiltrate centered around a follicle; (D) The amorphous basophilic material is composed of bacteria and inflammatory cell debris.

Ecthyma

- *S. aureus* and *Streptococcus pyogenes* most common causes
- Isolated or solitary crusted ulcers, often on the extremities
- Ulceration, sometimes with identifiable organisms overlying a diffuse neutrophilic dermal infiltrate.

Ecthyma Gangrenosum

- Usually presents with disseminated bullae and necrotic ulcers due to pseudomonas sepsis in critically ill patients (often fatal)
- Extensive epidermal necrosis with dermal infarction; inflammatory infiltrate is sparse, composed of lymphocytes and neutrophils around blood vessels
- Gram-negative bacilli may be visible within the dermis (light blue rods on H&E, bright red on Gram stain).

Erysipelas/Cellulitis

- *S. aureus* and *S. pyogenes* most commonly
- In contrast to cellulitis, erysipelas is a term used in cases with more dermal edema and lymphatic dilatation, sometimes with subepidermal blister formation.

Atypical Mycobacterial Infections

- Caused by *M. marinum, M. kansasii, M. fortuitum, M. chelonei, M. avium intracelluare* and *M. ulcerans*
- Necrosis and abscess formation dominate in early lesions, with progression to granulomatous inflammation in established infections; (Table 6.7).

THE DIFFUSE HISTIOCYTIC DERMATITIS PATTERN (TABLE 6.8)

Juvenile Xanthogranuloma and Adult Xanthogranuloma

- Yellow-brown or flesh-colored papules or nodules (sometimes simulating a Spitz nevus or mastocytosis) (Fig. 6.41A)
- Ill-demarcated aggregates of histiocytes with foamy, eosinophilic or vacuolated cytoplasm admixed with spindle cells and giant cells of Touton or foreign body type, lymphocytes, neutrophils and eosinophils (Figs 6.41B and C)
- When eosinophils are numerous, Langerhans cell histiocytosis should be excluded (using CD1a if necessary)
- Xanthogranulomas occurring in children and infants often termed "juvenile" xanthogranuloma (JXG).
- Histopathologic features usually identical to other xanthogranulomas
- Benign cephalic histiocytosis is likely a form of JXG that presents in infancy or early childhood as erythematous papules on the forehead and cheeks (and may involve other sites) and is composed of histiocytes with eosinophilic cytoplasm with xanthoma cells and multinucleated giant cells appearing in long-standing lesions (Figs 6.41A to C).

Reticulohistiocytoma and Multicentric Reticulohistiocytosis

Figures 6.42A and B show reticulohistiocytoma.

- Reticulohistiocytoma
- One or a few papules (reticulohistiocytoma) that most often arise on the face, ears and hands
- Multicentric reticulohistiocytosis
- Disseminated lesions associated with a destructive arthritis (arthritis mutilans) and intermittent fevers
- Both types have a female predominance
- Lesions of both are composed of histiocytes with eosinophilic slightly granular cytoplasm ("ground glass cytoplasm"), some of which are multinucleated and are PAS positive (Fig. 6.42B).

Xanthoma Disseminatum

- A rare condition that develops in young to middle aged adults with red or yellow papules nodules and plaques (Fig. 6.43A)
- Histopathologic appearance is similar to xanthogranulomas, with dermal aggregates of histiocytes with pale pink cytoplasm admixed with occasional xanthoma cells and multinucleated cells, as well as plasma cells and other inflammatory cells (Fig. 6.43B).

Generalized Eruptive Histiocytosis

Figures 6.44A and B show eruptive xanthoma.
- Very rare condition in which there is a generalized eruption of symmetrical crops of small tan to erythematous papules (Fig. 6.44A)
- Histiocytes have eosinophilic cytoplasm and lack the foamy cytoplasm of other histiocytosis.

Progressive Nodular Histiocytosis

- Very rare disease in which there are numerous papules composed of well demarcated collections of somewhat spindle shaped histiocytes with eosinophilic cytoplasm and occasional foamy xanthoma cells and Touton type giant cells.

Table 6.8: Diffuse histiocytic infiltrates			
Disease	Histopathologic Clues	Histochemical Stains	Clinical
Histoplasmosis *Histoplasma capsulatum var. capsulatum*	Diffuse sheets of macrophages with foamy appearing cytoplasm containing small round or ovoid yeast often surrounded by clear halo (pseudocapsule)	GMS (PAS often negative)	Mucosal ulcers, cutaneous nodules, plaques Often acquired by inhalation of soil contaminated by bird droppings; usually asymptomatic initially Hepatosplenomegaly, anemia, meningitis in disseminated disease Endemic to Southeastern and Midwestern US
Penicilliosis *Penicillium marneffei*	Diffuse infiltrate of macrophages admixed with lymphocytes Resembles histoplasmosis but organisms exhibit surface budding and septa formation	GMS PAS	Umbilicated papules (resembling molluscum contagiosum) and/or indurated plaques Fever, weight loss, lymphadenopathy common
Lepromatous leprosy *M. leprae*	Foamy macrophages containing aggregates of microorganisms ('globi')	AFB/Fite stain	Smooth patches, plaques, or nodules Leonine facies in some instances

Contd...

Disease	Histopathologic Clues	Histochemical Stains	Clinical
Leishmaniasis *Leishmania sp.*	In some cases may present with diffuse dermal histiocytic infiltrates (rather than discrete granulomas)	Giemsa stains nucleus purple and kinetoplast red to purple	Caused by various species of the Leishmania protozoas (unicellular parasites)
	Foamy macrophages containing microorganisms (amastigotes) that often aggregate at the periphery of the cytoplasm ('marquee sign')		Old World cutaneous form: L. tropica, L. major, L. aethiopica; acquired in Middle East, Africa, Asia, and meditarranean region
			Rural (moist) form: Papules that ulcerate with spontaneous healing in 6 months
			Urban (dry) form: Solitary nodule on face; persists for several years
			New World cutaneous and mucocutaneous form: L. brazilliensis and L. tropica
			Kala-azar is visceral leishmaniasis; cutaneous presentation is very rare but occasionally occurs as a papule or nodule at the site of the infecting bite
			Post-kala-azar dermal leishmaniasis is the development of macules, warty papules or nodules, usually on the face, that occurs up to 10 years after treatment for kala-azar
Malakoplakia	Diffuse sheets of histiocytes with abundant granular eosinophilic cytoplasm (von Hansemann cells)	Michaelis –Gutmann bodies stain with von Kossa calcium stain, PAS stain, and sometimes Perl's iron preparation	Soft plaques, nodules, sinuses, or polypoid lesions
	Michaelis-Gutmann bodies (lamellated, calcified basophilic spheres) within the cytoplasm		Skin lesions usually occur around genitals or perineurium
			May be caused by several types of bacteria, but *E. coli* is the most common culprit
Rhinoscleroma *Klebsiella rhinoscleromatis*	Macrophages with clear or vacuolated cytoplasm containing organisms ('Mickulicz cells')	Warthin-Starry stain highlights intracellular bacilli	Most commonly involves nasal and oral mucosa
	Plasma cells often prominent		Endemic in parts of Africa, Asia, and Latin America
			Swollen mucosa with purulent discharge
Xanthomas and xanthogranulomas	Diffuse sheets of histiocytes with foamy cytoplasm	CD68+ S100–	Yellow or brown papule
	Multinucleated cells with Touton configuration in xanthogranulomas		
Rosai-Dorfman disease	Macrophages with foamy cytoplasm admixed with plasma cells and lymphocytes	S100+ CD1a– Birbeck granules absent on electron microscopy	Red to yellow-red patches or plaques; may be multiple or solitary, systemic or skin limited
	Dense diffuse or nodular infiltrate of histiocytes, lymphocytes, plasma cells and neutrophils;		Massive lymphadenopathy with systemic disease
	Eosinophils are rare or altogether absent (helpful in excluding Langerhans cell histiocytosis)		

(GMS: Gomori methenamine silver; PAS: Periodic acid-Schiff; AFB: Acid-fast bacillus).

Xanthomas

- A spectrum of lesions with overlapping clinical and histopathologic features that are primarily differentiated by the anatomic site on which they occur and whether they are associated with hyperlipidemia (see Table 6.8).

- Several forms have distinctive clinical features (such as, the eyelid plaques of xanthelasma), and a few have distinctive histopathologic findings (for example, the extracellular lipid of eruptive xanthomas and the verrucous architecture of a verruciform xanthoma) (Figs 6.45A to C).

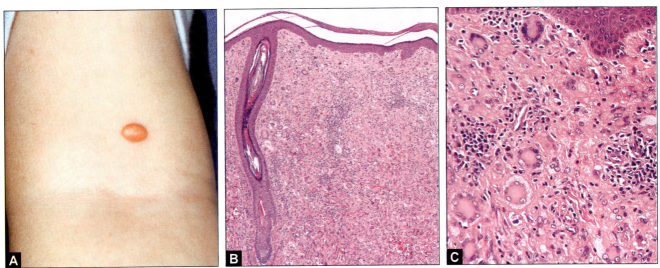

Figs 6.41A to C: Juvenile xanthogranuloma. (A) Diagnosis, smooth, dome-shaped, yellow-pink painless nodule on the forearm of a 10-month-old boy; (B) The dermis is filled by closely packed macrophages with numerous multinucleated giant cells; (C) Cells with rings of nuclei and an outer rim of vacuolated cytoplasm (Touton type giant cells) are characteristic.

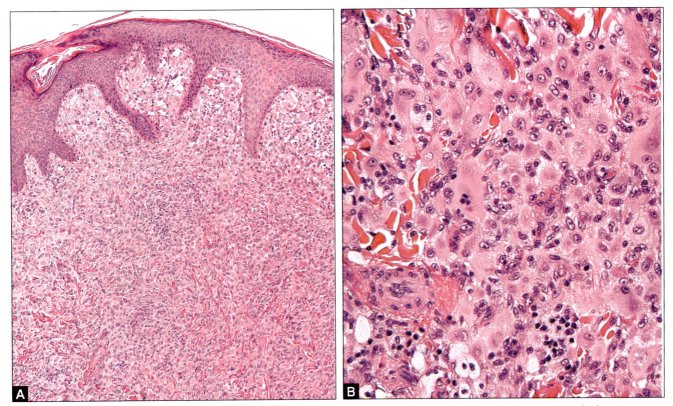

Figs 6.42A and B: Reticulohistiocytoma. (A) An aggregate of macrophages is present within the dermis; (B) At high power, the cells that compose a reticulohistiocytoma usually have finely granular eosinophilic cytoplasm (ground glass cytoplasm).

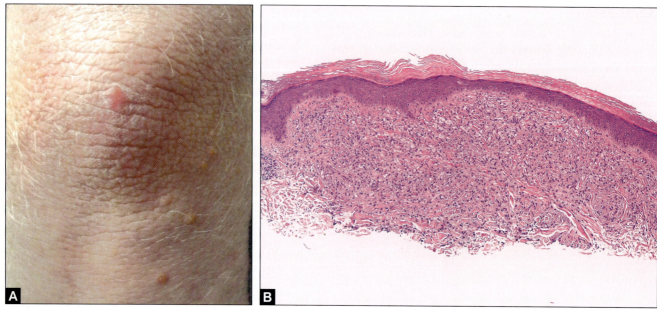

Figs 6.43A and B: Tuberous xanthoma. (A) Smooth papules over the joints; (B) The dermis contains macrophages filled with foamy cytoplasm.

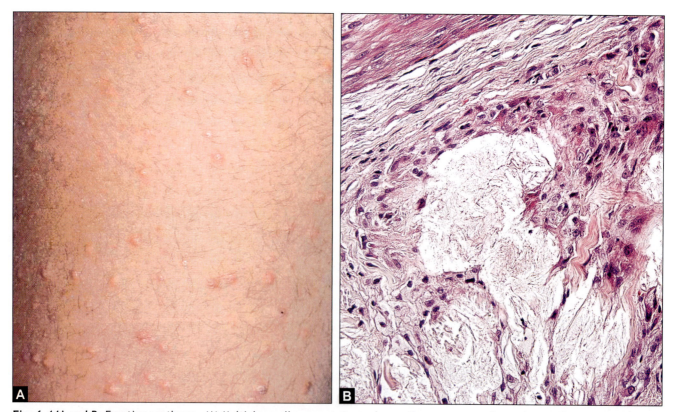

Figs 6.44A and B: Eruptive xanthoma. (A) Multiple small orange-tan papules on the upper arm of a patient with markedly elevated triglycerides; (B) Characteristic of eruptive xanthomas is the presence of extracellular lipid (or angular clefts where lipid had been present) and a mixed inflammatory infiltrate (features usually absent in other xanthomas).

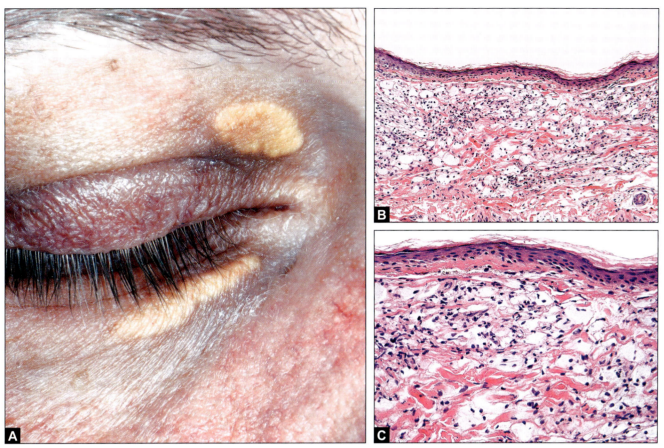

Figs 6.45A to C: Xanthelasma. (A) Smooth, yellow-orange plaques on the eyelid are the typical presentation; (B) Collections of macrophages filled with lipid occupy the dermis; (C) Note the lack of inflammatory cells and extracellular lipid.

Rosai-Dorfman Disease

■ *Criteria for diagnosis*

- Systemic or skin limited disease (cutaneous lesions are the same in both)
- Red to yellow-red patches or plaques; may be multiple or solitary
- Massive lymphadenopathy in patients with systemic disease
- Dense diffuse or nodular infiltrate of histiocytes, lymphocytes, plasma cells and neutrophils; eosinophils are rare or altogether absent (Figs 6.46A and B)
- S100+, CD1a–, absence of Birbeck granules on electron microscopy.

■ *Differential diagnosis*

- Xanthogranulomas and xanthomas
- Hemaphagocytic syndrome
- Histiocyte-rich infections
- Multiple myeloma
- Langerhans cell histiocytosis.

■ *Pitfalls*

- Emperipolesis of inflammatory cells is commonly cited as characteristic of Rosai-Dorfman disease but it is not specific and may be seen in xanthomas and xanthogranulomas (Fig. 6.46C)

- When the accompanying inflammatory infiltrate is dense it may obscure the characteristic histiocytic cells.

■ *Pearls*

- Fever, leukocytosis, hypergammaglobulinemia and elevated erythrocyte sedimentation rate in systemic cases
- Skin is the most common extranodal site of involvement; eyes, soft tissue, genitourinary tract, respiratory tract and nervous system may be involved
- Dense diffuse or nodular infiltrate of histiocytes, lymphocytes, plasma cells and neutrophils; eosinophils are rare or altogether absent
- Histiocytes in Rosai-Dorfman disease tend to have larger nuclei and more prominent nucleoli than in other histiocytoses
- Lymphoid aggregates with germinal centers and thick walled vessels surrounded by plasma cells are often seen at the periphery of the histiocytic nodules
- Dilated lymphatics may contain histiocytes.

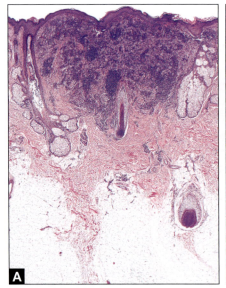 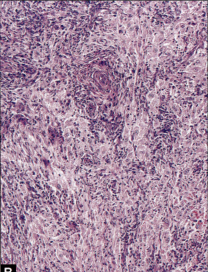 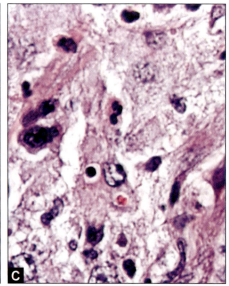

Figs 6.46A to C: Rosai-Dorfman disease. (A) A nodular and diffuse infiltrate of lymphoid cells is evident within the upper dermis; (B) The infiltrate contains numerous histiocytes with abundant, pale cytoplasm. Lymphocytes and plasma cells are also abundant; (C) So-called emperipolesis, histiocytes that contain apparently intact lymphocytes within their cytoplasm is usually seen in Rosai-Dorfman disease but can be found in many other histiocytic infiltrates as well.

Infectious Causes of Diffuse Histiocytic Infiltrates

Histoplasmosis

Figures 6.20A to E show histoplasmosis.
- Caused by two related fungi, *H. capsulatum* var. *capsulatum* and *H. capsulatum* var. *duboisii*
- The most common histopathologic pattern is diffuse aggregates of macrophages, some multinucleated containing small basophilic round or ovoid yeast surrounded by a clear halo
- Occasionally well-formed granulomas are seen
- Disseminated disease is uncommon but is seen in immunocompromised patients, especially those with HIV/AIDS
- Cutaneous lesions are rare (fewer than 10% of cases) and their clinical appearance varies markedly.

Penicilliosis

- Caused by the fungus *Penicillium marneffei*
- Endemic in Southeast Asia, Southern China, and Northeastern India
- Most patients are HIV positive
- Skin lesions are papules and nodules that may become ulcerated or umbilicate
- Organisms are typically numerous and fill the cytoplasm of histiocytes.

Lepromatous Leprosy

Lepromatous leprosy has been shown in Figures 6.47A to C.
- Caused by *M. leprae*
- Systemic infection with multiple symmetrical lesions that may involve much of the skin
- Firm nodular lesions with a predilection for the face and dorsal hands
- Facial lesions often cause loss of eyebrow hair
- Diffuse infiltration of the dermis by macrophages with foamy appearing cytoplasm (Fig. 6.47A)
- Large aggregates of bacilli may be present in histiocyte cytoplasm (globi)
- Fite stain (or Wade-Fite stain, a modified Ziehl-Neelsen stain) is best for highlighting organisms (6.47C).

Leishmaniasis

Figures 6.48A and B show leishmaniasis with a diffuse histiocytic infiltrate.
- Caused by various species of the *L. protozoas* (unicellular parasites)
- Old World cutaneous forms:
  - Caused by *L. tropica*, *L. major* and *L aethiopica* and acquired in Middle East, Africa, Asia and meditarranean region.
  - Rural (moist) form presents as papules that ulcerate with spontaneous healing in 6 months
  - Urban (dry) form presents as solitary nodule on face and has protracted course of several years.
- New World cutaneous and mucocutaneous form:
  - Caused by *L. brazilliensis* and *L. tropica*
- Kala-azar is visceral leishmaniasis; cutaneous presentation is very rare but occasionally occurs as a papule or nodule at the site of the infecting bite
  - Post-kala-azar dermal leishmaniasis is the development of macules, warty papules or nodules usually on the face that occur up to 10 years after treatment for kala-azar
- An infiltrate of dermal histiocytes, sometimes forming granulomas composed of epithelioid histiocytes is common to all forms
- The organisms (amastigotes referred to Donovan bodies) are found within the histiocytes
- Amastigotes have round basophilic nuclei and small basophilic rolike kinteoplast
- Giemsa stains nucleus purple and kinetoplast red to purple
- Differential diagnosis includes American trypanosomiasis (which may be difficult to differentiate on microscopic examination alone), histoplasmosis, rhinocleroma, granuloma inguinale, leprosy and atypical mycobacteria.

Trypanosomiasis

- Protozoal parasitic infection
- African forms
  - Eastern, Western and Central Africa
  - Caused by Tsetse fly bite transmission of *Trypanosoma gambiense* (Gambian form) and *T. rhodesiense* (Rhodesian form)
  - Trypanosomal chancre, a painful red-purple nodule develops at bite site
  - Rhodesian form more commonly produces skin lesions, typically a circinate eruption resembling erythema multiforme but lasts only a few hours after bite
  - Lymphadenopathy is common in Rhodesian form; urticaria, erythema nodosum and painful edema may develop
- American form (Chagas disease)
  - Southern U.S., Mexico, Central America; highest prevalence in Brazil

- Caused by reduviid bug bite transmission of *T. cruzi*
- The chancre (chagoma) is a very painful, erythematous indurated nodule which develops 5–17 days after bite
- Infections may spread to conjunctiva
- Variable course with fever, malaise, edema of face and extremities.
- Histopathologic features (both forms)
  - Ulcer flanked by epidermal hyperplasia
  - Underlying dermis is occupied by histiocytes, plasma cells, lymphocytes with marked edema and often necrosis
  - Vasculitis is common
  - Organisms are best seen on Giemsa stained sections.

Malakoplakia

- Soft plaques, nodules, sinuses or polypoid lesions
- Skin lesions usually occur around genitals or perineurium
- May be caused by several types of bacteria, but *E. coli* is the most common culprit
- Cause diffuse sheets of histiocytes with abundant granular eosinophilic cytoplasm (von Hansemann cells)
- Michaelis-Gutmann bodies; lamellated, calcified basophilic bodies are present within the cytoplasm and stain strongly with von Kossa calcium stain, PAS stain and sometimes Perl's iron preparations.

Rhinoscleroma

- Caused by *Klebsiella rhinoscleromatis*, a Gram-negative diplobacillus
- It is a severe chronic upper respiratory infection, usually in the nose
- The organisms fill histiocytes imparting a foamy appearance to the cytoplasm and often an eccentrically placed nucleus (Mickulicz cell)
- Lymphocytes and numerous plasma cells are also present.

Rhinosporidiosis

- Caused by *Microcystis aeruginosa* (formerly *Rhinosporidium seeberi*)
- In India and Sri Lanka, it usually occurs as a waterborne infection of the nasopharynx
- In the Southwestern United States, it is usually a dustborne infection that affects the conjunctiva and/or nasopharynx
- Lesions are usually polypoid nodules on the mucosa (Fig. 6.49A)
- Organisms are thick walled sporangia filled with endospores and are usually confined to the epithelium or submucosa of the polypoid lesion (Fig. 6.49B).

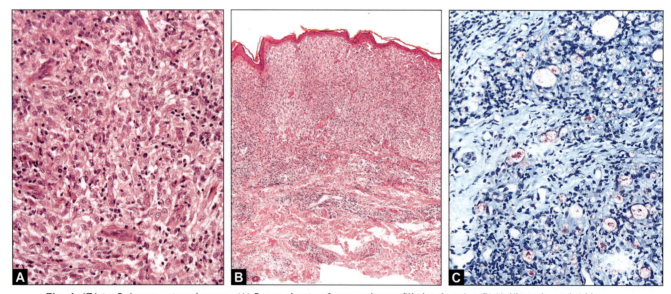

Figs 6.47A to C: Lepromatous leprosy. (A) Dense sheets of macrophages fill the dermis; (B) Unlike tuberculoid leprosy, discrete granulomas are not evident; (C) Wade-Fite stain can be used to highlight the organisms.

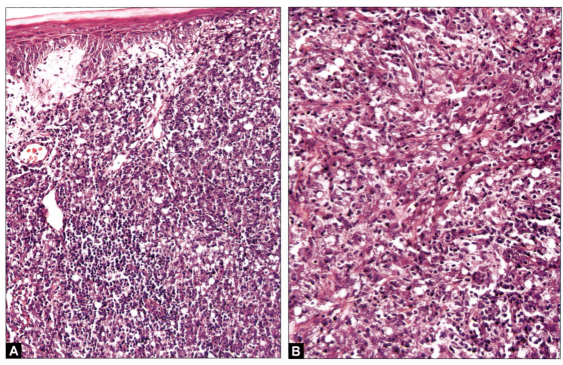

Figs 6.48A and B: Leishmaniasis with a diffuse histiocytic infiltrate. In some instances, the disease may present with diffuse histiocytic infiltrates of the dermis rather than with discrete granulomas (compare to Figures 6.25).

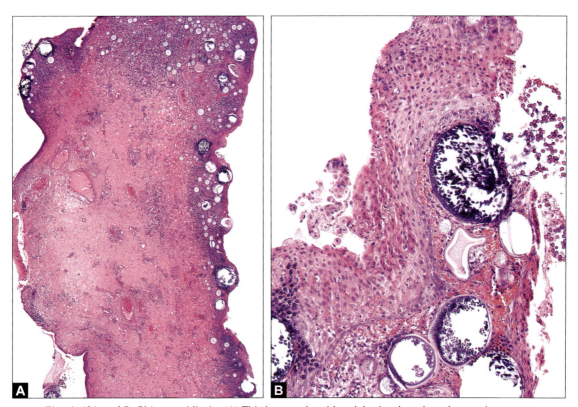

Figs 6.49A and B: Rhinosporidiosis. (A) This large polypoid nodule developed on the nasal mucosa; (B) The nodule contains numerous thick walled sporangia filled with endospores.

THE LYMPHOPLASMACYTIC DERMATITIS PATTERN (TABLE 6.9)

Hematolymphoid Neoplasms

- Any time a dense dermal infiltrate containing numerous lymphocytes and/or plasma cells is encountered, hematolymphoid neoplasms must be excluded
- Particularly, difficult to differentiate from reactive or infectious conditions are those hematolymphoid neoplasms that usually contain a mixture of inflammatory cells in addition to the neoplastic cells; lymphomatoid granulomatosis, lymphomatoid papulosis, cutaneous marginal zone lymphoma, leukemia cutis and cutaneous myeloma are notorious simulators of inflammatory and infectious conditions.
- See Chapter 15 for additional information regarding distinction of benign from neoplastic dermal infiltrates.

Infectious Causes of Lymphoplasmacytic Infiltrates

Secondary and Tertiary Syphilis

- Caused by the spirochete *T. pallidum*
- Although early lesions may show only superficial perivascular infiltrates, established lesions (usually papules or nodules clinically) contain dense dermal inflammatory infiltrates that almost always include numerous plasma cells
- Epidermal hyperplasia with thin elongated rete is common
- Granulomas may be present, especially in tertiary syphilis gummas
- Warthin-Starry silver stains or immunohistochemical stains for *T. pallidum* are useful in identifying organisms

Lymphogranuloma Venereum

- Caused by *Chlamydia trachomatis*
- Multiple genital ulcers with regional lymphadenopathy (nodes enlarged on both sides of Poupart's ligament produces the characteristic "groove sign")
- Lymphatic obstruction may occur, producing genital elephantiasis, rectal strictures or vegetative plaques
- Intracellular microorganisms (coccoid bodies) may occasionally be seen with Giemsa stain
- Differential diagnosis often includes chancroid (which also produces lymphadenopathy).

Chancroid

- Caused by *Hemophilus ducreyi*
- Genital ulcers appearing several days after sexual contact

- Ulcers with acanthosis
- Three relatively distinct "zones" of inflammation are often cited (but the appearance is neither specific nor sensitive):
  1. *Surface*: Ulcer with fibrin, neutrophils and erythrocytes
  2. *Mid-dermis*: Granulation tissue
  3. *Deep dermis*: Dense infiltrate of plasma cells lymphocytes.

Granuloma Inguinale

- Caused by *Calymmatobacterium granulomatis*
- Asymptomatic genital or perianal ulcers with abundant friable granulation tissue; sometimes lymphadenopathy
- Ulcers, sometimes flanked by marked pseudoepitheliomatous epidermal hyperplasia, overlying granulation tissue and mixed inflammation with histiocytes, plasma cells and sometimes neutrophilic microabscesses
- "Donovan bodies": Gram-negative microorganisms may be seen with Giemsa or Warthin-Starry stains
- Smear preparations (crushed tissue smeared on a slide) are more effective than tissue sections for identifying organisms.

Toxoplasmosis

- Obligate intracellular parasite (protozoan)
- Acquired from cat feces or eating undercooked meat from infected animals
- Up to 50% of the US. population may be asymptomatically infected, but infection is arrested early on in immunocompetent hosts; reactivation with progression may occur in immunocompromise and is the major source of disease
- May produce a mononucleosis like syndrome
- Macuolpapular erythematous rash usually on trunk and extremities (with sparing of palms and soles)
- Non-specific perivascular lymphoplasmacytic infiltrate in most cases
- Occasionally organisms seen as tachyzoites (round or crescentic intra- or extracellular organisms) extracellularly, intracellularly within pseudocysts or spherical extracellular pseudocysts filled with PAS+ bradyzoites.

Rhinoscleroma

- Occasionally, lymphocytes and plasma cells may predominate in rhinoscleroma (discussed previously), with the characteristic organism-filled histiocytes less conspicuous.

Disease	Histopathologic Findings	Histochemical Stains/IHC	Clinical
Syphilis *Treponema pallidum*	Psoriasiform epidermal hyperplasia Lichenoid lymphoplasmacytic infiltrate Macrophages and granulomas may be present Obliterative vacsculopathy sometimes Central ulcer often occurs in primary lesion	Treponema pallidum-specific IHC is available Warthin-Starry or Steiner stains may reveal spirochetes	*Primary* Painless papulonodular lesion that arises 3 weeks after exposure +/-Lymphadenopathy *Secondary* Disseminated macular or papulosquamous rash Hyperkeratotic palmoplantar lesions Fever and generalized lymphadenopathy *Tertiary* Nodules, ulcers, and gummatous skin and mucosal lesions Cardiovascular disease, aneurysms, neurologic disease, meningoencephalitis
Lymphomatoid granulomatosis (Lyg)	Lymphoplasmacytic infiltrate with granulomas, often centered on vessels (see Chapter 15)	IHC: CD20+ large B-cells ISH for EBER: EBV+ large B-cells	Cutaneous plaques, nodules Skin is second most common site (after lung)
Granuloma inguinale *Calymmatobacterium granulomatosis*	Ulcer +/– epithelial hyperplasia at border Macrophages, lymphocytes, and plasma cells 1-2 μm gram-negative organisms, often clustered within macrophages Smears made from crushed biopsy tissue are better than sections for visualizing organisms Organisms said to resemble 'safety-pins' with Warthin-Starry or Giemsa stains	Warthin-Starry, Steiner, or Giemsa stains	Genital ulcers, often with thick, friable granulation tissue in a serpiginous pattern Lymphadenopathy is usually minimal (compared to lymphogranuloma venereum; see below)
Lymphogranuloma venereum *Chlamydia trachomatis*	Epidermis normal or ulcerated Diffuse mixed suppurative granulomatous infiltrate		Multiple herpetiform genital ulcers Marked regional lymphadenopathy
Chancroid *Hemophilus ducreyi*	Ulcer with three zones: 1. *Superficial*: Neutrophils, erythrocytes, and fibrin aggregates 2. *Middle*: Granulation tissue 3. *Deep*: Plasma cells, lymphocytes, and microorganisms Microorganisms are Gram-negative bacilli Sometimes said to resemble a "school of fish"	Giemsa (Usually best seen on Giemsa-stained smear) Gram-stain (Gram negative bacilli)	Solitary, nonindurated, painful genital ulcer

Table 6.9: The lymphoplasmacytic (+/- granulomas) pattern

Contd...

Disease	Histopathologic Findings	Histochemical Stains/IHC	Clinical
Rhinoscleroma *Klebsiella rhinoslceromatis*	Organisms are Gram-negative coccobacilli Dense infiltrate of macrophages and plasma cells Some large macrophages containing numerous organisms are usually present (Mikulicz cells) Plasma cells may contain Russel bodies but are not specific	Best seen with Warthin Starry Gram Giemsa PAS	Usually occurs on nose but other parts of respiratory tract may be involved Nasal congestion, crusting, and discharge in early phases Deforming granulation tissue, hyperplasia, and scarring in later stage Most common in Central and South America, India, Indonesia, parts of the former Soviet Union, China, Africa

(IHC: Immunohistochemistry; ISH: In situ hybridization; EBER: Epstein-Barr virus-encoded small RNA; EBV: Epstein-Barr virus).

DERMAL INFESTATIONS AND ARTHROPOD BITE REACTIONS

Onchocerciasis

- Caused by the nematode *Onchocerca volvulus*
- Endemic in tropic Africa and Central and South America
- Larval forms are transmitted to humans by black fly bites (*Simulium*)
- Larvae develop into adult worms in the dermis and then produce microfilariae which migrate throughout the body (Figs 6.50A and B)
- Onchocerciasis is known as "river blindness" when microfilariae infiltrate the eyes and cause damage that may progress to blindness
- Most endemic areas are located along fast flowing rivers
- Adult worms produce tender, mobile dermal nodules with extensive fibrosis, commonly located over bony prominences
- Adult worms are found in groups within a fibrotic upper dermis beneath an acanthotic epidermis; microfilariae are often seen within gravid females
- Microfilariae infiltrate between collagen bundles of the dermis
- Inflammation (usually lymphocytes and eosinophils) is often mild, but degenerating organisms elicit a dense eosinophilic infiltrate.

Tungiasis

- Caused by Tunga penetrans, the sand flea or jigger flea
- Predominance is in Central and South America, Caribbean, Africa and Pakistan
- Highest prevalence is in impoverished areas
- Predilection for feet
- Pruritic painful white or erythematous nodule develops, often with a dark central punctum

- The bulk of the flea is usually contained within the epidermis; the proboscis extends into the dermis causing a mixed inflammatory infiltrate rich in lymphocytes, plasma cells and eosinophils
- The exoskeleton, hypodermal layer and developing eggs are the most easily identifiable structures (Fig. 6.51)
- In partial biopsies, fragments of the organisms may be mistaken for scabies mites or other arthropods.

Larva Migrans

- Most cases are caused by larval forms of the nematode *Ancylostoma braziliensis* (cat and dog hookworm)
- Most common in tropic regions, particularly coastal regions
- Larvae enter follicular ostia or acrosyringium, most commonly on feet
- Pruritic erythematous papules or papulovesicles develop at the site of penetration
- Larvae begin to migrate through the dermis several days later at a rate of 2–5 cm per day, producing distinctive erythematous serpiginous tracts (Fig. 6.52)
- Organisms are difficult to capture on biopsy since they precede the clinically visible tracts
- Often the findings are a "tunnel" within the superficial dermis with epidermal spongiosis and variably mixed inflammation, usually with eosinophils.

Schistosomiasis

Figures 6.53A and B show schistosomiasis.
- Caused by the trematode blood flukes *Schistosoma hematobium*, *Schistosoma mansoni* and *Schistosoma japonicum*
- Skin disease is uncommon and usually a minor feature of the disease
- Infestation by the aquatic cercarial form causes a pruritic erythematous urticarial rash known as "swimmer's itch" that usually resolves spontaneously

- Yellow river fever (Katayama disease) is caused by *S. japonicum* and produces erythema, macules, nodules, often accompanied by constitutional symptoms (fever, chills, arthralgias, etc.) and peripheral blood eosinophilia
- Lesions are often concentrated around genitalia, particularly in females
- Perirurethral lesions may result in perineal fistulas (watering can perineum)
- Organisms disseminate through vasculature and cause thrombosis, necrosis and inflammation
- Biopsy of involved skin may reveal adult worms within vessels of deep dermal veins or lymphatics
- Viable ova may be seen within abscesses containing neutrophils and eosinophils, and granulomas are sometimes present
- Dead ova usually calcify and elicit a granulomatous infiltrate.

Cysticercosis

- Cutaneous lesions are caused by the cylticerci of the adult pork tapeworm *Taenia solium*
- Ingestion of eggs leads to cysticercosis involving the skin, brain and eye

- Lesions present as solitary painless 1–2 cm nodules
- Viable organisms are lodged within the dermis without inflammation
- Degenerating organisms invoke a mixed inflammatory infiltrate that progresses to granulomas with fibrosis and calcified debris.

Scabies

- Caused by the mite *Sarcoptes scabiei* var. *hominis*
- Rarely is an intact scabies mite detected within biopsied skin, but serial sections may reveal mites, their excrement or their burrows in some cases (Fig. 6.54A)
- A dense dermal inflammatory infiltrate that includes many eosinophils is a clue to scabies infestation, particularly when there is evidence of excoriation and/or the history describes intense pruritus (Fig. 6.54B).

Tick Bite

- Tick bites often produce dense mixed dermal inflammatory infiltrates
- Mouth parts or occasionally the entire tick may be present (Figs 6.55A and B).

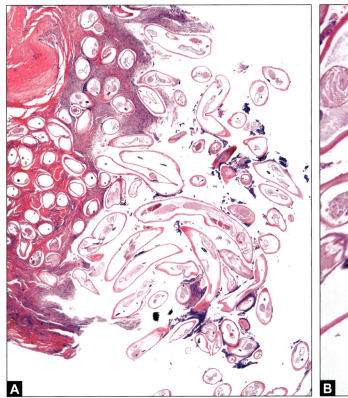
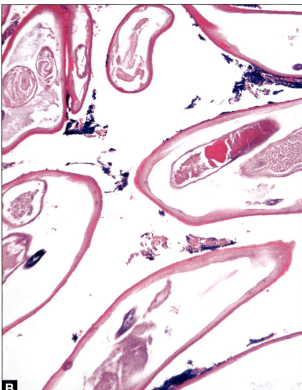

Figs 6.50A and B: Onchocerciasis. (A and B) Sections of an adult worm are present.

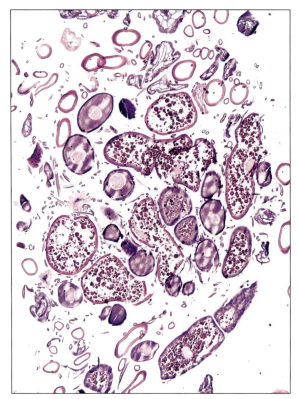

Fig. 6.51: Tungiasis. The exoskeleton, hypodermal layer and developing eggs are commonly recognizable.

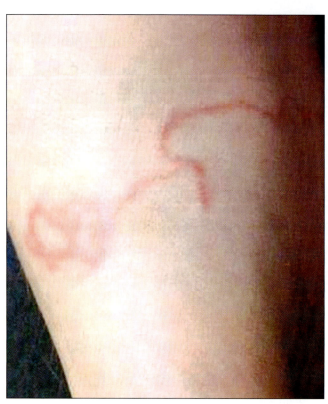

Fig. 6.52: Larva Migrans. A migrating serpiginous pink tract on the foot is the clinical presentation.

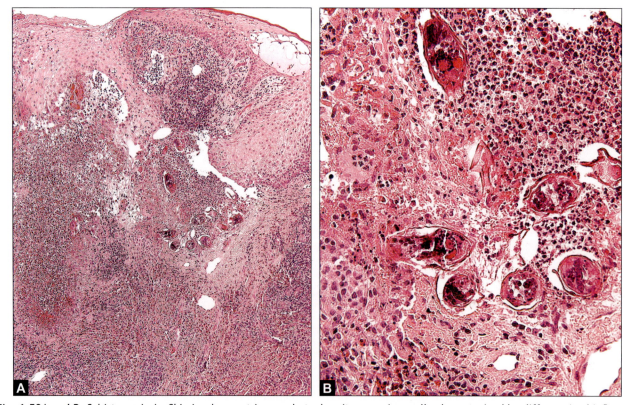

Figs 6.53A and B: Schistosomiasis. Skin involvement is rare, but when it occurs is usually characterized by diffuse mixed inflammation and abscess formation; (B) The organisms are evident within this dermal abscess.

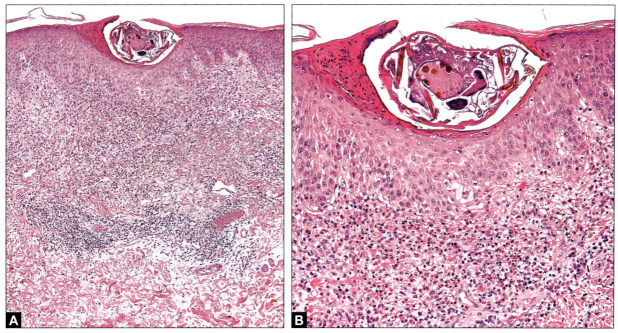

Figs 6.54A and B: Scabies infestation. (A) The scabies mite forms a burrow just beneath the stratum corneum; (B) If scabies infestation is suspected, serial sections may reveal the mite but a very dense dermal infiltrate of eosinophils suggests the possibility of scabies even when a mite cannot be found.

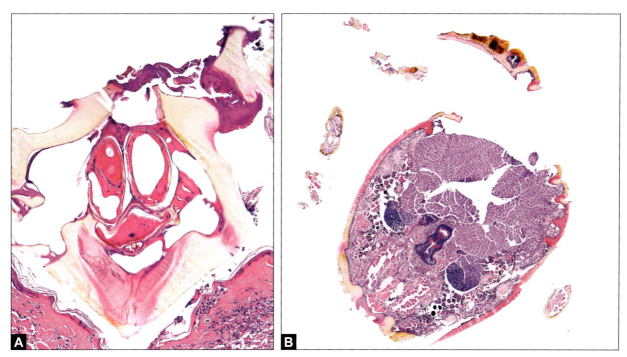

Figs 6.55A and B: Tick bite. (A) Retained tick mouth parts are occasionally seen within biopsies of the bite site; (B) Intact tick.

BIBLIOGRAPHY

1. Bonifaz A, Vázquez-González D, Tirado-Sánchez A, Ponce-Olivera RM. Cutaneous zygomycosis. Clin Dermatol. 2012;30 (4):413-9.

2. Motswaledi HM, Monyemangene FM, Maloba BR, Nemutavhanani DL. Blastomycosis: a case report and review of the literature. Int J Dermatol. 2012;51(9):1090-3.

3. Talhari S, Talhari C. Lobomycosis. Clin Dermatol. 2012;30(4): 420-4.

CHAPTER 7

The Vasculopathic Pattern

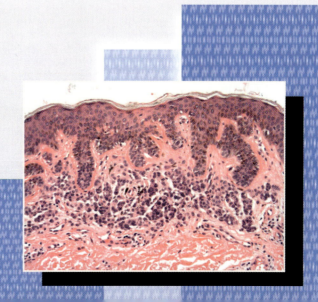

INTRODUCTION

Diseases of the cutaneous vasculature are caused by occlusion of vessels (occlusive vasculopathy) or inflammation (vasculitis). The general term "vasculopathy" encompasses both etiologies. Vasculitis is one of the two major vascular reaction patterns. Since, by definition, it implies inflammation, do not use it as a synonym for vasculopathy.

Approach the vasculopathic pattern by first determining whether it is primarily occlusive or inflammatory. Skin from an occlusive vasculopathy will contain congested blood vessels (vessels filled and expanded by red blood cells), intraluminal thrombi and generally lack inflammation. If inflammation is present, it should be sparse and composed mostly of lymphocytes and histiocytes. Neutrophils are almost always absent. The occlusive vasculopathies may be further subclassified.

If neutrophils or their remnants (leukocytoclastic debris) are present, the condition is a vasculitis. Skin biopsies usually include only the small vessels of the dermis (or occasionally a medium caliber vessel or two if subcutis is present), and in the vast majority, the predominant finding is a neutrophilic infiltrate in and around dermal postcapillary venules. This is known as leukocytoclastic vasculitis (LCV) and is discussed later. Leukocytoclastic vasculitis is not a diagnosis but a reaction pattern that can be caused by numerous conditions with diverse etiologies. Features that differentiate one cause from another are rarely evident and the final interpretation must often be "LCV" with a comment suggesting the most likely causes if any helpful clinical information is provided. Occasionally, however, the clinical presentation or the histopathologic findings are characteristic of specific subtypes of vasculitis, these features should be recognized.

Finally, vasculitis may be accompanied by diffuse dermal fibrosis (fibrosing vasculitis) or include macrophages or granulomas. These patterns are discussed in later in the chapter respectively.

THE OCCLUSIVE VASCULOPATHY PATTERN

The common histopathologic features of occlusive vasculopathy are vascular congestion, intraluminal thrombi and erythrocyte extravasation, but minimal inflammation in comparison to true vasculitis.

Occlusive vasculopathies have many causes and the histopathologic features are rarely diagnostic. Nevertheless, they may be categorized broadly into three groups:
1. Conditions that tend to cause petechiae or palpable purpura clinically and usually reveal vascular congestion and occasional intraluminal thrombi with mild red cell extravasation.
2. Conditions that can cause large ecchymotic areas, diffuse hemorrhage and/or necrosis, and often have more obvious vascular occlusion and destruction with extensive hemorrhage and diffuse necrotic areas.
3. Conditions with specific clinical and/or histopathologic features that allow a specific diagnosis or at least a narrower differential diagnosis.

The first two categories are best considered as groups of disorders with histopathologic and clinical features that often overlap. The conditions in the third category are discussed individually in order to emphasize the features that may allow a specific diagnosis.

Occlusive Vasculopathies with Minimal Vascular Damage

This pattern is most often associated with an underlying systemic coagulopathy. Common causes include Factor V Leiden mutation, protein C deficiency, anticardiolipin antibodies or antiphospholipid antibodies (Figs 7.1A and B). However, septic emboli (bacterial or fungal) may also produce occluded vessels with little or no inflammation (Figs 7.1C and D).

■ *Criteria for diagnosis*

- Petechiae or pigmented purpura clinically
- Dermal vessels that are congested and/or contain intraluminal fibrin thrombi
- A sparse perivascular lymphohistiocytic infiltrate sometimes, but no neutrophils or leukocytoclasis.

■ *Differential diagnosis*

- Other occlusive vasculopathies

■ *Pitfalls*

- The intraluminal fibrin thrombi are often sparse and sometimes confined to the deep dermis or subcutis (and therefore absent in superficial biopsies)
- The thrombi may be obscured by densely packed red cell aggregates since most are contained within congested blood vessels.

■ *Pearls*

- Search carefully for clues to a specific diagnosis (e.g. cholesterol crystals, microorganisms, calcifications; (see category 3, occlusive vasculopathies); if there are none, a diagnosis of "occlusive vasculopathy" is appropriate with a comment mentioning some of the differential diagnostic possibilities including the coagulopathies listed above.

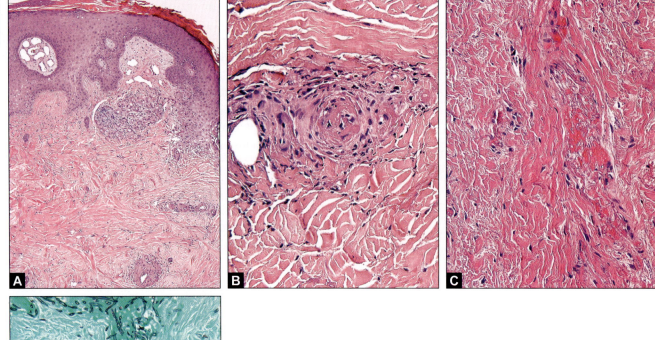

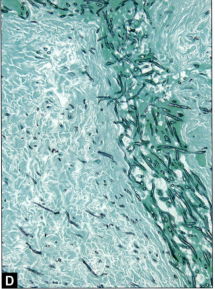

Figs 7.1A to D: Antiphospholipid antibody syndrome. (A) Dilated and congested vessels are the primary features on low power; (B) Close inspection reveals a few vessels occluded by fibrin thrombi; Fungal septic embolus. (C) Dusky macules appeared rapidly in this immunocompromised patient: at first glance, the vessel appears to contain a fibrin thrombus; (D) Grocott-Gomori methenamine silver stain shows a surprising number of angioinvasive fungi that are also present within the dermis.

Note the lack of inflammation, a feature that may be particularly common in immuno-compromised states

Severe Occlusive Vasculopathies (Vasculopathy with Extensive Vascular Damage, Hemorrhage and/or Necrosis)

More profound vascular damage can be caused by most of the conditions mentioned above in the first category, but severe occlusive vasculopathy is more often the result of coumarin/warfarin necrosis, thrombotic thrombocytopenic purpura and disseminated intravascular coagulation, especially when they are present as "purpura fulminans", a clinical syndrome of rapidly progressive, diffuse hemorrhagic skin necrosis (Figs 7.2A to C). Purpura fulminans is more common in children and tends to occur in association with infections, such as meningococcemia, scarlet fever or certain viruses.

Criteria for diagnosis

- Petechiae or pigmented purpura that evolve into large dusky ecchymotic or necrotic lesions, sometimes with blistering
- Blood vessels that are congested and contain intraluminal fibrin thrombi
- Extensive hemorrhage
- Necrosis in fully evolved lesions, especially in the setting of purpura fulminans.

Differential diagnosis

- Other occlusive vasculopathies
- Leukocytoclastic vasculitis (since neutrophils may appear in fully developed lesions).

Pitfalls

- Even in advanced lesions, intraluminal fibrin thrombi may be scattered or localized to the deep dermis or subcutis (and missed by superficial biopsies)
- Disseminated intravascular coagulation (especially with purpura fulminans presentation) may have a neutrophilic infiltrate simulating LCV.

Pearls

- Definitive diagnosis requires clinical correlation, e.g. suspected purpura fulminans or onset of lesions after starting coumadin therapy.

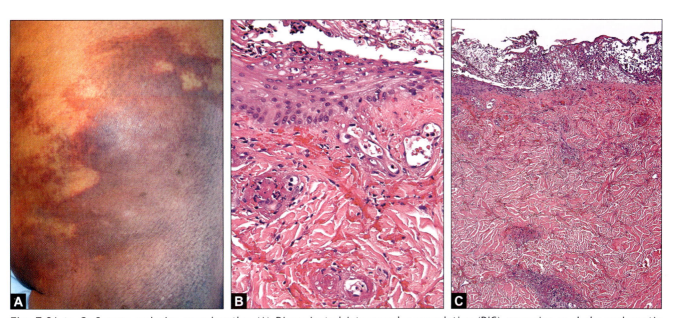

Figs 7.2A to C: Severe occlusive vasculopathy. (A) Disseminated intravascular coagulation (DIC) presening as dusky ecchymotic plaques; (B) Epidermal necrosis is the result of ischemia in this patient with disseminated intravascular coagulation; (C) There is vascular congestion and many vessels also contain fibrin thrombi.

Occlusive Vasculopathies with Characteristic Clinical or Histopathologic Features

Some occlusive vasculopathies have histopathologic features that may allow a specific diagnosis within the appropriate clinical scenario.

Livedoid Vasculopathy/Atrophie Blanche (Fig. 7.3A)

■ Criteria for diagnosis

- Livedo reticularis, a persistent red-blue mottling of the skin with a "net-like" pattern (Fig. 7.3B)
- Vessels with thick, "hyalinized" appearing walls (fibrinoid change) often with thrombi or occluded vessels
- Sparse perivascular lymphocytes and macrophages may be present but neutrophils and leukocytoclasis are absent
- Completely occluded vascular lumens, epidermal atrophy and dermal sclerosis in established lesions (corresponding to the atrophic scars of atrophie blanche seen clinically).

■ Differential diagnosis

- Cutis marmorata
- Other occlusive vasculopathies
- Stasis dermatitis
- Resolving LCV
- Amyloidosis

■ Pitfalls

- Biopsies from erythematous (red) areas often lack any abnormality

- Features may be similar to stasis dermatitis if fibrinoid thickening of vessel walls is not appreciated.

■ Pearls

- Livedoid vasculopathy is sometimes referred to as livedoid "vasculitis"; this is a misnomer since it is caused by occlusion rather than inflammation
- Fibrinoid thickening of blood vessels is a characteristic feature (generally absent in stasis dermatitis and most other vasculopathies)
- Common associations are autoimmune/connective tissue diseases, such as lupus erythematosus, and various causes of coagulopathy (Factor V Leiden mutation, protein C deficiency, etc.)
- The mottled pattern does not resolve with warming of the skin (unlike cutis marmorata)
- Ulceration may occur and healing lesions may scar and evolve into atrophie blanche (see below).

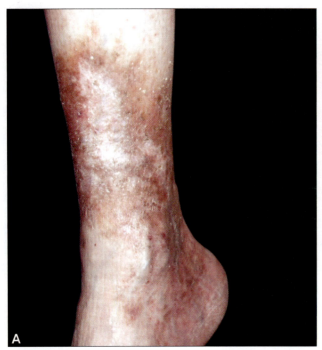

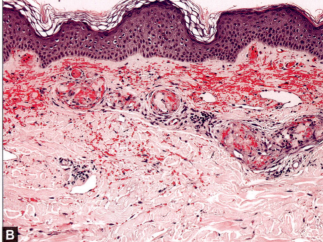

Figs 7.3A and B: Livedoid vasculopathy. (A) Purpura, atrophic white plaques are present on the dorsal foot; (B) This patient presented with the red-blue mottled pattern characteristic of livedo reticularis, the biopsy reveals vascular congestion, occasional thrombi and thickening of the vessel walls with little inflammation.

Cryoglobulinemia Type 1 (Figs 7.4A to C)

Criteria for diagnosis

- Purpuric, necrotic papules, livedo reticularis, acrocyanosis, digital necrosis, ulcers and Raynaud's phenomenon
- Amorphous thrombi that stain bright red with periodic acid Schiff (PAS)
- Confirmation that monoclonal IgG or IgM immunoglobulins are present.

Differential diagnosis

- Other occlusive vasculopathies.

Pitfalls

- Dilated congested vessels without obvious cryoglobulin thrombi are often present in the surrounding dermis
- Occasionally Type II and III may contain some PAS positive material.

Pearls

- Thrombi are pale pink on hematoxylin and eosin stain and bright red on PAS stain and often have a "cracked" or "fissured" appearance
- Type I cryoglobulinemia lacks the inflammation of Type II and III.
- Arthralgias, hepatosplenomegaly, lymphadenopathy and glomerulonephritis are common systemic associations.

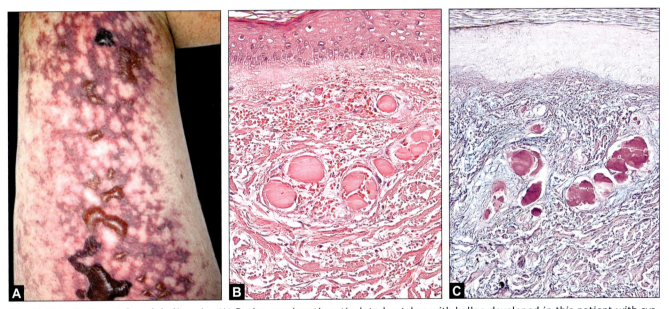

Figs 7.4A to C: Type 1 Cryoglobulinemia. (A) Dusky, eccyhmotic reticulated patches with bullae developed in this patient with systemic lymphoma; (B) Vessels are occluded by homogenous eosinophilic material—inflammation is absent in Type 1 cryoglobulinemia (unlike in Types II and III); (C) The intraluminal globules are bright pink in tissue stained with periodic acid-Schiff.

Cholesterol Emboli

Figure 7.5 shows clefts with tapered ends within an organized fibrin thrombus which are the characteristic finding.

■ Criteria for diagnosis

- Intraluminal emboli containing angular clefts surrounded by fibrin
- Dusky, purpuric or necrotic macules or plaques
- Predilection for the toes with cyanosis ("blue toes") initially and gangrenous necrosis in advanced or severe cases.

■ Differential diagnosis

- Other occlusive vasculopathies.

■ Pitfalls

- The thrombi containing the characteristic clefts are often few and sometimes only within deeper vessels, and may be easily missed, especially on superficial biopsies.

■ Pearls

- The angular clefts are an artifact of the dissolved cholesterol crystals
- Macrophages and/or a foreign body giant cell reaction may accompany the thrombi
- Elderly patients with atherosclerosis are most commonly affected
- A recent history of arterial catheterization is common and is a clinical clue to diagnosis
- Predilection for lower extremities
- Established lesions may be obliterated by fibrosis
- Arterial pulses are usually maintained, a clue that the ischemia is due to small vessel occlusion rather than thrombosis of major arteries.

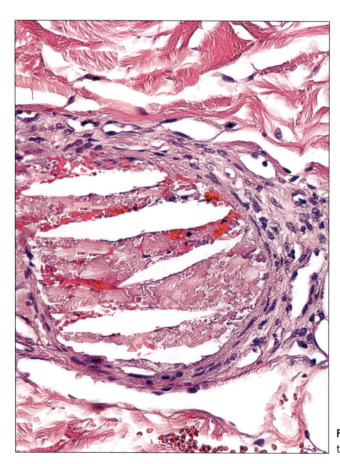

Fig. 7.5: Clefts with tapered ends within an organized fibrin thrombus are the characteristic finding.

Calciphylaxis (Figs 7.6A and B)

■ Criteria for diagnosis

- Painful violaceous indurated plaques that frequently form bullae, ulcers and scars
- Deep purple refractile calcium deposits within vascular lumens and walls that often fracture when sectioned
- Infarction and hemorrhage in established lesions, sometimes with a mixed inflammatory infiltrate.

■ Differential diagnosis

- Other occlusive vasculopathies
- Calcinosis cutis
- Medial calcific stenosis
- Pancreatic panniculitis.

■ Pitfalls

- Medial calcific sclerosis, a common expression of arteriosclerosis (Monckeberg's medial sclerosis) also contains calcium deposits within vessel walls
- Affected vessels may be few and are often found only in the deep dermis or subcutis
- Sectioning may destroy the calcium deposits, leaving behind only torn tissue.

■ Pearls

- Usually occurs with known renal disease and secondary or tertiary hyperparathyroidism
- An incisional biopsy including large quantities of subcutis allows the best chance at detecting the calcified thrombi
- Unlike calciphylaxis, the calcium in medial calcific sclerosis is confined within the vessel wall and does not encroach on the vascular lumen
- Unlike calciphylaxis, calcinosis cutis does not occlude vessels or cause infarction
- The "ghost cells" and extensive inflammation characteristic of pancreatic panniculitis are absent in calciphylaxis (and the clinical presentation is usually quite different)
- Fulminant sepsis and hypercoagulability are commonly associated with calciphylaxis, but the exact pathogenesis remains unclear
- Prognosis is usually poor even with parathyroidectomy, but an indolent "chronic form" has been described
- Obese people and female gender appear at increased risk.

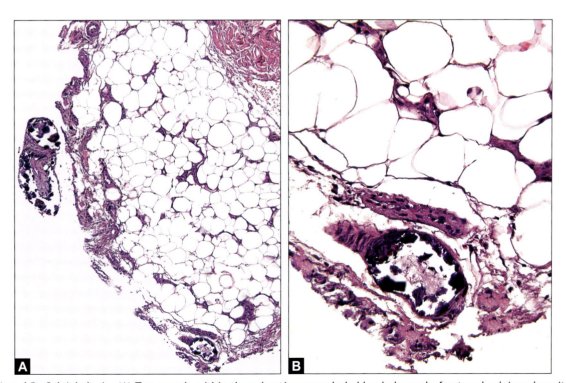

Figs 7.6A and B: Calciphylaxis. (A) Two vessels within the subcutis are occluded by dark purple fractured calcium deposits—notice that had the biopsy been just slightly more superficial, the diagnostic feature would have been absent; (B) The calcium deposits of calciphylaxis fill the vessel lumen, unlike those of medial calcific stenosis, which are localized to the vascular media and do not encroach on the lumen.

THE ACUTE VASCULITIS PATTERN

Leukocytoclastic Vasculitis (Hypersensitivity Vasculitis, Small Vessel Neutrophilic Vasculitis)

Leukocytoclastic vasculitis is the most common type of vasculitis encountered in the skin and may be a consequence of a vast array of disorders with many different etiologies. The histopathologic features alone rarely allow a specific diagnosis. The threshold for diagnosis varies greatly among dermatopathologists with some requiring only one histopathologic feature and others insisting on all criteria for definitive diagnosis (Figs 7.7A to E).

■ *Criteria for diagnosis*

- Clinically, lesions are most often bilateral and tend to involve the lower third of the legs, but may also occur on the buttocks and arms
- Lesions exhibit one of the three general patterns:
  - Small purpuric papules ("palpable purpura"), the most common manifestation
  - Edematous papules, urticarial papules, erythematous macules or pustules
  - Hemorrhagic blisters, livedo reticularis, erythematous nodules or ulcers (when deep vessels are involved)
- Histopathologic features of neutrophilic small vessel vasculitis, including:
  - Fibrin deposition in vessel walls
  - Neutrophils within and around small vessels
  - Leukocytoclasis (karyorrhectic nuclear debris).

■ *Differential diagnosis*

Leukocytoclastic vasculitis is a nonspecific reaction pattern that may occur in:
- nfections
  - Bacterial infections (including *Mycobacteria* and *Spirochetes*)
  - Rickettsial infections (including Rocky Mountain spotted fever and scrub typhus)
  - Fungal infections
  - Viral infections
- Immune complex-mediated diseases
  - Henoch-Schonlein purpura
  - Urticarial vasculitis

  - Cryoglobulinemias (Types II and III)
  - Serum sickness
  - Connective tissue and autoimmune diseases
  - Drug reactions
  - Paraneoplastic reactions
  - Behcet's disease
  - Erythema elevatum diutinum (early lesions)
  - Infection-induced immunologic injury (most often hepatitis B, hepatitis C and Streptococcal infections)
- Antineutrophilic antibody-associated diseases (ANCA-associated vasculitis)
  - Wegener's granulomatosis
  - Microscopic polyangiitis
  - Churg-Strauss syndrome
- Polyarteritis nodosa (PAN).

■ *Pitfalls*

- Histopathologic features vary with age of lesion sampled
- If criteria are applied too rigidly, early manifestations may be underdiagnosed
- In later lesions, lymphocytes may predominate over neutrophils
- Pustular variants (pustular vasculitis) or blistering (bullous vasculitis) may occur causing misinterpretation as a pustular or blistering disease
- In some cases, neutrophils appear to be distributed throughout the entire dermis rather than concentrated around vessels, simulating neutrophilic dermatoses, such as Sweet's disease and pyoderma gangrenosum
- Simulators include Schamberg's disease and other "purpuric dermatoses"
- "Palpable purpura" is not specific for vasculitis, as it may be seen in lichen aureus, pityriasis lichenoides and other disorders.

■ *Pearls*

- In most cases, "LCV" is a perfectly acceptable "line diagnosis" for a pathology report; a comment that definitive diagnosis requires clinical correlation and listing some of the common causes may be helpful, particularly if the clinician performing biopsy is not a dermatologist
- Occasionally, specific histopathologic findings and/or a characteristic clinical scenario allow a more precise diagnosis, and these features should be carefully sought before settling on the descriptive interpretation of LCV (e.g. urticarial vasculitis, Henoch-Schonlein purpura, septic vasculitis and cryoglobulinemia).

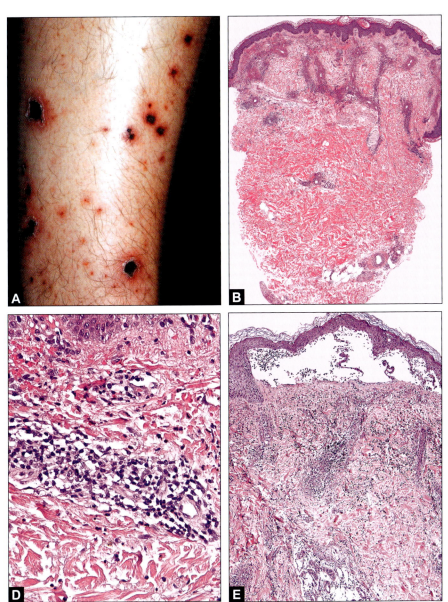

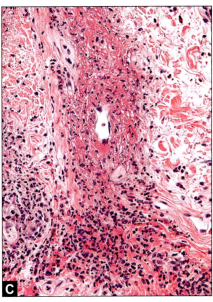

Figs 7.7A to E: Leukocytoclastic vasculitis. (A) Purpuric papules and nodules, some of which have ulcerated, covering the leg; (B) Inflammation and fibrin deposition surround vessels throughout the dermis; (C) Vessel walls are markedly thickened and the inflammation is centered within and around them; (D) In the later stages, lymphocytes may be as numerous as neutrophils; (E) Bullous type, when vascular damage is severe and necrosis develops, blistering may occur.

Urticarial Vasculitis

Urticarial vasculitis is a distinctive pattern if strictly defined, but like the other vasculopathic patterns it is not specific for any particular disease and may be idiopathic. Some regard it as merely an early manifestation of LCV. The major challenge is adhering to specific histopathologic criteria while keeping in mind that those criteria may often be subtle. Sometimes the only clues are small collections of leukocytoclastic debris around vessels and extravasated red blood cells (Figs 7.8A to C).

■ *Criteria for diagnosis*

- Wheals that persist for greater than 24 hours (often resolving with faint purpura or hyperpigmentation)
- Enlarged endothelial cells, dilated venules and an inflammatory infiltrate that vary in density and include neutrophils, eosinophils, mast cells and lymphocytes (Fig. 7.8B)
- Any evidence of vasculitis from small collections of perivascular dust and extravasated red cells to fully developed LCV.

■ *Differential diagnosis*

- Leukocytoclastic vasculitis
- Urticaria
- Mastocytosis, especially the telangiectasia macularis eruptiva perstans form
- Insect/arthropod bite reaction.

■ *Pitfalls*

- Urticarial papules are sometimes the presenting finding in LCV

- Vascular damage is often subtle, but may be indistinguishable from LCV in some examples.

■ *Pearls*

- The presence of just a few degenerated neutrophils (neutrophilic "dust") and extravasated red blood cells indicate urticarial vasculitis rather than urticarial (Fig. 7.8C)
- Approximately one-third of patients with urticarial vasculitis have decreased complement levels, an occasionally useful adjunctive diagnostic test
- Lupus erythematosus is a common cause and urticarial vasculitis may be the presenting sign of the disease
- Sjögren's syndrome and other autoimmune diseases are other causes
- Some cases are idiopathic
- Systemic findings are common, especially when there is hypocomplementemia and include fever, arthralgias, abdominal pain and lymphadenopathy, and may suggest a higher likelihood of an associated autoimmune disease.

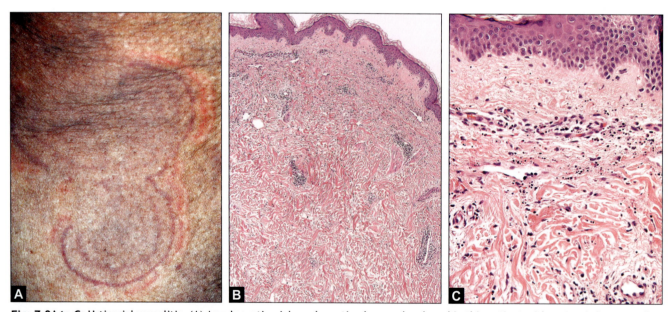

Figs 7.8A to C: Urticarial vasculitis. (A) Annular urticarial, ecchymotic plaques developed in this patient with systemic lupus erythematosus; (B) Features are often indistinguishable from leukocytoclastic vasulitis however, as pictured here, there may also be dilated venules and an interstitial inflammatory infiltrate that includes eosinophils, neutrophils and mast cells, as is seen in urticarial; (C) Although they may be mild, the perivascular neutrophils, neutrophilic "dust" and extravasated red blood cells indicate that genuine vascular damage has occurred.

Henoch-Schonlein Purpura (HSP) (Fig. 7.9)

▮ Criteria for diagnosis

- A history of one or more of the following:
  - Abdominal symptoms (e.g. colicky pain or hematochezia)
  - Hematuria or other evidence of glomerulonephritis
  - Arthritis
  - A history of recent upper respiratory infection
  - Leukocytoclastic vasculitis (usually presenting clinically as palpable purpura)
  - Perivascular deposits of IgA.

▮ Differential diagnosis

- The constellation of clinical findings with LCV and perivascular IgA deposition is virtually specific for HSP, although IgA deposition is sometimes found in LCV without the clinical features of HSP.

▮ Pitfalls

- Biopsies of lesions present for more than 48 hours often do not show the characteristic IgA deposition.

▮ Pearls

- Henoch-Schonlein purpura is by far the most common cause of vasculitis in children and young adults
- Overall it accounts for approximately 10% of all LCV.

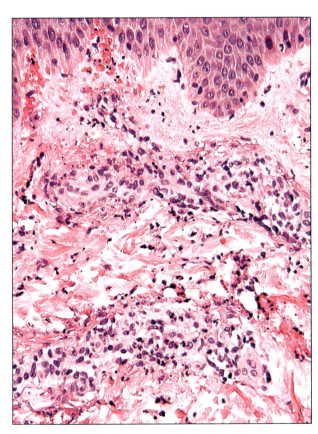

Fig. 7.9: Henoch-Schonlein purpura—the histopathologic features are identical to those of other causes of leukocytoclastic vasculitis.

Mixed Cryoglobulinemia (Types II and III)

■ *Criteria for diagnosis*

- Clinical features are commonly associated with mixed cryoglobulinemia, including purpura induced by cold exposure, arthralgias and weakness or presence of cryoglobulins demonstrated by laboratory methods
- An LCV is sometimes with hyalinized intraluminal thrombi.

■ *Differential diagnosis*

- Other types of LCV.

■ *Pitfalls*

- Without clinical history or laboratory confirmation, histopathologic findings are not specific enough to allow definitive diagnosis.

■ *Pearls*

- Hepatitis C virus infection is a common association
- Direct immunofluorescence may demonstrate perivascular IgM and/or complement deposition
- Evidence of systemic disease may be reported, including glomerulonephritis, neuropathy or pulmonary symptoms including hemoptysis and dyspnea
- Elevated rheumatoid factor and decreased C4 levels may be demonstrable
- Medium sized muscular vessels may be involved imparting a PAN appearance.

Septic Vasculitis (Figs 7.10A and B)

■ *Criteria for diagnosis*

- Clinical evidence of septicemia or virtually any other infection
- LCV that is sometimes florid but in some cases more subtle than other causes, with only minimal fibrin deposition and a scant inflammatory infiltrate.

■ *Differential diagnosis*

- Other causes of LCV.

■ *Pitfalls*

- Organisms are rarely identified, even with histochemical stains except in acute meningococcemia
- Patients with known infections are often receiving various drugs that have also been associated with LCV (e.g. sulfonamides and penicillin).

■ *Pearls*

- Approximately, 20% of LCV is associated with an underlying infection (including viruses)
- When vesicopustules are present, they may have a subtle gray "roof" indicative of necrosis.

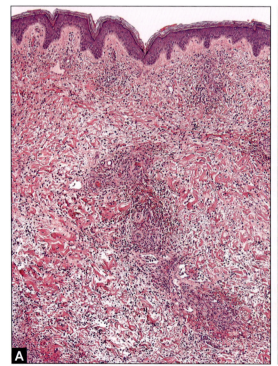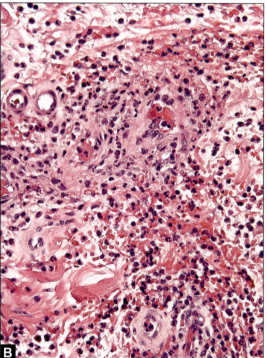

Figs 7.10A and B: Septic vasculitis. (A) There is marked inflammation around vessels in a pattern essentially identical to that of other causes of vasculitis; (B) Intraluminal thrombi are present, but organisms are not detectable—even with the aid of Gram staining, bacteria are rarely identifiable in bacterial sepsis (except in meningococcemia).

Microscopic Polyangiitis

▪ *Criteria for diagnosis*

- Systemic vasculitis with renal involvement (necrotizing glomerulonephritis with crescents) and often the lungs and skin
- Perinuclear anti neutrophil cytoplasmic antibodies (p-ANCA) or cytoplasmic anti neutrophil cytoplasmic antibodies (c-ANCA) (Fig. 7.11)
- Leukocytoclastic vasculitis.

▪ *Differential diagnosis*

- Other causes of LCV

- Polyarteritis nodosa
- Wegener's granulomatosis
- Churg-Strauss syndrome.

▪ *Pitfalls*

- Histopathologic features are sometimes indistinguishable from PAN.

▪ *Pearls*

- Most cases are associated with ANCAs unlike PAN, in which ANCAs are absent.

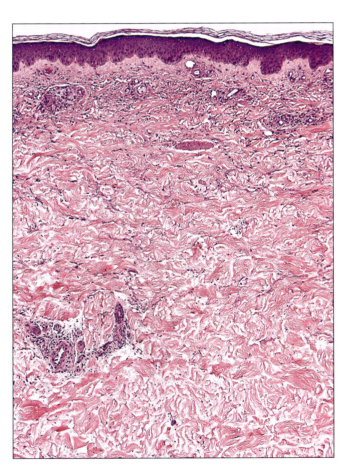

Fig. 7.11: Microscopic polyangiitis. Features are identical to most other causes of leukocytoclastic vasculitis, but this patient was positive for perinuclear anti neutrophil cytoplasmic antibodies and had lung and renal vasculitis.

Polyarteritis Nodosa

Classic PAN has numerous systemic symptoms; a "cutaneous type" has been proposed in which the features are mostly limited to the skin but remains controversial. In both the types, the histopathologic features are identical. The differential includes other causes of vasculitis. However, subcutaneous veins in the lower legs often have thick muscular layers with numerous intimal elastic fibers resembling the internal elastic lamina of an artery. Histopathologically, therefore, some cases can simulate thrombophlebitis, especially when there is extensive destruction of the vessel (Chen) (Figs 7.12A to D).

■ Criteria for diagnosis

- *Early lesions*: Leukocytoclastic vasculitis of small and medium-sized vessels
- *Late lesions*: Vessels with fibrointimal hyperplasia, thrombi, lymphohistiocytic inflammation and fibrosis
- Classic type
  - Constitutional symptoms (fever, malaise, weight loss, myalgias and arthralgias)
  - Hematuria, proteinuria, hypertension and azotemia
  - Myocardial infarcts and strokes
  - Subcutaneous nodules that may ulcerate
  - Ecchymoses and gangrenous necrosis of digits
  - Livedo reticularis, urticaria.
- "Cutaneous" type
  - Cutaneous lesions similar to those of classic type
  - Occasional involvement of muscle, peripheral nerve and joints but no systemic involvement
  - indolent but protracted course.

■ Differential diagnosis

- Wegener's granulomatosis
- Churg-Strauss syndrome
- Microscopic polyangiitis
- Thrombophlebitis

■ Pitfalls

- The characteristic medium-sized vessel vasculitis is often focal, localized to the subcutis and easily missed in small or superficial biopsies
- In some cases the vessel is almost completely destroyed or is obscure by dense inflammation; in this situation, reliable distinction from thrombophlebitis cannot be made histopathologically, since it is difficult to discern whether the vessel was an artery or a vein (veins within the subcutis may have muscular walls) (Figs 7.12C and D).

■ Pearls

- Small-vessel LCV may be present in the superficial dermis while necrotizing vasculitis may involve deeper vessels
- Clinically, thrombophlebitis usually presents as a solitary lesion, while there are multiple nodules in PAN.

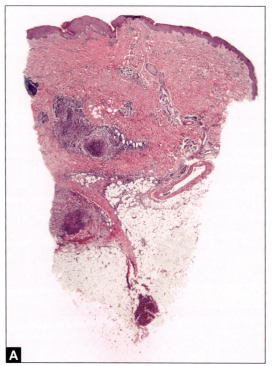 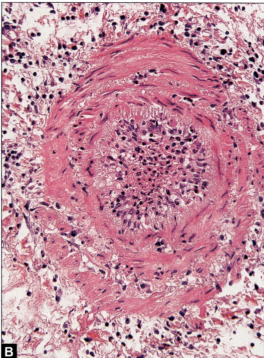

Figs 7.12A and B

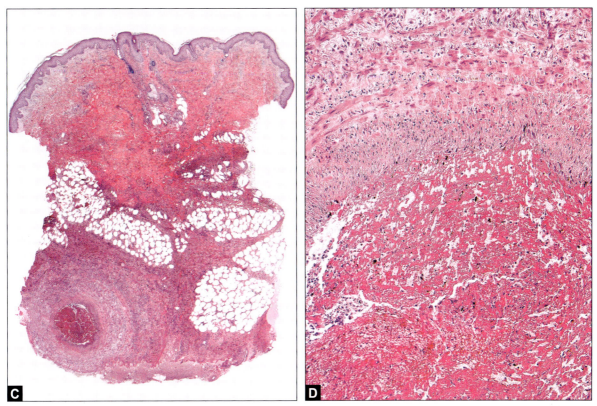

Figs 7.12A to D: Polyarteritis nodosa. (A) Medium caliber vessels within the subcutis are infiltrated by inflammatory cells, especially neutrophils, and are damaged or even entirely destroyed; (B) Neutrophils are present within and around the muscular vessel wall; (C) Thrombophlebitis. The low-power appearance is similar to that of polyarteritis nodosa; (D) Note that this vein has a muscular wall similar to that of a medium caliber artery.

THE FIBROSING VASCULITIS PATTERN

Erythema Elevatum Diutinum (Figs 7.13A to C)

■ *Criteria for diagnosis*

- Round or oval papules, nodules or plaques distributed symmetrically over joints, especially the dorsum of the hands, knees or elbows
- *Early lesions*: Red or violaceous papules and nodules that show LCV histopathologically
- *Fully evolved lesions*: Brown nodules or papules composed of a nodular and diffuse (but often sparse) infiltrate of neutrophils, lymphocytes, plasma cells and macrophages within a background of "wiry" collagen fibrosis
- Sparing of the papillary dermis ("Grenz zone") and periadnexal dermis.

■ *Differential diagnosis*

- *Early lesions*: Leukocytoclastic vasculitis
- *Established lesions*: Interstitial granulomatous dermatitis, localized chronic fibrosing vasculitis.

■ *Pitfalls*

- The findings, both clinically and histopathologically vary markedly with the course/duration of the lesions

- Lesions may be confused clinically with Sweet's syndrome, granuloma annulare or xanthomas.

■ *Pearls*

- Although early lesions are indistinguishable from LCV, none of the other causes of LCV progress to diffuse fibrosing dermatitis
- The sparing of the papillary dermis (Grenz zone) is a helpful clue, especially in evolving or established lesions
- The lesions are often histopathologically identical to granuloma faciale; only the anatomic site and distribution varies in most cases
- A significant number of patients have an underlying systemic disease, including infections, autoimmune disease or hematologic abnormalities
- An IgA gammopathy, either polyclonal or monoclonal, is often detected.

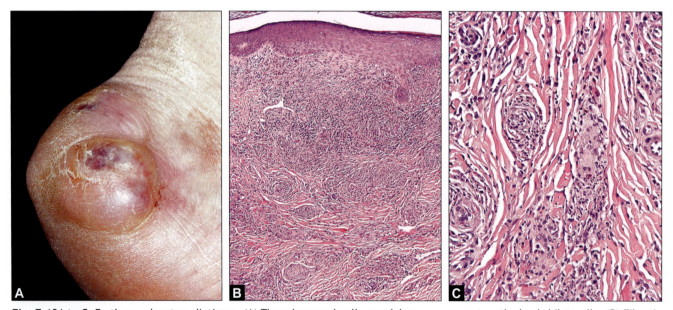

Figs 7.13A to C: Erythema elevatum diutinum. (A) These large red-yellow nodules were present on the heels bilaterally; (B) Fibrotic collagen bundles surround small blood vessels throughout the entire thickness of the dermis; (C) There is vasculitis that is predominantly neutrophilic, but scattered eosinophils are also evident.

Granuloma Faciale (Figs 7.14A and B)

■ *Criteria for diagnosis*

- Papules, plaques or nodules, often with dilated follicular ostia, localized to the face
- Histopathologic features (course, inflammatory infiltrate and fibrosis with spared papillary dermis) virtually identical to erythema elevatum diutinum, with the exception of dilated follicular ostia and a tendency for more eosinophils in granuloma faciale.

■ *Differential diagnosis*

- Leukocytoclastic vasculitis (early lesions)
- Erythema elevatum diutinum (differs by anatomic site).

■ *Pitfalls*

- Early lesions are indistinguishable from LCV (but LCV seldom if ever involves the face).

■ *Pearls*

- Granuloma faciale is histopathologically indistinguishable from erythema elevatum diutinum except that dilated follicular ostia are present (probably because the face contains numerous vellus follicles)
- Eosinophils are more likely to predominate in granuloma faciale.

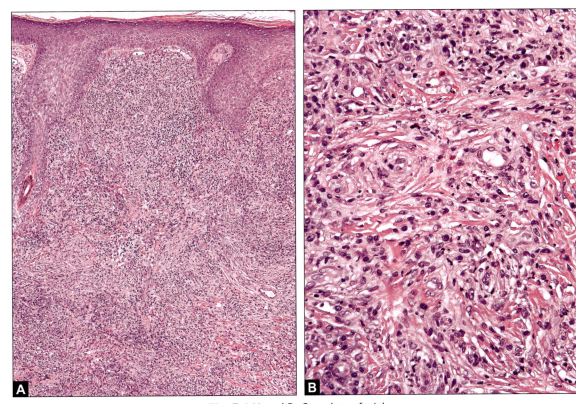

Figs 7.14A and B: Granuloma faciale

Localized Chronic Fibrosing Vasculitis
(Figs 7.15A and B)

■ *Criteria for diagnosis*

- Red-brown nodules resembling those of erythema elevatum diutinum, but usually solitary
- Histopathologic features virtually identical to those of erythema elevatum diutinum.

■ *Differential diagnosis*

- Erythema elevatum diutinum
- Chronic localized infections
- So called inflammatory pseudotumors.

■ *Pitfalls*

- Clinical description of the anatomic site and number and distribution of the lesion(s) is usually the only means of differentiation from erythema elevatum diutinum.

■ *Pearls*

- Similar to erythema elevatum diutinum, an underlying systemic illness may be present and there may be an associated IgA gammopathy.

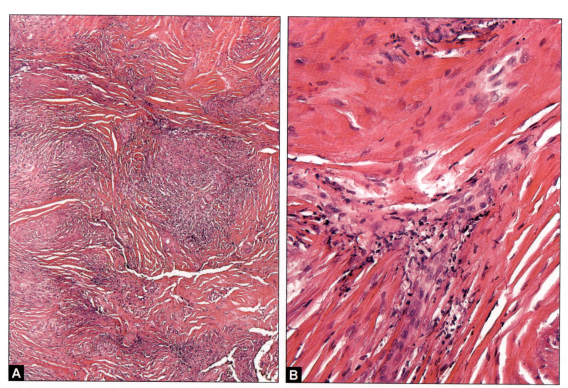

Figs 7.15A and B: Localized chronic fibrosing vasculitis. (A) Features are identical to those of erythema elevatum diutinum, with thick collagen bundles that often assume a lamellar pattern; (B) Throughout the dense collagen are collections of neutrophils emanating from small blood vessels. The distribution of the lesions and other clinical data are critical to making a specific diagnosis.

VASCULITIS WITH MACROPHAGES/GRANULOMAS

Wegener's Granulomatosis

■ *Criteria for diagnosis*

- Clinical evidence of necrotizing granulomatous vasculitis that produces infiltrates or cavitary lesions in the respiratory tract and glomerulonephritis of the kidneys (Fig. 7.16)
- Cytoplasmic anti neutrophil cytoplasmic antibodies positivity (present in approximately 80%)
- Cutaneous lesions (estimated to occur in 5–50% of patients) may be:
  - Purpuric with leukocytoclastic (small vessel) vasculitis
  - Subcutaneous nodules, ulcers or infarcts with medium sized vessel vasculitis
  - Necrotic plaques or ulcers over extensor surfaces (sometimes resembling pyoderma gangrenosum).

■ *Differential diagnosis*

- Other causes of LCV or medium sized vessel vasculitis
- Erythema elevatum diutinum
- Churg-Strauss disease.

■ *Pitfalls*

- In addition to LCV, cutaneous manifestations of Wegener's granulomatosis may include acneiform perifollicular and dermal granulomatous inflammation and palisaded neutrophilic and granulomatous inflammation (Comfere et al.)
- While necrotizing granulomatous inflammation is often cited as the characteristic finding in Wegener's granulomatosis; it is rare within cutaneous lesions and is usually found only in biopsies that include medium sized vessels
- Cutaneous lesions are occasionally the presenting feature
- Cytoplasmic anti neutrophil cytoplasmic antibodies may not be detectable until several weeks or even months into the course of the disease.

■ *Pearls*

- Predilection for middle-aged Caucasian males
- Leukocytoclastic vasculitis indistinguishable from other causes is the most common cutaneous finding; granulomatous vasculitis is much less common but is occasionally encountered
- Some have proposed the term "Wegener's syndrome" to emphasize that granulomas are not always identified and should not be required for diagnosis
- The granulomas are centered on vessels in Wegener's syndrome; in Churg-Strauss syndrome, the granulomas usually have a palisading appearance and surround granular debris rather than vessels.

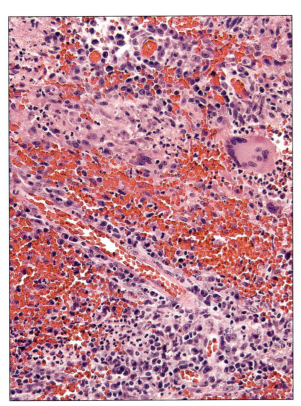

Fig. 7.16: Wegener's granulomatosis. Leukocytoclastic vasculitis is the most common cutaneous finding, but necrotizing granulomatous vasculitis, as shown here, is occasionally encountered.

Churg-Strauss Syndrome (Figs 7.17A and B)

■ *Criteria for diagnosis**

- Systemic
  - Asthma
  - Allergic rhinitis
  - Peripheral blood eosinophilia
  - Eosinophilic inflammation of viscera (e.g. eosinophilic pneumonia)
  - Systemic vasculitis
- Cutaneous (one or more of the following)
  - Palpable purpura
  - Livedo reticularis
  - Urticarial papules
  - Petechial hemorrhage, ecchymoses and hemorrhagic blisters
  - Subcutaneous nodules
- Histopathologic
  - Vasculitis resembling LCV but with numerous eosinophils
  - Diffuse dermal eosinophilia
  - Medium sized vessel vasculitis with eosinophilis
  - Palisading granulomas surrounding degenerating eosinophilic collagen bundles and degenerating degranulating eosinophils.

■ *Differential diagnosis*

- Other causes of LCV or medium sized vessel vasculitis, especially drug-related
- Other causes of dermal eosinophilic infiltrates (e.g. arthropod bite reaction, drug reactions)
- Other causes of palisading granulomatous dermatitis, especially rheumatoid nodule.

■ *Pitfalls*

- Cutaneous findings are not specific and without strong confirmatory clinical information, a specific diagnosis can rarely be made
- The palisading eosinophilic granulomas once thought to be specific for Churg-Strauss have since been demonstrated in numerous other conditions
- Lymphomas, particularly lymphomatoid granulomatosis and natural killer/T-cell lymphomas may also produce vasculocentric granulomas and necrosis (see Chapter 15).

■ *Pearls*

- Perinuclear anti neutrophil cytoplasmic antibodies positivity in approximately 70%; c-ANCA in about 7%
- The features must be assessed in constellation, since they vary greatly from case to case and over the course of the disease.

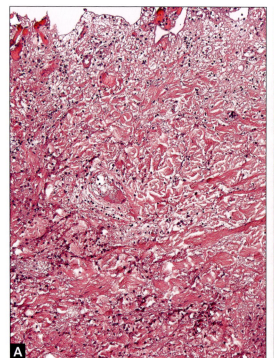 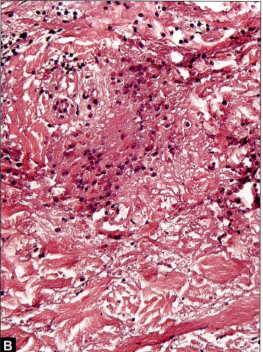

Figs 7.17A and B: Churg-Strauss syndrome. (A) When skin is involved the features may be indistinguishable from leukocytoclastic vasculitis, but there may be also be numerous eosinophils, as in the case shown here; (B) Occasionally, eosinophils and histiocytes may form vague palisades around aggregates of granular debris.

BIBLIOGRAPHY

1. Carlson JA. The histological assessment of cutaneous vasculitis. Histopathology. 2010;56(1):3-23.
2. Chen KR, Carlson JA. Clinical approach to cutaneous vasculitis. Am J Clin Dermatol. 2008;9(2):71-92.
3. Chen KR. The misdiagnosis of superficial thrombophlebitis as cutaneous polyarteritis nodosa: features of the internal elastic lamina and the compact concentric muscular layer as diagnostic pitfalls. Am J Dermatopathol. 2010;32(7):688-93.
4. Comfere NI, Macaron NC, Gibson LE. Cutaneous manifestations of Wegener's granulomatosis: a clinicopathologic study of 17 patients and correlation to antineutrophil cytoplasmic antibody status. J Cutan Pathol. 2007;34(10): 739-47.
5. Crowson AN, Mihm MC, Magro CM. Cutaneous vasculitis: A Review. J Cutan Pathol. 2003;30(3):161-73.
6. Russell JP, Gibson LE. Primary cutaneous small vessel vasculitis: approach to diagnosis and treatment. Int J Dermatol. 2006;45(1):3-13.
7. Smith JG Jr. Vasculitis. J Dermatol. 1995;22(11):812-22.
8. Wahl CE, Bouldin MB, Gibson LE. Erythema elevatum diutinum: clinical, histopathologic, and immunohistochemical characteristics of six patients. Am J Dermatopathol. 2005;27 (5):397-400.
9. Ziemer M, Koehler MJ, Weyers W. Erythema elevatum diutinum-a chronic leukocytoclastic vasculitis microscopically indistinguishable from granuloma faciale? J Cutan Pathol. 2011;38(11):876-83.

---

*The "criteria" are controversial and difficult to demonstrate clinically and histopathologically.

CHAPTER 8

Panniculitis

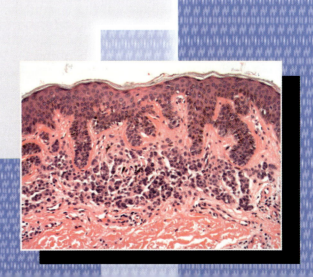

INTRODUCTION

Panniculitis can be subdivided into primarily lobular and primarily septal panniculitis. A primarily septal panniculitis is usually erythema nodosum. The septae can be involved in vasculitis and other dermal inflammatory processes can extend into the septae, such as morphea/scleroderma and necrobiosis lipoidica, but the primary septal panniculitis remains erythema nodosum. The differential diagnosis for lobular panniculitis is somewhat more extensive and can primarily be distinguished by examining the predominant cell type.

SEPTAL PANNICULITIS

Erythema Nodosum (Figs 8.1A to E)

■ *Clinical diagnosis*
- Subcutaneous red to violaceous nodules overlying shins.

■ *Criteria for diagnosis*
- Early lesion (Fig. 8.1A)
  - Hemorrhage
  - Edema within septae
  - Neutrophils within septae
- Established lesion (Figs 8.1B and C)
  - Fibrotic septae
  - Granulomatous inflammation
  - Miescher's radial granuloma (histiocytes and giant cells surrounding a cleft) (Fig. 8.1D).

■ *Differential diagnosis*
- Lipodermatosclerosis
- Vasculitis
- Factitial
- Erythema induratum
- Scleroderma.

■ *Pitfalls*
- The granulomatous inflammation in necrobiosis lipoidica can spill over into the septae.

■ *Pearls*
- Erythema nodosum never ulcerates
- Panniculitis below the knees is erythema nodosum until proven otherwise
- Erythema nodosum can be chronic (erythema nodosum migrans, subacute migratory panniculitis of Vilanoma).

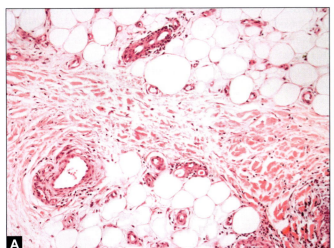
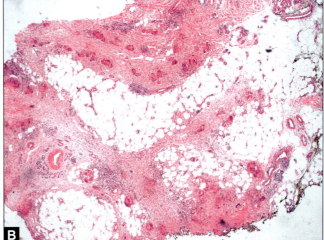

Figs 8.1A and B

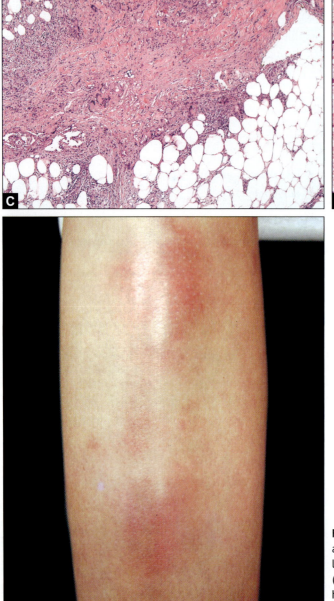

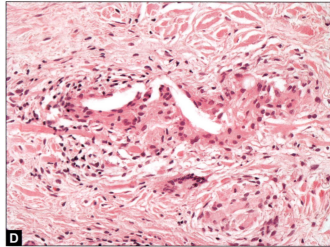

Figs 8.1A to E: Erythema Nodosum. (A) Early lesion: edema and mixed inflammatory infiltrate in septae and surrounding fat lobule; (B) Old lesion: fibrosis with giant cells in septae; (C) Fibrosis and giant cells in septae; (D) Miescher's granuloma: histiocytes surrounding cleft; (E) Clinical picture.
Courtesy: Dr Christie Regula.

Differential Diagnosis of Lobular Lymphocytic Panniculitis

- Subcutaneous T-cell lymphoma
- Lupus/connective tissue panniculitis
- Cold panniculitis.

Subcutaneous T-Cell Lymphoma (Figs 8.2A to C)

■ *Criteria for diagnosis*

- Atypical lymphocytes.

■ *Pearls*

- Two forms of subcutaneous T-cell lymphoma:
  - *Alpha beta type:* protracted course
  - *Gamma/delta T-cell phenotype:* rapidly fatal.

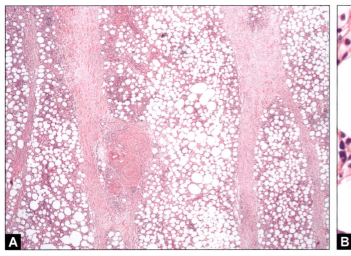

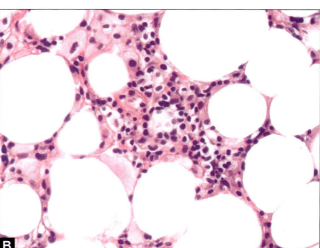

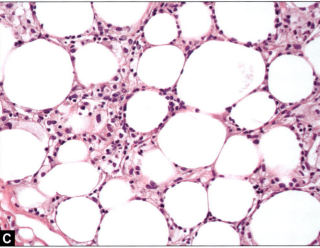

Figs 8.2A to C: Subcutaneous T-cell lymphoma. (A) Lobular lymphocytic panniculitis; (B) Atypical lymphocytes; (C) Atypical lymphocytes producing rim/circle around adipocyte.

Lupus Panniculitis (Figs 8.3A to D)

Criteria for diagnosis

- Lobular lymphocytic panniculitis with no atypical lymphocytes (Fig. 8.3A)
- Also look for:
  - Hyaline fat necrosis (Figs 8.3B and C)
  - Occasional calcification
  - Lymphocytic dust.

Pitfalls

- Missing the diagnosis of subcutaneous T-cell lymphoma (see prior).

Pearls

- The epidermal and dermal findings of lupus erythematosus are only present in approximately half of the cases.

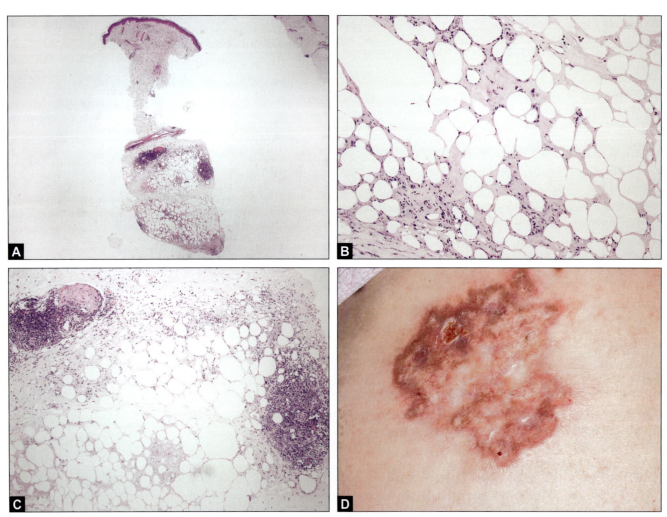

Figs 8.3A to D: Lupus panniculitis. (A) Lobular lymphocytic panniculitis with lymphoid aggregates; (B) Hyalin fat necrosis; (C) Hyalin fat necrosis with lymphoid aggregates; (D) Clinical picture.

Differential Diagnosis of Neutrophilic Panniculitis

- Pancreatic fat necrosis
- Infectious panniculitis
- Alpha one antitrypsin deficiency
- Subcutaneous Sweet's syndrome
- Pyoderma gangrenosum.

Pancreatic Panniculitis

▮ *Criteria for diagnosis*

- Neutrophilic panniculitis (Fig. 8.4A)
- Fat necrosis
- Ghost cells (Fig. 8.4B)

- Calcification
- Confirm presence of pancreatitis with serum amylase.

Infectious Panniculitis

▮ *Criteria for diagnosis*

- Special stains for infectious organisms—positive.

Alpha One Antitrypsin Deficiency

▮ *Criteria for diagnosis*

- Neutrophilic lobular panniculitis with focal areas of fat involvement
- Confirm with blood study for alpha one antitrypsin level.

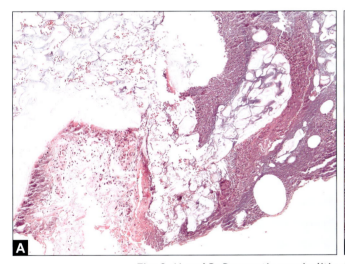 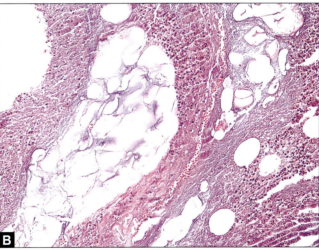

Figs 8.4A and B: Pancreatic panniculitis. (A) Necrosis with neutrophilic infiltrate; (B) Ghost cells, neutrophilic infiltrate and necrosis.

Color Atlas of Differential Diagnosis of Dermatopathology

Differential Diagnosis of Lobular Histiocytic Panniculitis

- Erythema induratum
- Erythema nodosum (spill over from septae)
- Factitial panniculitis
    - Inflammatory infiltrate polymorphous and does not fit any established category
    - Usually asymmetric and involves opposite extremity of patients dominant hand
- Infection
- Sarcoidosis or foreign object.

Infectious Panniculitis

■ *Criteria for diagnosis*

- Special stains or culture demonstrate infectious organisms.

Erythema Induratum/Nodular Vasculitis (Figs 8.5A and B)

■ *Clinical criteria for diagnosis*

- Panniculitis frequently involving the calf with ulceration.

■ *Histological criteria for diagnosis*

- Lobular panniculitis with mixed inflammatory infiltrate—histiocytes usually predominate (Fig. 8.5B).
- Associated with tuberculosis
    - Frequent vasculitis of small or medium sized blood vessels
    - Frequent necrosis
    - Clinically, predilection for calf
    - Lesions ulcerate.

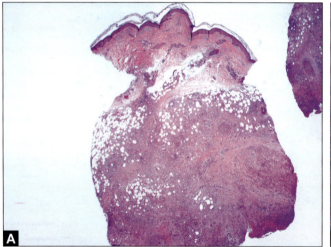
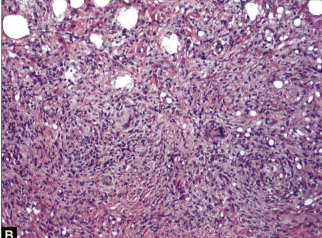

Figs 8.5A and B: Erythema induratum. (A) Lobular lymphohistiocytic panniculitis; (B) Lobular panniculitis with histiocytes and giant cells.

Subcutaneous Fat Necrosis of Newborn (Figs 8.6A to D)

Clinical criteria for diagnosis

- Indurated plaque or plaques in newborn baby
- Frequently located on cheeks, trunk, buttocks and thighs
- History of exposure to cold during delivery or birth.

Histologic criteria for diagnosis

- Lobular panniculitis with histiocytes
- Cleft like spaces in fat (Fig. 8.6C)
- Newborn baby.

Differential diagnosis

- *Sclerema neonatorum:* No inflammation
- *Post steroid panniculitis:* Older child.

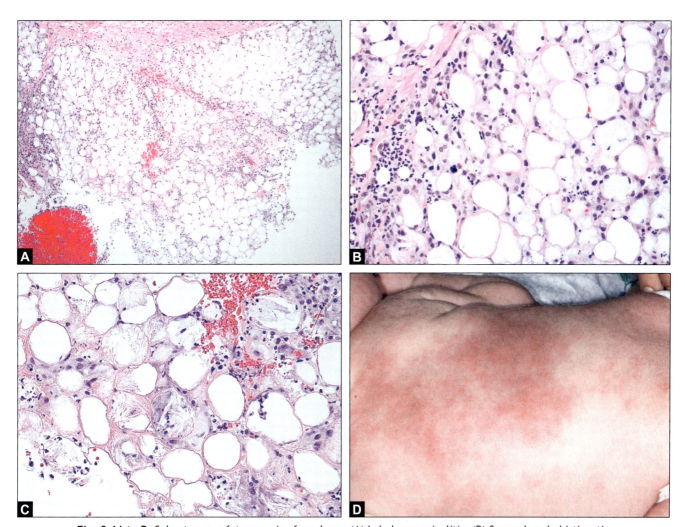

Figs 8.6A to D: Subcutaneous fat necrosis of newborn. (A) Lobular panniculitis; (B) Sparse lymphohistiocytic infiltrate; (C) Needle like clefts within adipocytes; (D) Extensive subcutaneous fat necrosis of newborn.

Calciphylaxis (Figs 8.7A to C)

■ *Criteria for diagnosis*

- Calcified blood vessels within subcutaneous septae (Fig. 8.7B)
- Extravascular calcification
- Majority of cases patients have renal disease
- Increased parathyroid hormone levels
- Ulcer may be present.

■ *Differential diagnosis*

- Arteriosclerosis (Buerger's disease).

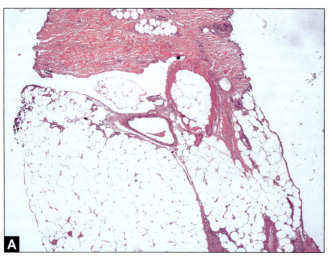

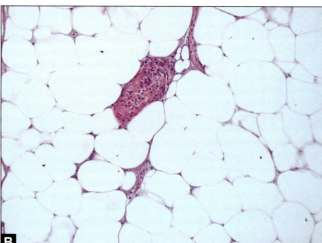

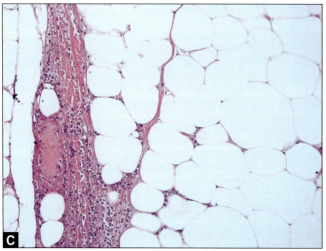

Figs 8.7A to C: Calciphylaxis. (A) Minimal inflammatory infiltrate; (B) Calcified blood vessel; (C) Calcification and sparse inflammatory infiltrate in fat septae.

Lipodermatosclerosis (Figs 8.8A to C)

Criteria for diagnosis

- Adipocytes vary in size and shape
- Few foam cells
- Minimal inflammation
- Cystic areas sometimes present (lined by hyalin like material from necrotic fat-imparting membranous appearance).

Differential diagnosis

- Traumatic fat necrosis.

Pitfalls

- Lipomembranous changes as seen in lipodermatosclerosis can be seen as sequelae of other panniculitides.

Pearls

- Diffuse involvement of lower leg often with fibrotic thickened fat septae in lipodermatosclerosis
- Traumatic fat necrosis usually localized occasionally encapsulated.

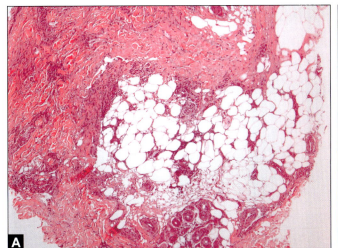

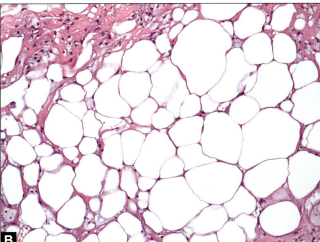

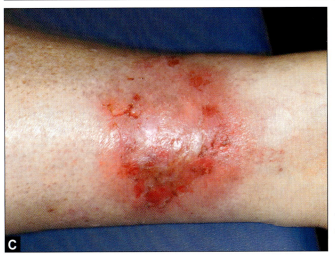

Figs 8.8A to C: Lipodermatosclerosis. (A) Fibrosis, minimal inflammation and fat cells with variation in size; (B) Small cystic areas within fat lobules with variation in size of adipocytes; (C) Clinical picture.

BIBLIOGRAPHY

1. Delgado-Jimenez Y, Fraga J, Garcia-Diez A. Infective panniculitis. Dermatol Clin. 2008;26(4):471-80.
2. Fraga J, Garcia-Diez A. Lupus erythematosus panniculitis. Dermatol Clin. 2008; 26(4):453-63.
3. Garcia-Romero D, Vanaclocha F. Pancreatic panniculitis. Dermatol Clin. 2008; 26(4):465-70.
4. Guhl G, Garcia-Diez A. Subcutaneous sweet syndrome. Dermatol Clin. 2008;26(4):541-51.
5. Kao GF, Resh B, McMahon C, et al. Fatal subcutaneous panniculitis-like T-cell lymphoma gamma/delta subtype (cutaneous gamma/delta T-cell lymphoma): report of a case and review of the literature. Am J Dermatopathol. 2008;30(6): 593-9.
6. Mascaro JM. Jr, Baselga E. Erythema induratum of bazin. Dermatol Clin. 2008;26(4):439-45.
7. Mitra S, Dove J, Somisetty SK. Subcutaneous fat necrosis in newborn-an unusual case and review of literature. Eur J Pediatr. 2011;170(9):1107-10.
8. Morrison LK, Rapini R, Willison CB, et al. Infection and panniculitis. Dermatol Ther. 2010;23(4):328-40.
9. Parveen Z, Thompson K. Subcutaneous panniculitis-like T-cell lymphoma: redefinition of diagnostic criteria in the recent World Health Organization-European Organization for Research and Treatment of Cancer classification for cutaneous lymphomas. Arch Pathol Lab Med. 2009;133(2):303-8.
10. Polcari IC, Stein SL. Panniculitis in childhood. Dermatol Ther. 2010;23(4):356-67.
11. Requena L, Yus ES. Erythema nodosum. Dermatol Clin. 2008;26(4):425-38.
12. Requena L, Yus ES. Panniculitis. Part I. Mostly septal panniculitis. J Am Acad Dermatol. 2001;45(2):163-83.
13. Requena L, Yus ES. Panniculitis. Part II. Mostly lobular panniculitis. J Am Acad Dermatol. 2001;45(3):325-61.
14. Sanmartin O, Requena C, Requena L. Factitial panniculitis. Dermatol Clin. 2008;26(4):519-27.
15. Valverde R, Rosales B, Ortiz-de Frutos FJ, et al. Alpha-1-antitrypsin deficiency panniculitis. Dermatol Clin. 2008;26(4): 447-51.

Color Atlas of Differential Diagnosis of Dermatopathology

CHAPTER 9

Fibrosing Dermatitis

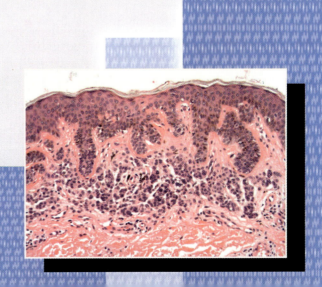

INTRODUCTION

Fibrosing dermatoses often are associated with other histologic reaction patterns. For example, morphea and scleroderma are associated with a superficial and deep lymphoplasmacytic infiltrate. Early lesions of lichen sclerosus demonstrate lichenoid tissue reaction. The presence of collagen changes can be used to narrow down the differential diagnosis considerably. Identifying whether the number of fibroblasts is increased or decreased provides important information, helpful in making a specific diagnosis.

DISEASES WITH DECREASED NUMBER OF FIBROBLASTS

Table 9.1: Differential diagnosis

Diseases with decreased number of fibroblasts-sclerosis:

- Morphea/Scleroderma/Atrophoderma (burn out morphea)
- Lichen sclerosus
- Eosinophilic fasciitis
- Radiation dermatitis
- Scleredema
- Borrelia fibroma
- Acrodermatitis atrophicans.

Diseases with increased number of fibroblasts-fibrosis:

- Scleromyxedema/Lichen myxedematosus
- Nephrogenic systemic fibrosis
- Erythema elevatum diutinum/Localized fibrosing vasculitis
- Scar
- Keloid
- Acne keloidalis (See Chapter 5 on folliculitis)
- Stasis dermatitis
- Lymphedema
- Neoplasms may occasionally mimic inflammatory fibrosis.
  - Dermatofibroma, Desmoplastic melanoma, etc

Morphea/Scleroderma

■ *Criteria for diagnosis*

Clinical criteria
- Indurated skin (Figs 9.1A and B)
  - Distinguishing between morphea and systemic scleroderma is performed on clinical not pathologic grounds
  - Scleroderma involves the fingers whereas fingers are usually spared in morphea
  - Scleroderma is associated with Raynaud's phenomena
  - Morphea not associated with renal or systemic disease.

Histopathological criteria
- Early lesions (Figs 9.1C and D)
  - Inflammatory infiltrate, perivascular and interstitial lymphocytes, plasma cells and eosinophils
- Established lesion (Figs 9.1E and F)
  - Sclerotic collagen bundles
  - Lymphoplasmacytic infiltrate-frequently centered on dermal subcutaneous junction
  - Loss of adipocytes around eccrine glands
- Old lesions (Fig. 9.1G)
  - Minimal to no inflammation
  - Normal appearing skin requiring clinical path correlation.

■ *Differential diagnosis*

See Table 9.1

■ *Pitfalls*

- Erythema migrans can have a superficial and deep lymphoplasmacytic infiltrate but collagen changes should be lacking.

■ *Pearls*

- Decreased CD34 expression can be helpful in diagnosis
- Old lesions of morphea are also called atrophoderma.

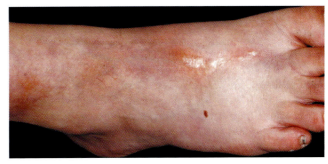

Fig. 9.1A

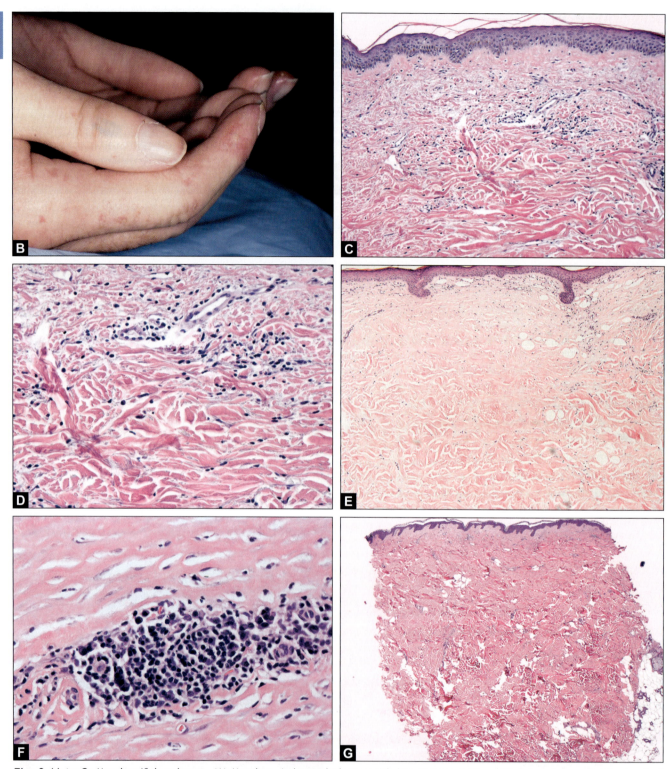

Figs 9.1A to G: Morphea/Scleroderma. (A) Morphea—indurated plaque with hyperpigmentation; (B) Scleroderma—involvement of hands with sausage like fingers and distal infarcts; (C) Unremarkable epidermis: dermis contains perivascular and interstitial inflammatory infiltrate; (D) Close up on perivascular and interstitial infiltrate—(Note presence of mucin as can be seen in collagen vascular diseases); (E) Established lesion with sclerotic collagen budles; (F) Established lesion with lymphoplasmacytic infiltrate along dermal subcutaneous junction; (G) Old lesion—Note rectangular/square shaped biopsy due to increased collagen—otherwise looks like normal skin.

Lichen Sclerosus

■ *Criteria for diagnosis*

Clinical criteria
- Hypopigmented white patches (9.2A and B).

Histological criteria
- Band like lymphocytic infiltrate (Fig. 9.2C)
- Homogenized collagen bundles (Fig. 9.2D).

■ *Differential diagnosis*

See Table 9.1

■ *Pitfalls*

- In early lesions of lichen sclerosus, the inflammatory infiltrate can be lichenoid resembling lichen planus.

- The epidermis can either be acanthotic or atrophic in lichen sclerosus
- The collagen changes in radiation dermatitis can mimic the changes seen in lichen sclerosus.

■ *Pearls*

- Lichen sclerosus, not involving genital skin, may be an early edematous variant of morphea
- A thickened basement membrane zone is a clue to lichen sclerosus.

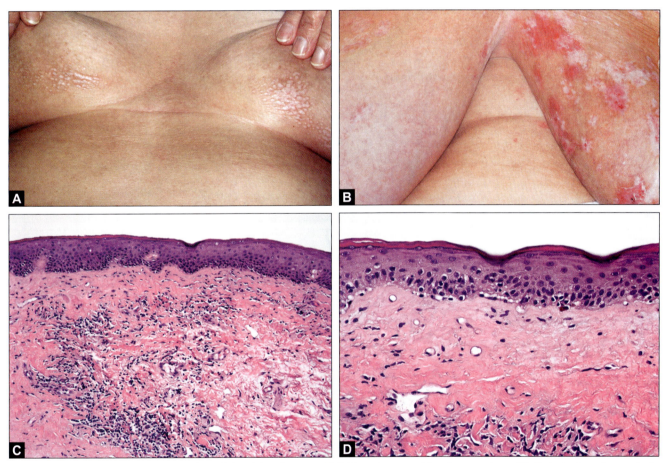

Figs 9.2A to D: Lichen sclerosus. (A) Porcelain white plaques; (B) White plaques with a few erosions; (C) Early lesions demonstrate band like lymphocytic infiltrate; (D) Older lesions developed homogenized collagen bundles that push the band like lymphocytic infiltrate downward.

Chronic Radiation Dermatitis

■ *Criteria for diagnosis*

Clinical criteria (Fig. 9.3A)
- History of radiation exposure.

Histological criteria (Figs 9.3B and C)
- Atrophic epidermis
- Telangiectasias
- Radiation fibroblasts
- Homogenized collagen bundles and elastic tissue.

■ *Differential diagnosis*

Erythema Ab Igne and Table 9.1

■ *Pitfalls*

- Lichen sclerosus (see above).

■ *Pearls*

- Altered elastic fibers deep within the dermis clue to radiation dermatitis (sunlight does not penetrate very deep (Fig. 9.3D)
- Inflammation is lacking (unless acute radiation dermatitis).

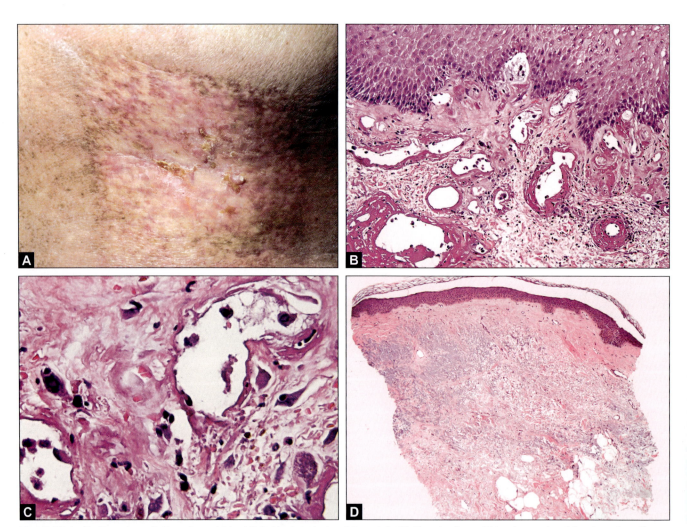

Figs 9.3A to D: Chronic radiation dermatitis. (A) Reticulated atrophic patch (B) Ectatic shaped blood vessels with sclerotic collagen bundles; (C) Higher power demonstrates bizarre shaped "radiation" fibroblasts; (D) Note absence of adnexal structures and elastic fibers deeper in the dermis than would be expected for actinic damage.

Scleromyxedema/Lichen Myxedematosus/Papular Mucinosis

■ *Criteria for diagnosis*

Clinical criteria (Figs 9.4A and B)

- Symmetrical papules predominating on upper extremities and sun exposed skin
- Scleromyxedema also presents with indurated skin.

Histological criteria (Figs 9.4C and D)

- Increased fibroblasts
- Increased collagen
- Mucin deposition
- Band like lymphoplasmacytic infiltrate.

Laboratory

- Paraproteinemia (IgG lambda most common).

■ *Differential diagnosis and potential pitfall*

- Histology of nephrogenic systemic fibrosis can look similar.

■ *Pearls*

- Nephrogenic systemic fibrosis usually does not involve the face.

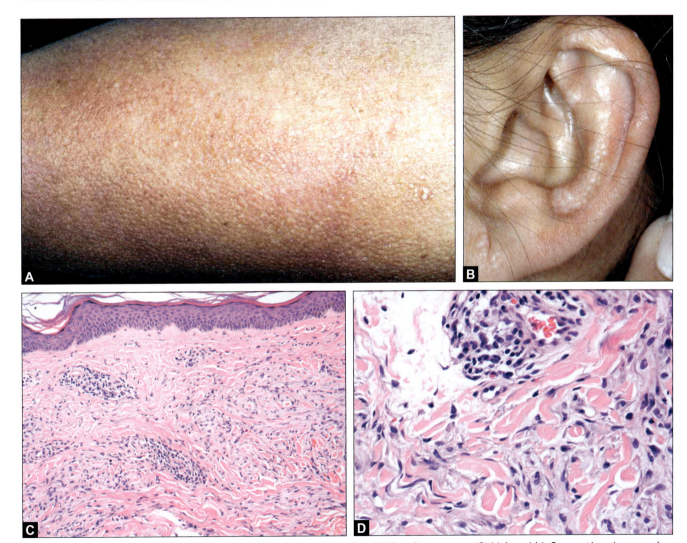

Figs 9.4A to D: Scleromyxedema. (A) Minute papules on extremity; (B) Papules on ears; (C) Lichenoid inflammation, increased number of fibroblasts, and mucin deposition; (D) Increased number of fibroblasts and mucin.

Nephrogenic Systemic Fibrosis

■ *Criteria for diagnosis*

Clinical criteria (Fig. 9.5A)
- Renal insufficiency or failure
- History of scan using gadolinium.

Histological criteria (Figs 9.5B to D)
- Increased number of CD34 staining fibroblasts
- Mucin deposition
- Inflammation is minimal.

■ *Differential diagnosis and pitfall*
- Scleromyxedema (see above)
- Scleroderma-decreased number of fibroblasts.

■ *Pearls*
- Presence of significant inflammation millitates against diagnosis

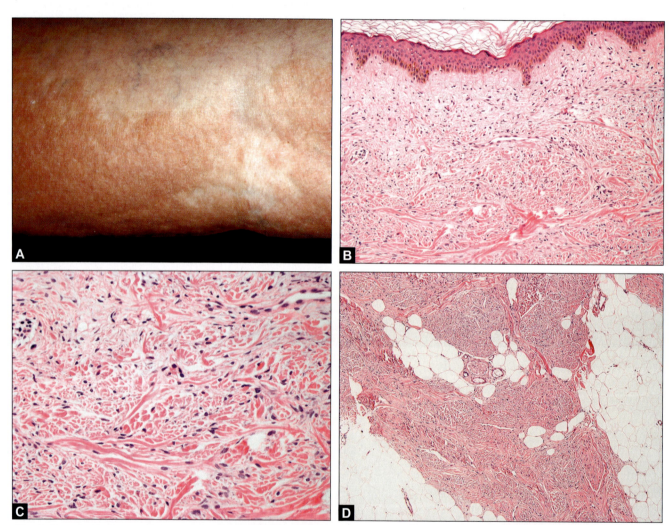

Figs 9.5A to D: Nephrogenic systemic fibrosis. (A) Clinical: Indurated plaques; (B and C) Increased fibroblasts and mucin as in scleromyxedema, but, unlike scleromyxedema, no inflammatory cells; (D) Fibrous tracks extend into subcutaneous tissue.

Erythema Elevatum Diutinum

■ *Criteria for diagnosis*

Clinical criteria

- Symmetrical red to brown colored plaques and nodules
- Extensor surfaces (Fig. 9.6A).

Histological criteria (Figs 9.6B and C)

- Early lesions are identical to leukocytoclastic vasculitis
- Well-developed lesions:
  - Vasculitis no longer present
  - Increased number of fibroblasts and collagen
  - Sprinkling of neutrophils and nuclear dust
- Old lesions:
  - Same as well-developed lesions along with foam cells.

■ *Differential diagnosis*

- Leukocytolastic vasculitis
- Localized Fibrosing vasculitis
- Granuloma Faciale

■ *Pitfalls*

- Old lesions can resemble dermatofibromas (fibrous histiocytoma).

■ *Pearls*

- The histological features of localized fibrosing vasculitis and granuloma faciale can be identical.

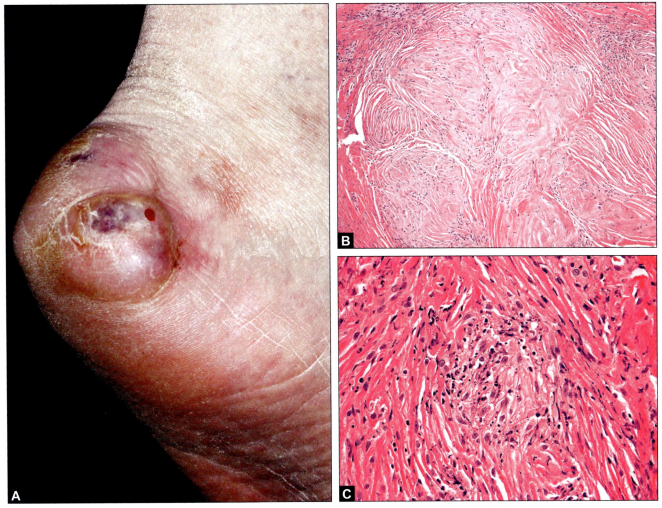

Figs 9.6A to C: Erythema elevatum diutinum. (A) Crusted nodule on heel; (B) Dermal fibrosis with characteristic clefting between collagen bundles; (C) Neutrophils and nuclear dust between collagen bundles is clue to diagnosis.

Stasis Dermatitis

■ *Criteria for diagnosis*

Clinical criteria (Fig. 9.7A)

- Dermatitis in lower extremities
- Frequently associated with edema and varicose veins
- Petechiae and purpura may be present
- May ulcerate.

Histological criteria (Figs 9.7B and C)

- Spongiosis and parakeratosis
- Lobular proliferation of blood vessels within the dermis
- Increased number of fibroblasts
- Extravasated erythrocytes
- Hemosiderin deposition.

■ *Differential diagnosis and pitfall*

Mucin can be found in stasis dermatitis (Fig. 9.7D) resembling pretibial myxedema but in pretibial myxedema the mucin does not extend into the papillary dermis.

■ *Pearls*

Stasis dermatitis is frequently clinically misdiagnosed as cellulitis.

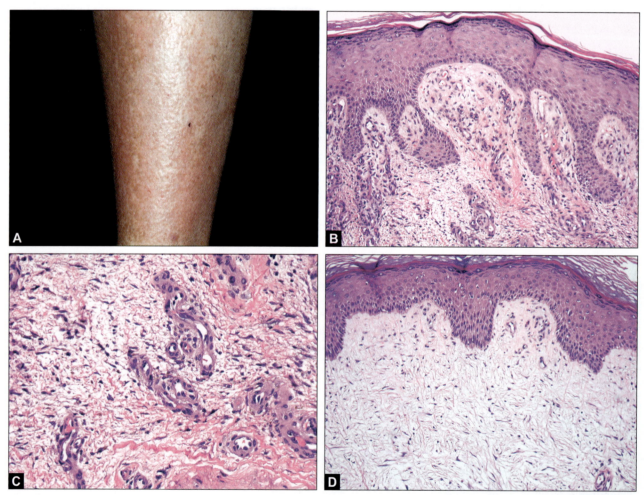

Figs 9.7A to D: Stasis dermatitis. (A) Eczematous plaque on lower extremity with hemosiderin deposition; (B) Lobular proliferation of blood vessels associated with increased number of fibroblasts and epidermal acanthosis; (C) High power demonstrates blood vessels with prominent endothelial cells, increased number of fibroblasts and hemosiderin; (D) Dermal edema and mucin present simulating pretibial myxedema.

BIBLIOGRAPHY

1. Aberer E, Klade H, Hobisch G. A clinical, histological, and immunohistochemical comparison of acrodermatitis chronica atrophicans and morphea. Am J Dermatopathol. 1990;13(4):334-41.

2. Helm KF, Gibson LE, Muller SA. Lichen sclerosus et atrophicus in children and young adults. Pediatr Dermatol. 1991;8(2): 97-101.

3. Marshall K, Klepeiss SA, Ioffreda MD, et al. Scleromyxedema presenting with neurologic symptoms: a case report and review of the literature. Cutis. 2010;85(3):137-40.

4. Miteva M, Romanelli P, Kirsner RS. Lipodermatosclerosis. Dermatol Ther. 2010;23(4):375-88.

5. Skobieranda K, Helm KF. Decreased expression of the human progenitor cell antigen (CD34) in morphea. Am J Dermatopathol. 1995;17(5):471-5.

6. Somach SC, Helm TN, Lawlor KB, et al. Pretibial mucin. Histologic patterns and clinical correlation. Arch Dermatol. 1993;129(9):1152-6.

7. Wahl CE, Bouldin MB, Gibson LE. Erythema elevatum diutinum: clinical, histopathologic, and immunohistochemical characteristics of six patients. Am J Dermatopathol. 2005;27(5):397-400.

8. Wilford C, Fine JD, Boyd AS, et al. Nephrogenic systemic fibrosis: report of an additional case with granulomatous inflammation. Am J Dermatopathol. 2010;32(1):71-5.

9. Young EM, Barr RJ. Sclerosing dermatoses. J Cutan Pathol. 1985;12(5):426-41.

CHAPTER 10

The Depositional Pattern

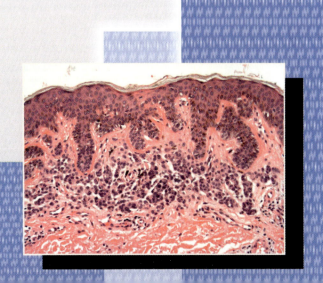

INTRODUCTION

The common denominator of the heterogeneous group of conditions that produce the depositional pattern is the accumulation of abnormal biologic materials, metabolic by-products or a cutaneous material that is normal in its composition, but abnormal in distribution or amount. Some, such as gout and calcinosis, are readily recognizable and the differential diagnosis is limited. More difficult are deposits of amorphous eosinophilic material (hyaline deposits) and acid glycosaminoglycans (mucin). Approach cutaneous depositions by assigning them first to one of these categories, as discussed below, and then narrowing the differential diagnosis by considering the clinical features. Depending on the presentation, further evaluation may be required by histochemical techniques (e.g. a Congo red stain for amyloid or an Alcian blue stain to detect subtle accumulation of glycosaminoglycans).

DEPOSITS OF AMORPHOUS EOSINOPHILIC MATERIAL ("HYALINE" DEPOSITION)

AMYLOIDOSES

Systemic Amyloidoses

Systemic Light Chain Amyloidosis (Primary Systemic Amyloidosis, Myeloma-Associated Systemic Amyloidosis)

Criteria for diagnosis

- Clinical presentation as "waxy" papules and plaques, often with petechiae, purpura or ecchymosis
- Macroglossia and hardening of oral mucosa
- Clinical history of myeloma or plasma cell dyscrasia (or exclusion of other possible causes of amyloidosis) (Fig. 10.1A)
- Deposition of amorphous, homogeneous, pale eosinophilic material
- Localization around blood vessels, adnexa and fat cells in early lesions
- Diffuse, cracked or fissured deposits involving entire dermis in later lesions
- Bright pale green birefringence when Congo red stained sections are viewed with polarized light.

Differential diagnosis

- Other amyloidosis (either systemic or skin-limited)
- Colloid milium
- Lipoid proteinosis.

Pitfalls

- Periorbital area is the most common location of deposits
- The plasma cell dyscrasia or other myeloma may be occult or subclinical
- Light microscopic features are not specific.

Pearls

- Deposits are abnormal aggregates of monoclonal immunoglobulin light chain (more commonly lambda than kappa type)
- Kidneys, liver and heart are commonly involved

- Skin lesions occur in up to 30–40% of cases
- May occur in patients with known myeloma, but may also be the presenting feature of an occult plasma cell dyscrasia.

Systemic Amyloid A Amyloidosis (Secondary Systemic Amyloidosis)

Criteria for diagnosis

- Visible cutaneous lesions are rarely seen, if ever seen, fat biopsy is performed to confirm clinical suspicion of systemic amyloidosis
- Deep biopsy of abdominal fat containing amyloid deposition around adipocytes of subcutis (amyloid rings) and/or eccrine coils
- Congo red stain positive
- Loss of Congo red reactivity after treatment of tissue with potassium permanganate (unlike amyloid L (AL), which is unaffected by potassium permanganate).

Differential diagnosis

- Systemic light chain amyloidosis.

Pitfalls

- Identification of amyloid is highly dependent on sampling, which is often performed using needle "cores"
- Less than 70% of samples are diagnostic.

Pearls

- An underlying chronic disease is almost always present
- Commonly associated chronic inflammatory diseases include autoimmune diseases, such as rheumatoid arthritis, psoriasis, etc
- Chronic infectious diseases include leprosy, bacterial endocarditis, etc
- Kidney, liver and spleen are affected far more severely than skin, but are less amenable to biopsy (hence the abdominal fat approach)
- Rectal biopsies may be attempted; these reveal submucosal perivascular amyloid.

Hemodialysis-Associated Amyloidosis (Systemic Beta-2 Microglobulin Amyloidosis)

■ Criteria for diagnosis

- Small, shiny lichenoid papules on the trunk and arms in patients on long-term hemodialysis
- Amorphous eosinophilic amyloid deposits, similar to AL chain amyloid in distribution and course.

■ Differential diagnosis

- Other types of systemic and skin-limited amyloidosis
- Injection site related-amyloidosis.

■ Pitfalls

- Differentiation from other types of amyloid may be difficult without clinical history of dialysis.

■ Pearls

- Cutaneous lesions are rare and have been reported as subcutaneous masses on the buttocks, multiple lichenoid papules and "wrinkled" appearing skin on the hands and fingers
- Clinical history is obviously crucial.

Cutaneous Amyloidoses

Macular Amyloidosis

■ Criteria for diagnosis

- Irregularly pigmented macules (sometimes with a "rippled" pattern)
- Small globules of amorphous pale or dull pink material within widened dermal papillae
- Melanophages within the papillary dermis.

■ Differential diagnosis

- Other types of systemic and skin-limited amyloidosis
- Postinflammatory hypermelanosis
- Juvenile and adult type colloid milium
- The "normal skin" differential.

■ Pitfalls

- Amyloid deposition may be subtle, especially in early lesions of macular amyloidosis (Fig. 10.1B)
- Postinflammatory hyperpigmentation is often the clinical impression and may be the histopathologic one, if the amyloid globules are inconspicuous
- Features of lichen simplex chronicus are superimposed on some lesions.

■ Pearls

- Upper back and scapular area are the most common sites, breast and buttocks occasionally

- Most often occurs in women who are middle-aged or older
- Predilection for darker-skinned people, especially those from the Middle East, Asia, Central and South America
- Anatomic site and clinical description of lesions are clues that should prompt careful examination for subtle amyloid deposition
- History of repetitive friction/irritation in some cases (Fig. 10.1B)
- Closely related or identical to lichen amyloidosis [both are formed of amyloid K; (see lichen amyloidosis)].

Lichen Amyloidosis

■ Criteria for diagnosis

- Pruritic hyperkeratotic papules and plaques on the shins or rarely, the extensor surfaces of the arms
- Small globules of amorphous pale or dull pink material within expanded dermal papillae
- Melanophages
- Epidermal hyperplasia and compact hyperorthokeratosis (indicative of superimposed lichen simplex chronicus).

■ Differential diagnosis

- Other types of systemic and skin-limited amyloidosis
- Postinflammatory hypermelanosis
- Stasis dermatitis

■ Pitfalls

- As in macular amyloidosis, the earliest manifestations may be subtle (Fig. 10.1B)
- Melanophages may be interpreted as post-inflammatory hyperpigmentation
- Subtle features in lesions on the shins (the most common site) may be obscured by stasis change
- Superimposed lichen simplex chronicus may dominate the histopathologic findings.

■ Pearls

- Lichen amyloidosis differs from macular amyloidosis only by anatomic site and the more pronounced features of lichen simplex chronicus
- The amyloid in both types is often termed amyloid K and seems to be the result of altered keratin derived from individual necrotic epidermal keratinocytes (presumably due to repetitive irritation/trauma) (Fig. 10.1B).

Nodular Amyloidosis

Figures 10.1C to F show nodular amyloidosis.

■ Criteria for diagnosis

- Waxy appearing pink to brown papules and nodules
- Predilection for the trunk, extremities and genital area, but may also involve face including periorbital region (a favored site of systemic light chain amyloidosis)

- Histopathologic features similar or identical to systemic light chain/myeloma-associated amyloid
- Plasma cells are often present at the periphery of the amyloid nodule (Fig. 10.1E).

■ *Differential diagnosis*

- Skin involved by systemic light chain/myeloma-associated amyloidosis
- Skin deposits of other systemic amyloidoses.

■ *Pitfalls*

- The histopathologic features are identical to those of skin involved by systemic light chain/myeloma-associated amyloidosis, including lambda light chain composition of the amyloid.

■ *Pearls*

- The diagnosis should prompt evaluation for underlying systemic amyloidosis, myeloma or plasma cell dyscrasia
- Only 7% of the patients develop systemic amyloidosis
- The amyloid is presumably produced by localized plasma cell aggregates
- The plasma cells have been shown to be monoclonal in some cases, polyclonal in others
- A monoclonal paraproteinemia is sometimes discovered, but is of uncertain significance
- Some cases have been associated with lymphomas, autoimmune diseases and other systemic disorders.

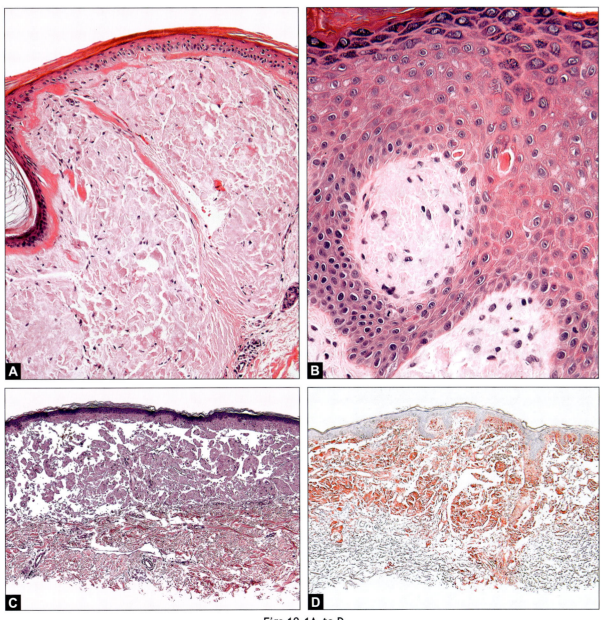

Figs 10.1A to D

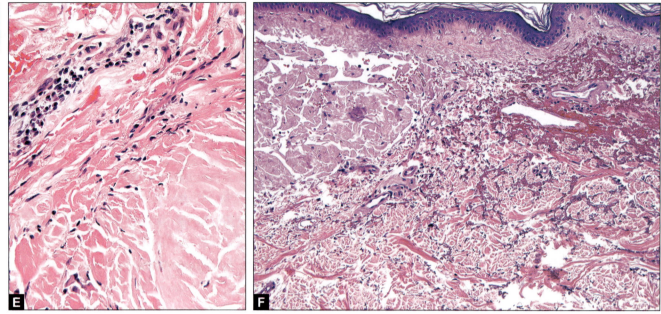

Figs 10.1A to F: (A) Systemic amyloidosis. The dermal collagen is almost entirely by amyloid in this biopsy from a patient with myeloma; (B) Lichen amyloidosis. The amyloid deposits in lichen amyloidosis (and macular amyloidosis) are usually superficial and may be subtle. Note the hypergranulosis that suggests chronic rubbing; (C) Nodular amyloidosis. Amyloid occupies the papillary dermis in this example. The characteristic "cracking" artifact is marked in this example; (D) Nodular amyloidosis, Congo red stain. Amyloid deposits usually have a dark red color when stained with Congo red. Polarization should demonstrate a pale green birefringence; (E) Plasma cells are usually apparent around or within the amyloid deposits; (F) The amyloid deposits within blood vessel walls, making them fragile and prone to hemorrhage.

Juvenile Colloid Milium

■ Criteria for diagnosis

- Flesh-colored, yellow or light brown papules, sometimes becoming confluent that present in childhood (before puberty)
- Nodules of amorphous dull pink material with a cracked or fissured appearance located in the papillary dermis that lift or impinge upon the overlying epidermis
- Congo red positive with bright green birefringence on polariscopic examination.

■ Differential diagnosis

- Nodular amyloidosis
- Systemic amyloidosis.

■ Pitfalls

- The histopathologic appearance may be very similar to nodular amyloidosis.

■ Pearls

- Very rare
- The so-called "colloid" material is histopathologically and chemically identical to amyloid and probably represents amyloid K (the type deposited in macular and lichenoid amyloidosis)
- The etiology is unknown, but an abnormal reaction to sun damage in genetically predisposed individuals has been postulated.

Adult Colloid Milium (Papular Elastosis)

Criteria for diagnosis

- Flesh-colored, pale yellow, translucent, dome-shaped papules, nodules or plaques on sun-exposed skin containing gelatinous material
- Nodular deposits of amorphous eosinophilic material with cracks and fissures (usually identical to amyloid) located within sun-damaged skin with extensive solar elastosis (Figs 10.2A and B)
- Material is periodic acid-Schiff diastase positive and Congo red positive, but does not label with antibodies directed against keratin and does not demonstrate immunoglobulin or complement deposits (Fig. 10.2B).

Differential diagnosis

- Various types of amyloid.

Pitfalls

- Histopathologically, may be virtually identical to nodular amyloid
- Exhibits the same bright green birefringence with Congo red staining as amyloid.

Pearls

- Occurs on sun-exposed skin, particularly the face, ears, neck and dorsum of the hands
- Predilection for middle-aged males
- Solar elastosis is almost always present and is usually marked.
- Despite its similarities to juvenile colloid milium and amyloid, the amorphous material in adult type colloid milium is made up of aggregated actinically damaged elastin fibers (hence the suggested designation, "papular elastosis").

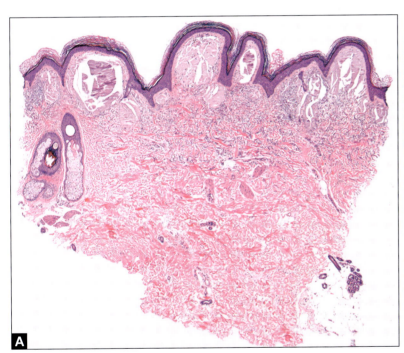 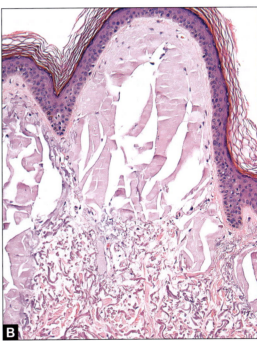

Figs 10.2A and B: Adult colloid milium. (A) The upper dermis contains cracked hyaline deposits that are virtually indistinguishable from amyloid; (B) There is usually solar elastosis around and beneath the colloid deposits. The material cannot be reliably differentiated from amyloid on H and E stains, but it does not label with antibodies directed against keratin nor contain identifiable immunoglobulin or complement deposits.

Acid glycosaminoglycans (dermal mucin) are normal components of the dermis produced by fibroblasts. Hyaluronic acid is the major component; chondroitin sulfate and heparin are other components. Cutaneous mucinoses are disorders in which dermal fibroblasts overproduce these substances, probably in response to cytokines or immunoglobulins. These activated fibroblasts often assume triangular and stellate shapes. Since hyaluronic acid absorbs water, its increase is accompanied by edema, causing the thickened skin characteristic of these diseases.

Discussed here are mucinous and myxoid depositions that tend to be generalized rather than localized. Localized conditions, such as digital myxoid pseudocyst and focal mucinosis, are discussed in Chapter 14. While it shares some elements of the pathogenesis of scleromyxedema and related conditions, scleredema is discussed in Chapter 1, since the findings are usually so subtle that it resembles other conditions within the "normal skin" as differential diagnosis.

LICHEN MYXEDEMATOSUS

Figures 10.3A and B show lichen myxedematosus and scleromyxedema.

Lichen myxedematosus is a term that encompasses a spectrum of related disorders that may be broadly subdivided into one of the two major types:

1. Scleromyxedema (generalized lichen myxedematosus)
2. Localized lichen myxedematosus.

Numerous clinical variants have been described, but the histopathologic features are common to all forms and consist essentially of a subtle increase in dermal fibrocytes/fibroblasts and glycosaminoglycans (mucin).

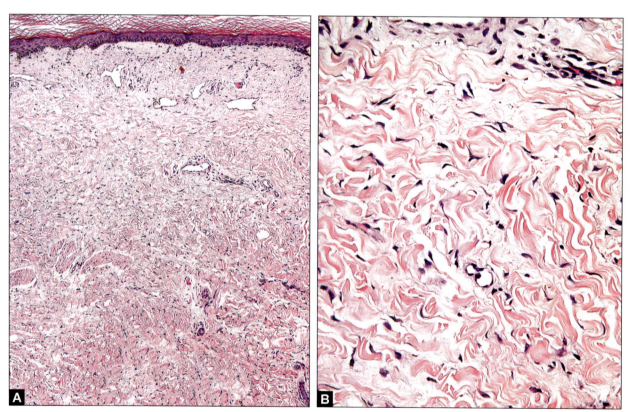

Figs 10.3A and B: Lichen myxedematosus/Scleromyxedema. (A) The dermis is fibrotic and there is subtle separation of the collagen bundles in some regions; (B) There is an increased complement of fibroblasts within the dermis, some of which have stellate contours. There is also increased separation of the collagen bundles.

Color Atlas of Differential Diagnosis of Dermatopathology

Scleromyxedema (Generalized Lichen Myxedematosus)

■ *Criteria for diagnosis*

- Indurated skin and small lichenoid papules (often with a "waxy" texture) that tend to coalesce into infiltrated plaques
- Monoclonal gammopathy (usually IgG lambda type)
- Normal thyroid function.

■ *Differential diagnosis*

- Nephrogenic systemic fibrosis
- Scleredema

■ *Pitfalls*

- Nephrogenic systemic fibrosis may be identical to scleromyxedema histopathologically
- Superficial biopsies will not contain the diagnostic features.

■ *Pearls*

- Alcian blue or colloidal iron stains may be helpful in detecting the often subtle deposition of dermal glycosaminoglycans (dermal "mucin")
- Lesions tend to present symmetrically on the distal extremities and progress to involve the trunk and face
- Established disease is characterized by sclerosis, sclerodactyly and contractures
- Systemic involvement may occur
- Clinical history, i.e. exposure to gadolinium, may be necessary to differentiate scleromyxedema from nephrogenic systemic fibrosis.

Localized Lichen Myxedematosus

■ *Criteria for diagnosis*

- Multiple clinical presentations and subtypes, but discrete papules that are flesh colored to slightly erythematous are features common to virtually all of the variants
- Histopathologic features are identical to scleromyxedema.

■ *Differential diagnosis*

- Scleromyxedema (generalized form)
- Connective tissue diseases
- Other mucinoses.

■ *Pitfalls*

- Like its generalized counterpart, the localized form of lichen myxedematosus may be subtle, shallow biopsies may not include the diagnostic features and nephrogenic systemic fibrosis cannot be reliably differentiated on microscopic examination.

■ *Pearls*

- Histopathologic examination alone does not allow distinction from generalized disease/scleromyxedema or differentiation of the various clinical subtypes.

PRETIBIAL MYXEDEMA (LOCALIZED MYXEDEMA)

Localized myxedema is most often encountered on the anterior lower extremities, hence the common designation "pretibial" myxedema, but it may also occur on the thighs, upper extremities and face.

■ *Criteria for diagnosis*

- Indurated yellow or erythematous plaques and diffusely thickened skin on the anterolateral aspect of the legs
- Mucin deposition within the reticular dermis with an uninvolved papillary dermis (Fig. 10.4)
- Collagen bundles that are thin and widely separated
- No appreciable increase in fibroblasts (Fig. 10.4).

■ *Differential diagnosis*

- Scleromyxedema
- Scleredema

■ *Pitfalls*

- Although it is associated with autoimmune hyperthyroidism (Graves' disease), the myxedema often precedes the diagnosis.

■ *Pearls*

- Alcian blue, pH 2.5 will highlight the mucin deposition
- Epidermal hyperplasia with hyperkeratosis may be present
- Diagnosis should prompt evaluation for Graves' disease.

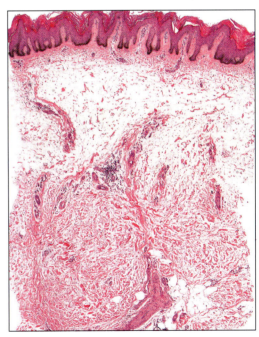

Fig. 10.4: Pretibial myxedema. The mid reticular dermis is markedly expanded by glycosaminoglycan deposition. Note that the papillary dermis is uninvolved and there is no appreciable increase in fibroblasts. The epidermal hyperplasia and hyperkeratosis seen here is present in some cases, but others may have a normal or even thinned epidermis.

GOUT (AND PSEUDOGOUT) (FIGS 10.5A TO E)

■ *Criteria for diagnosis*

- *Acute*: Monoarticular arthritis of small joints of the hands and feet (classically the big toe) associated with soft tissue swelling, skin erythema and sometimes fever
- *Chronic*: Firm nodules overlying joints, usually pale yellow, white or flesh-colored that may produce material resembling moist white chalk (Fig. 10.5A)
- Dermal and subcutaneous deposits of amorphous or crystalline material that are usually amphophilic or slightly basophilic, when fixed in formalin; brown-green to pale gray crystals when fixed in alcohol (Fig. 10.5B)
- Elevated uric acid levels.

■ *Differential diagnosis*

- Pseudogout, which is deposition of calcium pyrophosphate rather than urate
- Granulomatous reactions to other depositions or infections, if crystals or clefted spaces are inconspicuous or if there is palisading inflammation.

■ *Pitfalls*

- Biopsies of early lesions may contain only small urate deposits that may be mistaken for other depositions or various causes of granulomatous inflammation

- A palisaded arrangement of inflammatory cells around the periphery of the deposits is not uncommon and may simulate a palisading granulomatous condition at first glance (Fig. 10.5C)
- Urate crystals are usually evident if the specimen is fixed in alcohol; they dissolve in the water-diluted formalin used in routine processing.

■ *Pearls*

- Most common in middle-aged and elderly males
- May be precipitated by excessive intake of alcohol, purine-rich foods, medications (especially diuretics and cyclosporine), renal disease, lymphoproliferative disorders and chemotherapy
- Alcohol fixation will preserve some of the urate crystals, but the diagnosis must be suspected clinically or upon gross examination since even brief exposure to dilute formalin will dissolve many of the crystals (Fig. 10.5D)
- The diagnosis is often made without alcohol fixation since the crystals leave characteristic cleft-like spaces and the clinical presentation is often stereotypical.

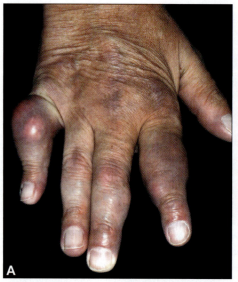
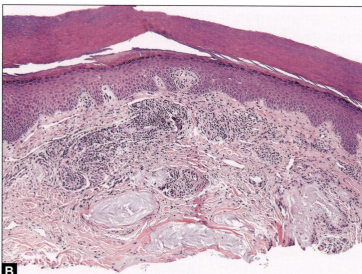

Figs 10.5A and B

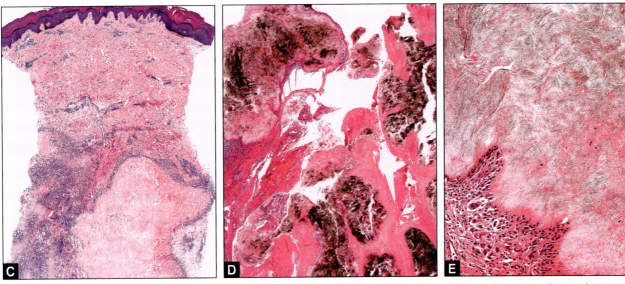

Figs 10.5A to E: Gout. Firm nodules are present over the joints of the fingers in this example of long-standing tophaceous gout. Note the resemblance to rheumatoid arthritis (Fig. 6.32A); (B) Early lesions may consist of relatively small aggregates of amorphous basophilic material in the dermis; (C) This large urate deposit is surrounded by granulomatous inflammation and resembles other lesions characterized by palisading granulomatous inflammation; (D) When alcohol is used as the fixative, the dark brown urate crystals are preserved; (E) The crystals are thin and distributed in a feather-like pattern.

CALCINOSIS CUTIS (AND OSTEOMA CUTIS)

Calcinosis cutis describes the presence of nodular calcium deposits within the skin. Multiple conditions result in calcinosis cutis, resulting in the proliferation of supposed "variants", all of which are poorly named. The etiology can only occasionally be determined by microscopic examination alone, and in most cases, "calcinosis cutis" is the most accurate diagnosis a histopathologist can provide. Osteoma cutis simply describes bone generation that often occurs concomitantly with calcinosis within many of the same scenarios (Fig. 10.6A).

There are essentially two settings in which the clinical features are distinctive. These include:

1. "Dystrophic calcification", which may occur in autoimmune connective tissues diseases, such as scleroderma, dermatomyositis or CREST syndrome (calcinosis, Raynaud's phenomenon, esophageal dysfunction, sclerodactyly, and telangiectasia), congenital diseases such as Ehlers-Danlos disease and pseudoxanthoma elasticum (Fig. 10.6B).

2. So-called "metastatic calcification", (another misleading term) used to describe deposition of calcium due to elevated serum calcium levels, usually in the setting of renal disease, hyperparathyroidism, protein C deficiency or hypervitaminoses A or D.

Beyond these, numerous terms are used to describe what is essentially a common entity, namely calcification in response to trauma or inflammation, recent or remote (and remembered or not) (Fig. 10.6C). Ironically, "dystrophic" is a more accurate descriptor for these entities. Examples include the various subtypes of "idiopathic calcinosis," which when encountered in the scrotal skin of children and young adults is designated "idiopathic scrotal calcinosis", but receives different names when it occurs at other sites, e.g. "subepidermal calcified nodule" or "tumoral calcinosis" when the nodules are large and occur over a bony prominence. The best approach may be to adopt a single term, localized calcinosis to encompass all of the above (Fig. 10.6D).

Although calciphylaxis results from calcium deposition, the main feature is tissue necrosis due to vascular occlusion. It is therefore discussed within the context of the other vasculopathies in Chapter 7 (Figs 7.6A and B).

■ *Criteria for diagnosis*

- Discrete, firm nodules of variable size in any location, composed of calcium, sometimes associated with granulomatous inflammation (Fig. 10.6E)
- No evidence of an existing calcium-producing neoplasm (e.g. pilomatricoma).

■ *Differential diagnosis*

- Other depositional diseases, rarely
- Pilomatricoma or trichilemmal cyst with extensive calcification.

■ *Pitfalls*

- Occasionally, pilomatricomas that are partially sampled have only small epithelial components or are disrupted by inflammation, may simulate calcinosis cutis; careful search for epithelial elements and trichilemmal keratin is warranted in this situation.

■ *Pearls*

- A von Kossa stain may be used if there is any doubt about whether the deposited material is calcium.

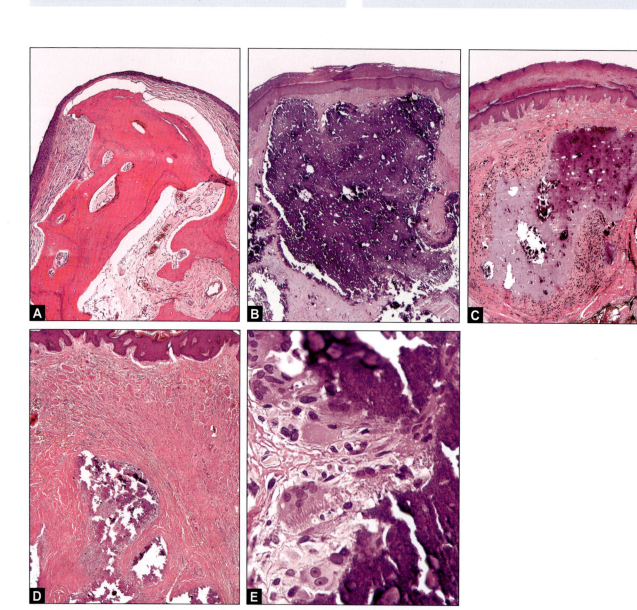

Figs 10.6A to E: (A) Osteoma cutis. The dermis contains bone tissue that imparts a nodular configuration to the skin; (B) Calcinosis cutis (dystrophic type). This lesion was one of several nodules that developed in a patient with dermatomyositis; (C) Localized calcinosis. The calcium deposition is accompanied by evidence of trauma, namely the black carbon fragments and fibrosis; (D Localized calcinosis (idiopathic scrotal calcinosis). This nodule occurred within the scrotal skin of a 10-year-old. The numerous small smooth muscle bundles within the surrounding dermis are a clue to the anatomic site; (E) Calcinosis cutis (dystrophic type). The refractile purple calcium deposits may be surrounded by granulomatous inflammation.

CHAPTER 11

The Melanocytic Tumors

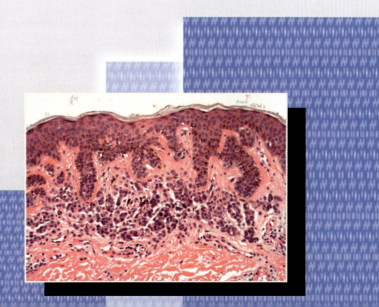

INTRODUCTION

Neoplastic melanocytes vary markedly in their appearance. The first step in diagnosis of a melanocytic neoplasm, therefore, is to be certain that the lesional cells are indeed melanocytes. Given their potential for cytologic variability, even experienced dermatopathologists have confused melanocytes for histiocytes, epithelial cells and Schwann cells to name few examples. Fortunately, the melanocytes of most nevi and melanomas are readily recognizable as such, but mistaking a melanocytic neoplasm for something else entirely is obviously an embarrassing (and potentially disastrous) pitfall.

The next step is determining the distribution of the melanocytes. Are they confined to the epidermis (junctional), the dermis and epidermis (compound) or localized predominantly within the dermis (intradermal)? The simple determination of melanocyte distribution allows the differential diagnosis to be narrowed considerably.

Determining whether the neoplasm is benign or malignant is the final step and unfortunately a very difficult one in some cases. As mentioned above, melanocytes may vary markedly in their cytologic features. Some malignant melanomas are composed of cells that differ only slightly from their benign counterparts. Conversely, benign nevi may be composed partly or entirely of cells that are larger and more pleomorphic than those of some melanoma variants. Architectural features have almost as great a potential for overlap. Therefore, consider the entire constellation of architectural and cytologic features before arriving at a diagnosis, and only then after the clinical description has been carefully considered.

Neoplasms that are relatively small, symmetrical, well-demarcated and composed predominantly of melanocytes that are small, and when present in the dermis exhibit "maturation" (progressive diminution in size and density within the dermis) are almost always benign nevi. The major exception to this rule is the rare, but dreaded "nevoid" melanoma, which may exhibit almost all of these features (but can usually be differentiated by the presence of numerous mitotic figures).

Conversely, neoplasms that are broad, lack symmetry, circumscription and are composed of melanocytes with obvious cytologic atypia and mitotic figures are usually malignant melanomas.

Tumors composed of melanocytes that are spindled, fusiform or epithelioid, may be either nevi or melanomas and for practical purposes should be considered together as a separate class. They include presumably benign neoplasms including Spitz's nevus, Reed's nevus, Seab's nevus (so-called "deep penetrating nevus"), some variants of blue nevus and Mihm's nevus (so-called "pigmented epithelioid melanocytoma"). However, some melanomas exhibit architectural and cytologic properties that overlap with the nevi in this category ('Spitzoid melanomas, for example) and unfortunately, histopathologic features, even in constellation, are sometimes unreliable predictors of biological potential in a significant number of these tumors and some may even prove to be "low-grade" or indolent forms of melanoma that have the capacity to involve regional lymph nodes, but rarely pursue an aggressive course.

The organization of most textbooks presumes that one first decides outright, whether a melanocytic neoplasm is benign (nevus) or malignant (melanoma). Since, this is not always straightforward, especially for novices, we once again advise a pattern analysis approach in which the architecture and cytologic features are assessed first and then the constellation of findings are interpreted within the clinical context to determine whether the lesion is benign, malignant or occasionally indeterminate.

When architectural and cytologic features are considered together, six basic patterns emerge:
1. Junctional neoplasms composed of cytologically banal melanocytes
2. Junctional neoplasms composed of cytologically atypical melanocytes
3. Compound or intradermal neoplasms composed of cytologically banal melanocytes
4. Compound or intradermal neoplasms composed of melanocytes that are spindled and/or epithelioid: Spitz's nevus and Reed's nevus
5. Predominantly dermal tumors composed of pigment synthesizing melanocytes: The "Blue nevus" variants
6. Compound or intradermal neoplasms composed of markedly atypical melanocytes.

Obviously, the definition of a "banal" melanocyte is subjective, but this is precisely why cytologic properties must be interpreted within the context of architecture. Recognition of these patterns encourages the generation of a differential diagnosis prior to arriving at a final diagnosis and in our experience, lessens the likelihood of falling victim to one of the many pitfalls presented by melanocytic tumors.

CYTOLOGICALLY BANAL MELANOCYTES CONFINED TO THE EPIDERMIS

Simple Lentigo

■ *Criteria for diagnosis*

- Well-demarcated and symmetrical pigmented macule (usually less than 5 mm in greatest dimension that persists in the absence of sun exposure)
- A slightly increased number of cytologically banal melanocytes confined to the basal layer of an epidermis that has elongated, bulbous rete and uniform hyperpigmentation (Fig. 11.1A)
- An absence of melanocytic nests.

■ *Differential diagnosis*

- Solar lentigo
- Ephelis (freckle)
- Early junctional nevus.

■ *Pitfalls*

- Melanocytic nest s differentiate a junctional nevus from a simple lentigo, but nests may be small and sparse in some nevi and not present in every tissue section (Fig. 11.1B).

■ *Pearls*

- Lentigo simplex may represent the earliest stage in the evolution of lentiginous melanocytic nevi
- An ephelis (common "freckle") fades or disappears entirely in the absence of continued sun exposure
- Solar lentigo (lentigo maligna) is often larger, less circumscribed and have more severe solar elastosis than a simple lentigo
- Multiple or widespread lentigines are a feature of Laugier-Hunziker syndrome, Peutz-Jeghers syndrome, Carney complex, and the LEOPARD (lentigines, electrocardiograph abnormalities, ocular hypertelorism, pulmonary stenosis, abnormal genitalia, retarded growth and deafness) and LAMB syndromes.

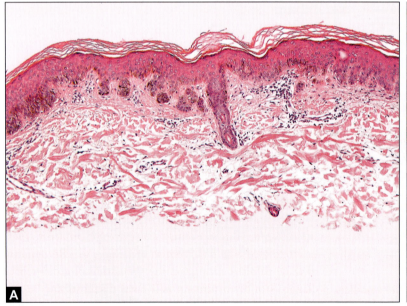
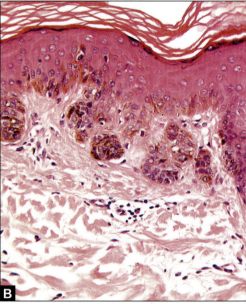

Figs 11.1A and B: Simple lentigo. (A) The epidermal rete are elongated and bulbous, and there is a uniform increase in melanin pigmentation. Note the absence of dermal solar elastosis. This biopsy was from a 5-year-old child; (B) Although an increase in the number of melanocytes is usually detectable with immunohistochemical methods, they are relatively inconspicuous and evenly spaced. The elongated rete are populated mostly by keratinocytes that contain increased melanin pigment.

Mucocutaneous Lentigo (Melanotic Macules)

■ *Criteria for diagnosis*

- A pigmented macule on the oral mucosa, vermillion border of the lip, genitalia or conjunctiva (Fig. 11.2A)
- Well-defined borders
- Increased, but uniformly distributed melanin hyperpigmentation (Fig. 11.2B).

■ *Differential diagnosis*

- Mucosal nevi (including blue nevi)
- Postinflammatory hyperpigmentation
- Mucosal melanoma
- Deposits of pigment other than melanin (e.g. "amalgam tattoos" of oral mucosa).

■ *Pitfalls*

- The increased density of melanocytes may be subtle or occasionally not appreciable in some sections (Fig. 11.2C)

- The hyperpigmentation may be difficult to appreciate histopathologically.

■ *Pearls*

- Bulbous rete may be absent, but acanthosis is often present
- The lesions are essentially a mucosal counterpart of the simple lentigo
- Multiple lentigines on the oral mucosa or vermillion border of the lip are commonly encountered in Peutz-Jeghers syndrome
- The so-called "ink spot lentigo" (reticulated lentigo) is a variant in which pigmentation is particularly dense and often imparts a very dark brown or black color clinically; the histopathologic correlate is markedly increased basilar pigmentation and often, melanin within the dermis and within dermal macrophages (melanophages).

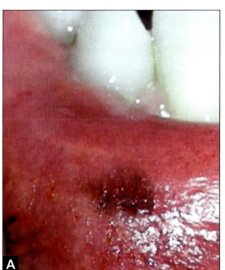

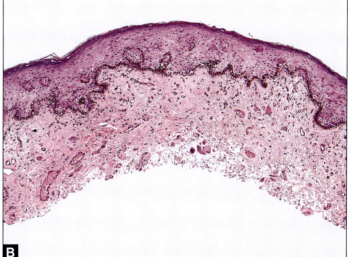

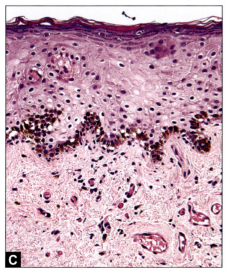

Figs 11.2A to C: Mucocutaneous lentigo (labial melanotic macule). (A) Most are evenly pigmented brown macules; (B) The epidermal rete is elongated and bulbous and there is a uniform increase in melanin pigmentation. Note the absence of dermal solar elastosis. This biopsy was from a 5 year-old child; (C) Although an increase in melanin pigment is evident, the number of melanocytes is normal or only slightly increased.

Solar Lentigo (Figs 11.3A to D)

Criteria for diagnosis

- A tan to dark brown macule that persists in the absence of sun exposure (Fig. 11.3A)
- Variable circumscription and size (some exceed 5 mm or even several centimeters and not all are well-demarcated) (Fig. 11.3A)
- Elongated epidermal rete, some with bulbous or anastomosing tips, with basal layer hyperpigmentation (Fig. 11.3B).

Differential diagnosis

- Early seborrheic keratosis (may evolve from solar lentigo)
- Pigmented actinic keratosis
- Early stage or histologically subtle melanoma in situ, lentigo maligna type.

Pitfalls

- Lentigo maligna type melanoma in situ may arise around or within a solar lentigo, but small samples of large pigmented lesions may not include the melanoma component.

Pearls

- A solar lentigo with keratinocyte atypia is not uncommon and in some cases this may warrant the diagnosis of "solar lentigo and pigmented actinic keratosis"
- The solar lentigo is often biopsied to "rule out" lentigo maligna/melanoma in situ, but if the biopsy represents a small sample of a larger lesion or the clinical information lacks a description of the lesion's size and appearance, definitive exclusion of melanoma in situ is not possible in some cases.

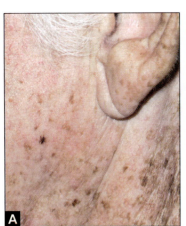
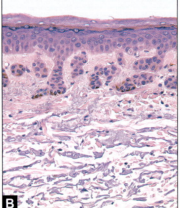
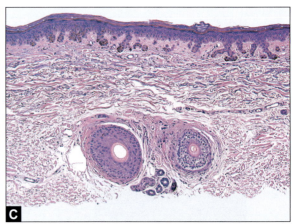
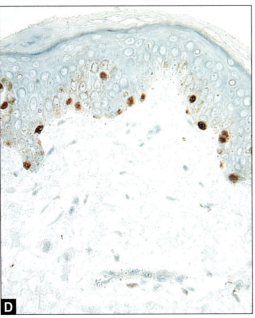

Figs 11.3A to D: Solar lentigo. (A) The lesions are often multiple, as in this patient, and occur on sun-damaged skin as brown macules of varying size and pigmentation; (B) Like a simple lentigo, the epidermal rete are elongated and bulbous, and there is a uniform increase in melanin pigmentation. Evidence of sun damage (solar elastosis) is readily apparent, however; (C) The bulbous, long rete may be sectioned tangentially, causing them to be discontiguous within a given profile. This sometimes results in confusion with melanocytic nests; (D) Immunohistochemistry for MITF demonstrates that the number of melanocytes is increased relative to normal skin, but the melanocytes are distributed as single cells rather than nested. Most are uniformly spaced, but some irregularly spacing occurs, especially in severely sun-damaged skin.

Junctional Melanocytic Nevus

■ *Criteria for diagnosis*

- A symmetrical and uniformly pigmented macule
- An increased number of single melanocytes confined to the basal layer of the epidermis arranged as single cells but also within nests (Fig. 11.4)
- Variability in the size and shape of melanocytes in some cases, but a lack of the cytologic atypia, usually encountered in melanoma in situ (Fig. 11.4).

■ *Differential diagnosis*

- Solar lentigo and simple lentigo
- Lentigo maligna
- Junctional atypical melanocytosis.

■ *Pitfalls*

- Nests may be inconspicuous in evolving or small junctional nevi, causing confusion with a lentigo

- Junctional nevi that are very broad (greater than 6 mm), have cytologic atypia or arise on sun-damaged skin should be examined carefully to exclude subtle presentations of melanoma in situ.

■ *Pearls*

- Solar lentigo and simple lentigo may be precursors of junctional nevi
- Junctional nevi, in turn, may progress to involve the underlying dermis
- If biopsied very early in their course, lentiginous growth may predominate significantly over nested growth and the lesional borders may be indistinct
- "Ordinary" junctional nevi are not uncommon, but many of those that are biopsied are of Clark's type and exhibit dermal fibroplasia, some cytologic variability and a lymphohistiocytic infiltrate within the papillary dermis.

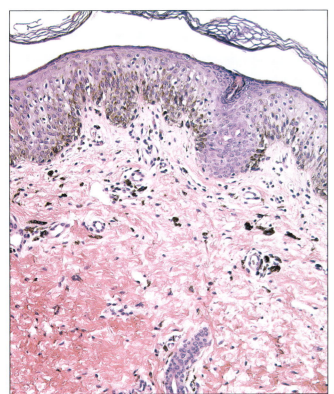

Fig. 11.4: Junctional melanocytic nevus. Although some authors seem to label all junctional nevi as "Clark's nevi" or "dysplastic nevi", there exists a subset in which the features that define those types are absent, such as this example. Melanocytes are increased and many appear to be distributed as single cells, but cytologicatypia, bridging nests and other features of Clark's/dysplastic nevi are absent.

Junctional Atypical Melanocytosis

("Atypical Junctional Melanocytic Proliferation," "Atypical Solar Lentigo")

■ Criteria for diagnosis

- Ill-defined pigmented macule resembling a lentigo or a lentigo maligna clinically
- An increased number of melanocytes confined to the basal layer and disposed as single cells that are unevenly spaced and approach contiguity in some foci but do not form nests (Fig. 11.5A)
- The melanocytes lack the degree of cytologic atypia usually encountered in melanoma in situ.

■ Differential diagnosis

- Junctional nevus
- Solar intraepidermal melanocytosis (SIM)
- Melanoma in situ
- Pigmented actinic keratosis
- Solar lentigo.

■ Pitfalls

- Because the melanocytes are small and distributed singly, they may be difficult to appreciate without the aid of immunohistochemical stains (Fig. 11.5B).

■ Pearls

- This term implies the possibility of an early melanoma in situ and should be reserved for situations in which the lentiginous growth of melanocytes exceeds that of a solar lentigo or Clark's nevus, but does not quite fulfill the criteria for lentigo maligna or lentiginous melanoma even after multiple sections and/or immunohistochemical stains have been examined.

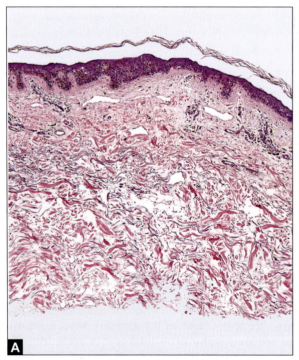 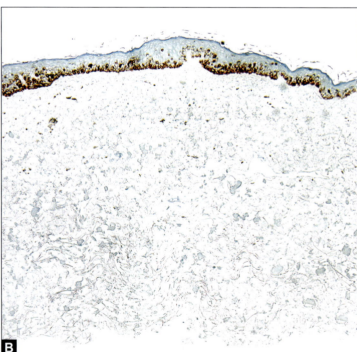

Figs 11.5A and B: Junctional atypical melanocytosis. (A) The epidermis contains an increased number of melanocytes confined to the basal layer. They are disposed as single cells that are unevenly spaced. Although they may approach contiguity in some foci, such areas are usually small and nests are absent by definition; (B) Often, immunohistochemical stains for melanocytes (such as MITF or Melan-A/Mart-1) are helpful in determining the exact degree of melanocytosis.

Persistent Nevus (Recurrent Nevus)

■ *Criteria for diagnosis*

- Melanocytes arranged as single cells and/or irregularly shaped and unevenly distributed nests along the dermoepidermal junction (and often within the dermis if the pre-existing nevus was compound) (Fig. 11.6A)
- Scar tissue within the dermis
- Localization of the atypical architecture to the scarred area.

■ *Differential diagnosis*

- Recurrent melanoma
- Partially regressed malignant melanoma
- Partially regressed nevus.

■ *Pitfalls*

- May be mistaken for melanoma, if scar is not appreciated or scar cannot be differentiated from the dermal fibrosis that occurs within regressing melanomas (Fig. 11.6B)
- Simulates melanoma with regression and in some cases the two are indistinguishable, if clinical history of trauma or a prior biopsy at the site is lacking.
- Partial sampling may not include the melanocytic lesion in the non-scarred area and definitive exclusion of recurrent/persistent melanoma requires examination of this component.

■ *Pearls*

- Recurrent persistent nevus is a common simulator of melanoma
- Clinical history of a prior biopsy at the site is helpful, but may not be available (the clinician may not know if the site was biopsied and patients themselves may not remember)
- A persistent melanocytic proliferation that resembles melanoma must be confined to the area of the scar; if it extends beyond the scar, melanoma must be carefully excluded or the lesion must be re-excised in its entirety
- If the same degree of atypia involves skin adjacent to the scar, persistent/recurrent melanoma is more likely
- If possible, evaluate the original biopsy in conjunction with the recurrent lesion
- Clark's nevi are the most type of nevus to persist/recur, but other types also recur and the type of original nevus often cannot be determined by examination of the recurrent lesion alone
- Repopulation of the skin by lesional melanocytes located within adnexal structures lying beyond the sections examined is the most likely explanation when a neoplasm that appears to have been excised completely recurs.

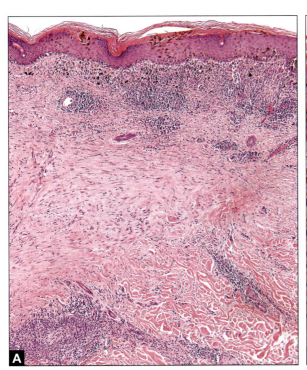 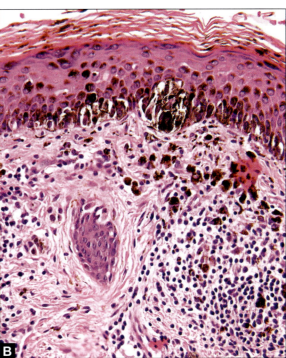

Figs 11.6A and B: Persistent/Recurrent nevus. (A) Note the irregular distribution of melanocytes along the dermoepidermal junction directly overlying a scar. Near the bottom of the image, small residual nevus cells are present in a congenital distribution along an eccrine duct within the reticular dermis; (B) The junctional component of persistent/recurrent nevi may closely resemble the disordered architecture of a melanoma. Identifying the underlying scar is crucial.

Atypical Intraepidermal Melanocytosis

■ Criteria for diagnosis

- An increased number of single melanocytes confined to the basal layer of the epidermis that are unevenly spaced, but not confluent, nested or present in the dermis (Fig. 11.7A)
- Lesional borders that cannot be reliably distinguished either clinically or histopathologically
- Solar elastosis
- Few, if any melanophages in the underlying dermis.

■ Differential diagnosis

- Lentigo maligna
- Junctional atypical melanocytosis
- Solar lentigo
- Pigmented actinic keratosis

■ Pitfalls

- Atypical intraepidermal melanocytosis (AIM) can contain melanocytes that are as cytologically atypical as those of lentigo maligna; in such cases, only architecture (confluence of cells and nesting in lentigo maligna) allows distinction
- Atypical intraepidermal melanocytosis can complicate diagnosis and margin evaluation in lentigo maligna since it may occur within the skin adjacent to lentigo maligna and even "merge" with it.

■ Pearls

- Atypical intraepidermal melanocytosis is a descriptive term for a diffuse increase in the complement of melanocytes as a consequence of chronic sun exposure and actinic damage; it is not a diagnosis per se and a comment explaining its meaning should be included in the report
- Atypical intraepidermal melanocytosis is a histopathologic finding, that is not clinically detectable as a discrete lesion and is usually an incidental finding adjacent to other lesions in sun-damaged skin (Fig. 11.7B)
- In some cases, determining where a lentigo maligna ends and AIM begins is virtually impossible and the distinction may be somewhat arbitrary
- Unlike lentigo maligna, in AIM melanophages are rare or altogether absent
- By definition, AIM contains atypical melanocytes, it occurs in sun-damaged skin and therefore, implies at least some increased risk of melanoma
- Re-excision of AIM is not indicated, since by definition, the process lacks clinically identifiable borders and may be extensive, involving much of a patient's actinically-damaged skin.

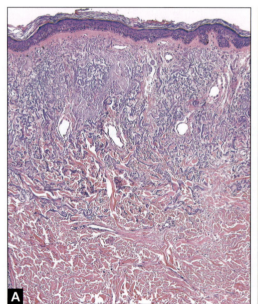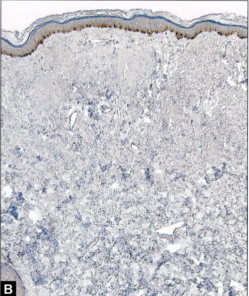

Figs 11.7A and B: Atypical intraepidermal melanocytosis. (A) There is an increased number of single melanocytes confined to the basal layer of the epidermis that are unevenly spaced but not confluent, nested or present in the dermis. Solar elastosis is invariably present; (B) The melanocytosis, highlighted here with Melan-A/Mart-1 does not have a "border" that can be reliably distinguished either clinically or histopathologically (differentiating it from atypical intraepidermal melanocytosis). It is essentially a melanocytosis that is an incidental finding in severely sun-damaged skin.

Melanoma In Situ, Lentigo Maligna Type

■ *Criteria for diagnosis*

- Broad, variably pigmented macules with irregular borders on sun-damaged skin of adults (Fig. 11.8A)
- Atypical melanocytes (often angulated or spindled as well as round) arranged in contiguity along the basal layer of the epidermis, mostly as single cells, but also in small irregularly shaped and unevenly distributed nests (Fig. 11.8B)
- Malignant melanocytes are not present within the dermis
- Solar elastosis of the underlying dermis.

■ *Differential diagnosis*

- Lentiginous melanoma
- Junctional Clark's dysplastic nevus
- Solar lentigo
- Solar intraepidermal melanocytosis (SIM)
- Pigmented actinic keratosis/squamous cell carcinoma in situ.

■ *Pitfalls*

- May arise in contiguity with a solar lentigo; partial biopsies may include only the solar lentigo and "miss" the adjacent lentigo maligna
- May have "skip" areas—regions where the melanoma has regressed partially or entirely, that complicate diagnosis in partially sampled lesions
- Skip areas make assessment of margins difficult in excisions
- Extension of atypical melanocytes along rete and adnexal epithelium is common in lentigo maligna; tangentially sectioned rete and adnexal epithelium may produce the false impression of dermal involvement (see lentigo maligna melanoma) and inflammation within the underlying dermis (a common finding) may make it difficult to exclude melanocytes within the dermis
- Extension into the dermis (lentigo maligna melanoma) commonly has a "desmoplastic" appearance—the neoplastic cells are spindled and the surrounding dermis is sclerotic, and may be mistaken for scar tissue (see desmoplastic melanoma).

■ *Pearls*

- Epidermal atrophy is common; solar elastosis is required by definition
- Extension of atypical cells along adnexal epithelium is common in lentigo maligna
- Cytologic atypia varies and may be mild to marked, including multinucleated giant cells
- Junctional nests, if present, usually vary markedly in size and shape and are unevenly spaced (Fig. 11.8C)
- A dermal lymphohistiocytic infiltrate with melanophages is common
- Pagetoid spread may occur, but is usually less extensive than in superficial spreading melanoma
- Dermal invasion—lentigo maligna melanoma, typically occurs within long-standing lesions
- Regression is common; its presence at an excision margin is an indication for re-excision
- Large excisions are sometimes examined using tangential margins, but since lentigo maligna often has ill-defined borders, perpendicular margins are preferred, when possible, because they allow melanocyte density at the margins to be compared with the central areas in which the tumor is most obvious.

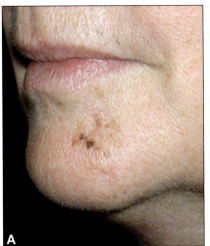 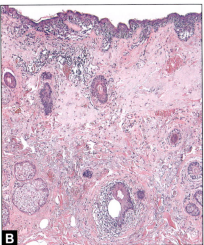 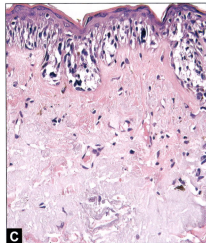

Figs 11.8A to C: Melanoma in situ, lentigo maligna type. (A) The lesions usually present on the face or other chronically sun-exposed skin and have irregular borders and, often, variability in pigmentation; (B) Melanocytes are arranged predominantly along the basal layer of the epidermis. There is usually overt cytologic and architectural atypia, and solar elastosis is present by definition. The dermis is not involved. If it is, the diagnosis is lentigo maligna melanoma; (C) Occasionally there are relatively well-formed nests, but their irregular spacing and distribution, within the context of other features characteristic of lentigo maligna, aid in their recognition as part of the melanoma.

Melanoma (In Situ Other than Lentigo Maligna) Type (Figs 11.9A to E)

■ *Criteria for diagnosis*

- An increased number of intraepidermal melanocytes with cytologic atypia (Fig. 11.9A)
- Broad areas in which lentiginous growth of single melanocytes predominates over melanocytes arranged in nests (Fig. 11.9B)
- Melanocytes within the spinous and granular cell layers ("pagetoid" distribution), in some cases (Fig. 11.9A)
- A lack of actinic damage, epidermal atrophy and other features that would favor melanoma of lentigo maligna type.

■ *Differential diagnosis*

- Recurrent persistent nevus
- Squamous cell carcinoma in situ
- Extramammary Paget's disease (EPD)
- Junctional variants of Clark's nevus and Spitz's nevus
- Melanoma in situ arising within a nevus.

■ *Pitfalls*

- Squamous cell carcinoma and extramammary Paget's disease are well known simulators of melanoma in situ and their distinction from melanoma in situ may require immunohistochemistry for keratins and melanocytic markers (Figs 11.9C and E)
- A dermal component may not be appreciable in partial biopsies of larger lesions.

■ *Pearls*

- When in doubt, Ber-Ep4 (positive in extramammary Paget's disease) and a pan-cytokeratin (positive in squamous cell carcinoma in situ) should be used in conjunction with melanocytic markers to differentiate lesions with a "pagetoid" pattern (Figs 11.9C and E)
- Examine the dermis carefully for a scar that might suggest recurrent persistent nevus rather than melanoma in situ (see persistent/recurrent nevus).

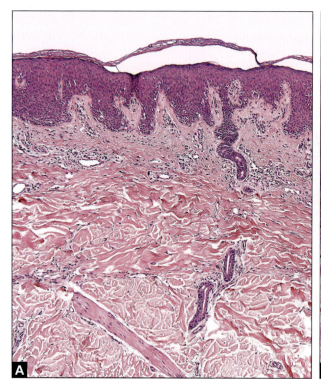
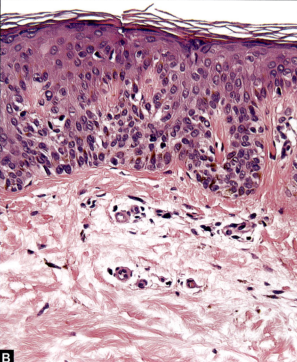

Figs 11.9A and B

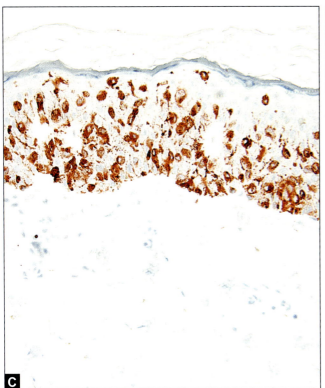

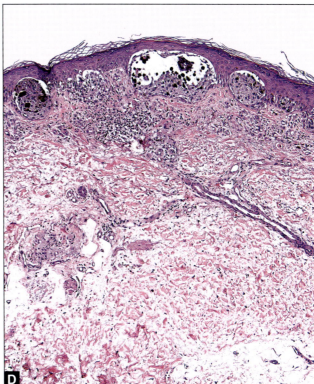

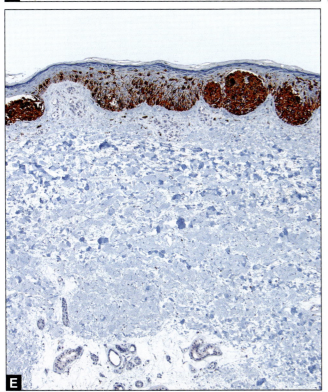

Figs 11.9A to E: Melanoma in situ (other than lentigo maligna). (A) Atypical melanocytes are present within the epidermis. They are often distributed above the basal layer, and solar elastosis is absent, features that aid in the distinction from lentigo maligna; (B) There are typically broad regions in which the melanocytes are arranged as single cells without obvious nests; (C) In some cases it may be difficult to determine the degree and distribution of melanocyte overgrowth. Melanocytes markers (Melan-A/Mart-1 in this image) are helpful in this regard; (D) Nests may be evident in some cases, but they are irregularly shaped and usually composed of cells with obvious atypia; (E) Again, when in doubt, immunohistochemistry for melanocytic markers may help highlight the single cell growth around the nests and occult melanocytes within the upper levels of the epidermis (Melan-A/Mart-1).

COMPOUND OR INTRADERMAL NEOPLASMS THAT ARE CYTOLOGICALLY BANAL

Criteria that Suggest a Benign Nevus

The criteria are:
- A small, symmetrical, evenly pigmented papule or nodule with even borders on clinical examination (Fig. 11.10A)
- A balanced* (or symmetrical) silhouette at scanning magnifi-cation; an inflammatory infiltrate, if present, should be symmetrical as well (Figs 11.10B and C)
- Well-demarcated lateral borders (especially when delimited by nests on both sides) (Fig. 11.10D)
- Melanocytes arranged in nests predominating over those disposed as single cells (Fig. 11.10E)
- Melanocytes arranged in small nests, cords and single cells within the dermis
- Relative uniformity of cell morphology, density and architecture across the horizontal plane, i.e. the lesion looks the same from side to side (Fig. 11.10C)
- "Maturation", i.e. progressive diminution in the size of nests and the size of individual cells within the vertical plane (from the dermoepidermal junction toward the reticular dermis or "superficial to deep")(Figs 11.10F and G)
- "Dispersion", i.e. a progressive increase in the distance between nevus cells within the vertical plane (Figs 11.10F and G)
- Melanocytes that (relatives to those of melanoma) are small and monomorphous with round, regular nuclear contours, evenly dispersed chromatin and inconspicuous nucleoli.
- Few (if any) mitotic figures.

*While "symmetry" has historically been the descriptor of a benign nevus, "balance" is more accurate, since even the most banal nevi are never truly perfectly symmetrical. Few biological processes, even perfectly normal ones, result in perfect symmetry.

Note that eight of the ten criteria are primarily architectural. Given the aforementioned potential for cytologic variability among melanocytes, architectural features are the most reliable.

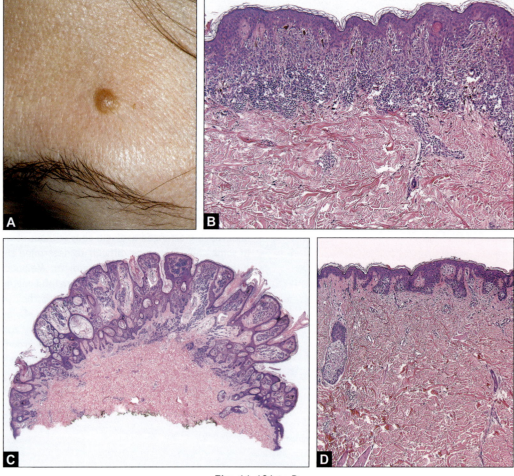

Figs 11.10A to D

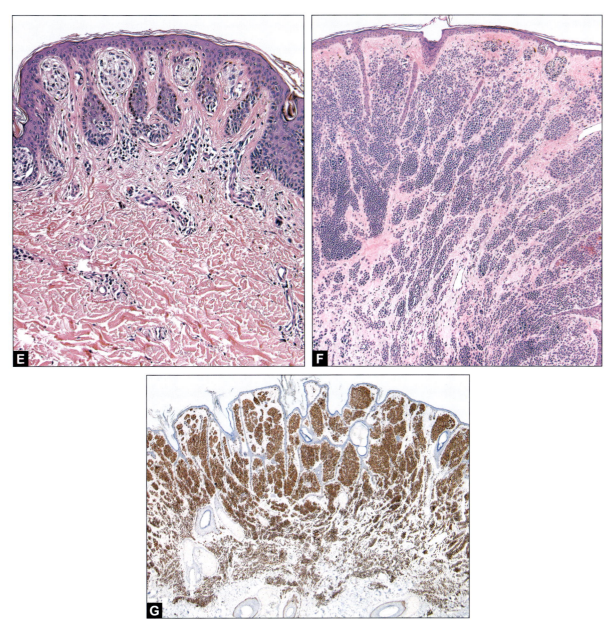

Figs 11.10A to G: Features of a benign nevus. (A) The clinical appearance is invaluable in helping to establish that a melanocytic lesion is benign. This typical nevus (Miescher's pattern) is relatively small, has uniform rounded borders, and is evenly pigmented; (B) When an inflammatory infiltrate is present, it too should be balanced, meaning that it is esse tially uniform in its distribution across the entire lesion; (C) The silhouette at scanning magnification is balanced, or rel tively "symmetrical", meaning that the overall distribution of melanocytes is of equal density within the horizontal plane (from side to side), and nests are arranged relatively evenly; (D) Benign lesions are typically well-demarcated at their peripheral borders. A particularly helpful clue is when nests are present at either edge. There should not be a lentiginous component that is significantly greater at one peripheral border than at the other; (E) Melanocytes arranged in nests generally predominate over those distributed as single cells. Note that the nests are relatively uniform in size and spacing; (F) Within the vertical plane of a banal compound nevus there is usually a progressive diminution in the size of nests and the size of individual cells. Note also that the spacing of the cells increases near the base of the lesion, i.e. there are fewer melanocytes near the base, a feature often referred to as "dispersion"; (G) Here, "maturation" and "dispersion" are highlighted with immunohistochemistry for MITF.

Exceptions to the criteria

- Nevoid melanoma is a rare morphological pattern of melanoma, which may closely simulate ordinary compound nevi; in some cases, only recognition of an increased mitotic index leads to close inspection and the correct diagnosis (compare Figure 11.10C, a benign nevus, to Figure 11.42C, a nevoid malignant melanoma) (Fig. 11.11A)

- The junctional component of an otherwise banal nevus may occasionally appear "disorganized" (nests vary in shape and spacing) or contain a larger number of cells distributed as solitary units (lentiginous growth). This must not be over-interpreted as signifying melanoma or melanoma arising within a nevus (Fig. 11.11B)

- One or two mitotic figures may occasionally be found within the upper portion of an otherwise banal compound nevus and are of no clinical significance

- Nevi on acral skin may have extensive lentiginous growth and contain melanocytes within the spinous layer, but this should not be interpreted as evidence of melanoma (see below) (Fig. 11.11C)

- Nevi on genital skin, on the breast and on the ear may exhibit "atypical" features including a disorderly appearance to the junctional component (see below)

- Nevi in infants may contain significant "pagetoid spread" of melanocytes that is of no consequence, if the other features favor a nevus (Fig. 11.11D)

- Some otherwise ordinary compound nevi contain dilated vascular spaces and an edematous stroma, numerous mature adipocytes or homogenized dense dermal collagen (desmoplastic nevus); these features are without significance

- Neural differentiation or "neurotization"—nevus cells that become small and spindle shaped within the deep dermis, is common in the Miescher and Unna variants of compound nevi

- Nevus cells occasionally have a "balloon cell" appearance— abundant pale cytoplasm and distinct cell borders (Fig. 11.11E)

- "Ancient change"—nevus cells with larger, more pleomorphic nuclei, is occasionally seen; their presence within a nevus with otherwise typical morphologic features is of no consequence and the lack of mitotic figures is helpful in excluding melanoma (Fig. 11.11F).

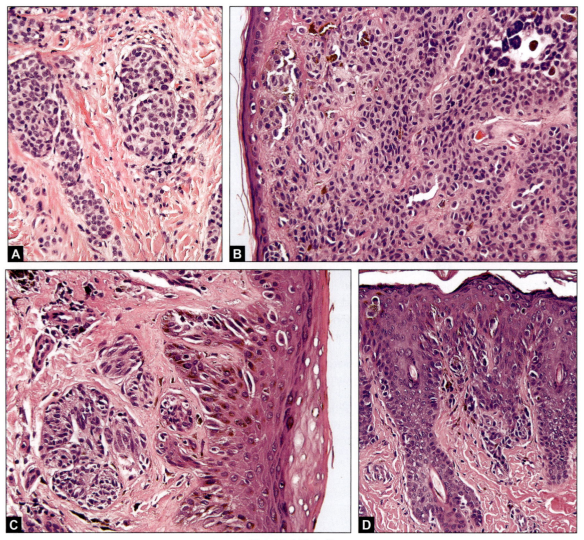

Figs 11.11A to D

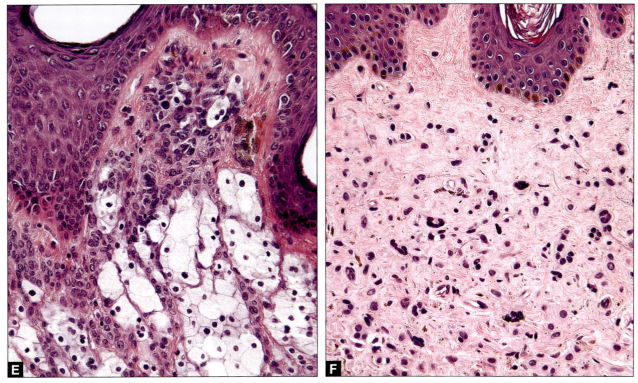

Figs 11.11A to F: (A) Nevoid melanoma. Rarely, melanomas may closely resemble nevi, even to the extent of having some maturation and dispersion. See also Figure 11.42; (B) Nevus with atypical junctional cells. In this typical Miescher's nevus there are regions in which the junctional component consists of irregularly spaced single melanocytes and nested melanocytes. In addition, a cluster of multinucleated cells is present at the bottom right. These findings can be dismissed within the context of a nevus that is otherwise typical; (C) Acral nevus. Nevi occurring on acral skin, particulary the hands and feet, may have a more disorganized appearing intraepidermal component, including lentiginous growth and melanocytes that are distributed within the upper levels of the epidermis; (D) Congenital nevus in an infant. Melanocytes are evident within the epidermis to the level of the granular layer, but within the context of a congenital pattern nevus (usually a Mark's nevus, sometimes a Zitelli's nevus) in an infant, this finding is of no concern; (E) Nevus with "Balloon cells". Copious pale or clear cytoplasm may develop in melanocytes both benign and malignant. If the nuclei appear banal and the architecture and other features are those of a nevus, however, they are of no particular concern; (F) Nevus with degenerative atypia ("Ancient change"). Occasionally a nevus may exhibit cellular pleomorphism with marked variability in nuclear size and odd nuclear shapes. This is not indicative of malignancy. An absence of mitotic figures is a reassuring finding when in doubt.

Classification of Melanocytic Nevi

Currently, no uniformly accepted classification system exists for nevi and numerous types, subtypes, and variants have been proposed. While, many have abandoned the eponymous designations, to us this system, originally advocated by Ackerman, makes the most sense for three reasons: (1) attempts to use "descriptive" terminology have not clarified matters at all, for example, the use of the term "spindled and or epithelioid nevus" has been proposed as a substitute for "Spitz's nevus". Multiple different types of nevi are composed of cells that are spindled and/or epithelioid, however, so this term greatly oversimplifies the constellation of features necessary to make a diagnosis of a Spitz's nevus; (2) these descriptive terms are long and clumsy by comparison to a simple two-word eponymous designation and in our experience, potential for confusing clinicians (and histopathologists) increases proportionally to the number of

words used to convey a diagnosis; (3) eponyms have been retained for some nevi (Spitz's nevus being the primary example), but abandoned for others, further complicating matters. It is our opinion that a classification should strive for consistency and no consistency results, when eponyms are used for some types, while clinical features or histopathologic characteristics are used for others.

While, some types of nevi do seem more prone to be associated with melanoma than others, many clinicians now seem to regard only so-called "dysplastic nevi" as having a tendency to harbor an evolving melanoma. In fact, in the experience of many dermatopathologists, the features of pre-existing nevi seen within many melanomas are at least as likely to have a congenital pattern nevi (Zitelli and Mark's nevi) as a "dysplastic" (Clark's) nevus. Therefore, we have included commonly used terms in parantheses, but emphasize the eponyms suggested by Ackerman for simplicity and uniformity.

The Common Subtypes of Compound and Intradermal Nevi

Miescher's Nevus (Common Plaque-like Nevus) (Figs 11.12A to D)

■ Criteria for diagnosis

- Clinically, symmetrical papule or dome-shaped nodule, often flesh-colored or only slightly pigmented (Fig. 11.12A)
- Nevus cells arranged predominantly within nests along the dermoepidermal junction and as nests, syncytia, cords and single cells that extend into the reticular dermis, often with neurotization of the cells at the base of the lesion.

■ Differential diagnosis

- Other types of nevi
- Nevoid melanoma
- Melanoma arising within a nevus.

■ Pitfalls

- Some "architectural disorder" of the junctional component may occur
- Cells along the junction may be large, sometimes with multinucleated forms (Fig. 11.12C)
- Trauma or chronic "irritation" may accentuate cytologic and architectural disorder or produce fibrosis that may simulate regression.

■ Pearls

- Most common on the face, particularly in women (Fig. 11.12D)
- May be compound or intradermal.

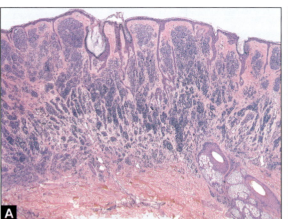
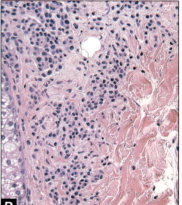
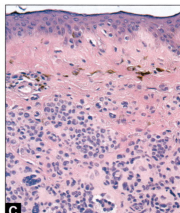

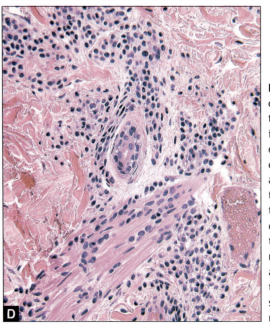

Figs 11.12A to D: Miescher's nevus. (A) The nevus has a smooth, dome-shaped contour due to the expansion of the dermis by melanocytes. Correlate this histopathologic appearance with the clinical image of a Miescher's nevus shown in Figure 11.10A; (B) The melanocytes become progressively smaller and increasingly separated from one another with increasing distance from the epidermis. This is often referred to as "maturation". Note that the nuclei are approximately the same size as those of adjacent mature sebaceous cells at the top of the field but are less than one half that size near the base. Cells at the deepest aspect of the nevus are separated by dermal collagen bundles and distributed singly rather than as nests (dispersion); (C) Often, the cells along the junction or within the upper dermis may be large, epithelioid or even multinucleated. These findings are of no concern when the remaining features are those of a benign nevus; (D) These nevi, especially those that occur on the face, often have "congenital" features, namely nevus cells that closely surround adnexal structures. They may even be present within the smooth muscle bundles of an arrector pili muscle, as they are in this field.

Unna's Nevus (Common Polyploid Nevus) (Figs 11.13A to D)

Criteria for diagnosis

- Clinically, symmetrical verrucous, papillomatous and sometimes polypoid papule, variably pigmented, with a predilection for the back and intertriginous areas (Fig. 11.13A)
- Exophytic, polypoid projections of the papillary dermis occupied by melanocytes in nests, syncytia, cords and single cells, sometimes with neurotization (Fig. 11.13C)
- Melanocytes within the epidermis are arranged as discrete nests at the base of rete, but lentiginous growth may also be present.

Differential diagnosis

- Other types of nevi
- Nevoid melanoma
- Melanoma arising within a nevus.

Pitfalls

- Architectural disorder and cytological variability of the junctional component may occur, especially in those occurring in intertriginous sites.

Pearls

- Most common on the back and in intertriginous areas
- May be compound or intradermal.

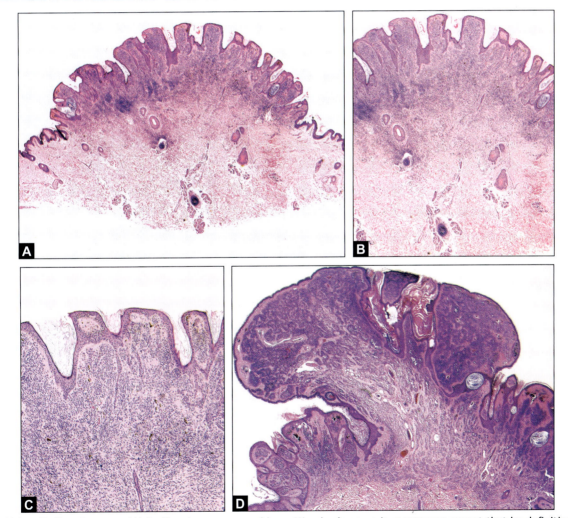

Figs 11.13A to D: Unna's nevus. (A) An Unna's nevus resembles a Miescher's nevus in many ways except that by definition it has a verrucous, papillomatous or polypoid architecture; (B) There is progressive maturation and dispersion of the nevus cells within the base; (C) The exophytic papillomatous projections are occupied by melanocytes in nests, small syncytia aggregates, cords, and single cells; (D) Some Unna's nevi have polypoid or even pedunculated growth.

Zitelli's Nevus (Common Congenital Pattern Nevus, Superficial Type)

Criteria for diagnosis

- Clinically, symmetrical, slightly raised plaque
- Nevus cells within adnexal structures and/or concentrated around them (Fig. 11.14A)
- Melanocytes that extend between individual collagen bundles of the reticular dermis (Fig. 11.14B)
- Melanocytes are primarily nested along the dermoepidermal junction and form nests, syncytia, cords and single cells within the dermis with an "adnexocentric" pattern (Figs 11.14A and C).

Differential diagnosis

- Clark's nevus
- Malignant melanoma arising within a nevus.

Pitfalls

- In infants, melanocytes disposed as single cells and nests are often present within the spinous and granular cell layers.

Pearls

- Despite the "congenital features", few are actually present at birth; however most appear within the first two decades
- Some have features ("shouldering") identical to those of a Clark's nevus
- When histopathologic features of a "pre-existing nevus" are seen in association with malignant melanomas, they often resemble this type of nevus
- The frequency with which melanoma arises within Zitelli's nevi is unknown (since they share features with Clark's nevi and often only small portions of residual nevus are seen within the "background" of the melanoma).

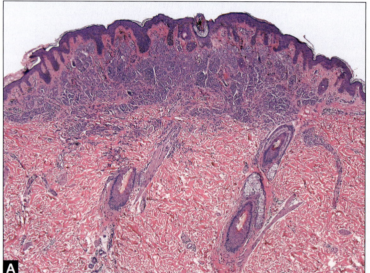
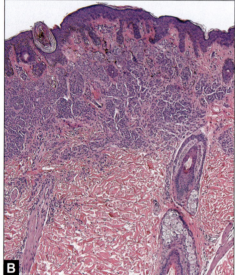
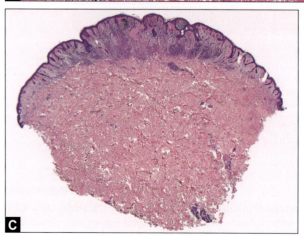

Figs 11.14A to C: Zitelli's nevus. (A) The melanocytes within the reticular dermis are almost always found in close association with adnexal structures, especially pilosebaceous units; (B) There is maturation and dispersion of the melanocytes within the reticular dermis; (C) Zitelli's nevi are also known as the superficial type of congenital pattern nevi. In addition to growth along the dermo-epidermal junction, they also contain melanocytes that extend into the reticular dermis.

Mark's Nevus (Congenital Pattern Nevus, Deep Type) (Figs 11.15A to E)

■ Criteria for diagnosis

- A broad (usually several centimeters), variably pigmented plaque, that may be smooth, papillomatous or undulating
- Melanocytes in nests and single cells along the dermoepidermal junction, throughout broad regions of the entire dermis (not restricted to periadnexal areas), sometimes with extension along fibrous septa into the subcutis (Figs 11.15B and C).

■ Differential diagnosis

- Diffuse variant of neurofibroma (when a junctional component is absent)
- Melanoma arising within a nevus.

■ Pitfalls

- Examples that lack a junctional component may simulate the diffuse form of neurofibroma

- Cytologic variability, a disorderly appearing junctional component, one or two mitotic figures or large intradermal nodules that may simulate melanoma arising within the nevus
- In the first year of life, melanocytes disposed as single cells and nests are often present within the spinous and granular cell layers, simulating melanoma.

■ Pearls

- Increasing risk for melanoma with increasing size
- When very large (20 centimeters or more), there is a significant risk for the development of melanoma
- Intraepidermal spread of melanocytes is very common in young patients, particularly in infants (Fig. 11.15D)
- Some are removed in staged excisions and regrowth of the persistent nevus within the scar from prior excision may simulate melanoma (see persistent nevus).

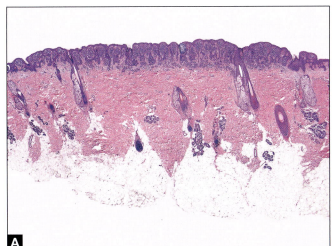 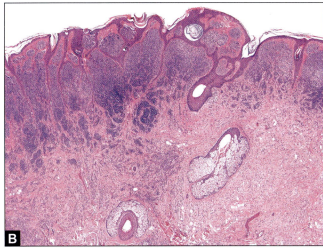

Figs 11.15A and B

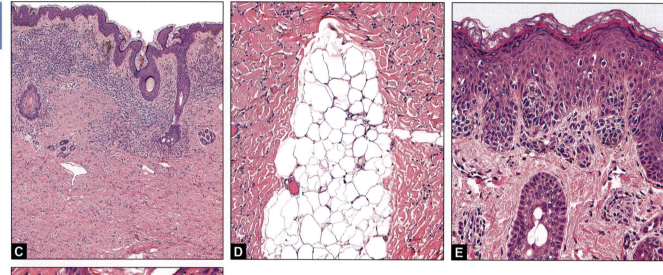

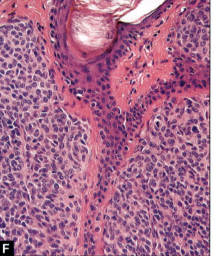

Figs 11.15A to F: Mark's nevus. (A) Like Zitelli's nevi, these are also considered to have a congenital pattern. Usually, however, they are much broader; (B) In addition, nevus cells extend more deeply into the dermis, and often they are distributed diffusely between reticular dermal collagen bundles; (C) In this field, melanocytes are most conspicuous around adnexa, but the smaller cells distributed diffusely through the reticular dermis between individual collagen bundles are also nevus cells; (D) Melanocytes may extend very deeply into the reticular dermis and even the subcutaneous layer. The small cells extending into the fibrous septa of the subcutis in this field are nevus cells; (E) In infants, it is not uncommon for melanocytes to be distributed within the upper levels of the epidermis; (F) Two mitotic figures are present within the superficial nests of this congenital nevus on the scalp of a young girl. The remainder of the nevus was entirely characteristic of a Mark's nevus, and in this context, an occasional mitotic figure is of no significance.

Clark's Nevus (Dysplastic Nevus) (Figs 11.16A to H)

■ Criteria for diagnosis

- A flat macule or slightly raised mamillated plaque that is larger than most "common" nevi (at least 5 mm) with irregular pigmentation and ill-defined "fuzzy" borders
- Melanocytes within the epidermis that vary moderately in size and shape and are distributed in a lentiginous pattern (single cells along the sides of epidermal rete and the epidermis between adjacent rete) and irregularly shaped "bridging" nests (Figs 11.16A to C)
- Melanocytes confined to the dermoepidermal junction (junctional variant) or extending into the papillary dermis as nests, cords or single cells (compound variant) (Fig. 11.16D)
- Extension of the intraepidermal component beyond the dermal component ("shouldering") when compound (Fig. 11.16E)
- Fibrosis or sclerosis of the papillary dermis, accentuated around the sides of rete ("concentric fibroplasia") or at their base ("lamellar fibroplasia") (Fig. 11.16F)
- Lymphohistiocytic inflammation within the papillary dermis.

■ Differential diagnosis

- Zitelli's nevus
- Malignant melanoma (superficial spreading type or lentiginous type)
- Melanoma arising within a nevus.

■ Pitfalls

- When cytologic or architectural abnormalities are pronounced ("dysplasia"), differentiation from melanoma arising within a nevus or lentiginous melanoma may be very difficult.

■ Pearls

- When histopathologic features of a "pre-existing nevus" are seen in association with malignant melanomas, they often resemble this type of nevus, suggesting that like Zitelli's nevi, Clark's nevi may have a greater risk of giving rise to melanoma than other nevus variants
- A traumatized (or "irritated") nevus may have a few melanocytes above the basal layer, but this should not be misinterpreted as melanoma
- Some melanomas have been convincingly documented to arise within pre-existing Clark's nevi
- On the face, except around the hairline, Clark's nevi are very uncommon and melanoma (especially lentigo maligna melanoma) must be very carefully excluded
- In severely sun-damaged skin, distinction between a Clark's nevus and lentigo maligna melanoma may be very difficult
- On occasions in elderly patients, what appears to be a Clark's nevus may in fact be a lentiginous melanoma.

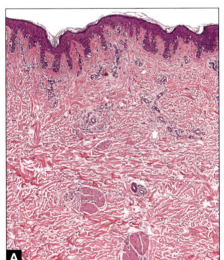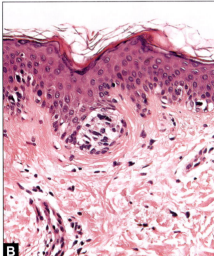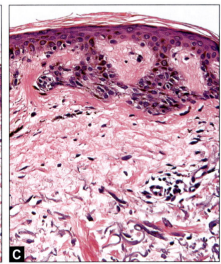

Figs 11.16A to C

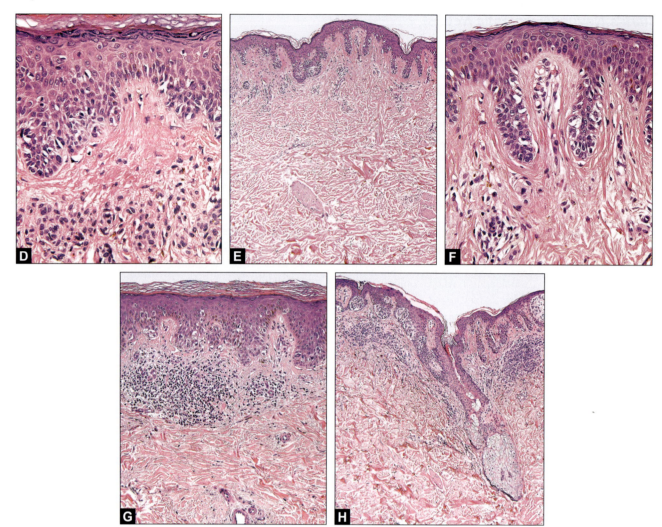

Figs 11.16A to H: Clark's nevus (Dysplastic nevus), Junctional pattern. (A) Melanocytes are increased in number along the dermoepidermal junction. Most are present within the basal layer of the epidermis. Some of the cells are arranged within nests, but other are distributed as solitary units. When significant portions of the nevus are composed of singly disposed melanocytes, this is referred to as a "lentiginous pattern"; (B) The nevus cells vary in size, shape, and nuclear chromatin density, but the cytologic atypia is usually less than that of malignant melanomas; (C) Clark's nevus (Dysplastic nevus). Bridging of melanocytic nests at the dermoepidermal junction is a characteristic feature; (D) Clark's nevus (Dysplastic nevus), Compound pattern. In compound variants of Clark's nevi, there are dermal nevus cells, many of which are identical to their intraepidermal counterparts. When compound, the nevus cells within the upper dermis may be relatively similar in size and morphology to those within the epidermis. In some cases, maturation and dispersion are less obvious than in nevi with a Zitelli's or Unna's pattern; (E) Clark's nevus (Dysplastic nevus). "Shoulders" are characteristic of Clark's nevi, meaning that intraepidermal nevus cells extend peripherally beyond the nevus cells within the dermis. In this image, the dermal component is present within the left one-third of the field, while the intraepidermal component (the "shoulder") extends far beyond it to the right; (F) Clark's nevus (Dysplastic nevus), Junctional pattern. Lamellar fibrosis of the papillary dermis is a helpful clue to the diagnosis of a Clark's nevus; (G) Inflammatory cells distributed along the junction are a common finding; (H) Clark's and Zitelli's patterns in combination. This lesion has the cytologic and architectural features of a Clark's (dysplastic) nevus, including bridging of nests and cytoatypia, but the dermal component has a Zitelli pattern (superficial congenital pattern) in which nevus cells extend into the reticular dermis in close association with adnexal structures.

Nevus Spilus (Figs 11.17A to C)

■ Criteria for diagnosis

- A large macule with varying pigmentation, imparting a "speckled" or "spotted" appearance clinically
- Histopathologically, a nevus with a lentiginous pattern that appears discontiguous due to "skip" areas—regions in which the nevus is either inconspicuous or altogether absent (Fig. 11.17A).

■ Differential diagnosis

- Partially regressed malignant melanoma or regressed nevus
- Two or more adjacent nevi.

■ Pitfalls

- In some cases, histopathologic features do not allow definitive distinction between a nevus with regression or multiple discrete nevi located in close proximity to one another

- Partial sampling is common in nevus spilus, since they are often large and partially regressed melanoma or melanoma arising within a nevus may be difficult to exclude.

■ Pearls

- The clinical impression of a nevus spilus by an experienced dermatologist in conjunction with the typical histopathologic findings is the most reliable means of making the correct diagnosis
- Unlike partially regressed melanoma, the "skip" areas of a nevus spilus do not exhibit fibrosis of the papillary dermis, effacement of the normal epidermal rete architecture or a complete absence of junctional melanocytes.

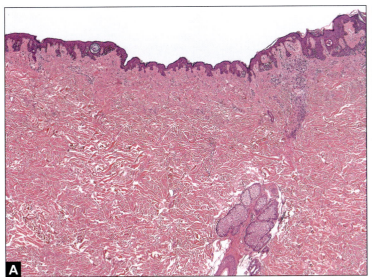
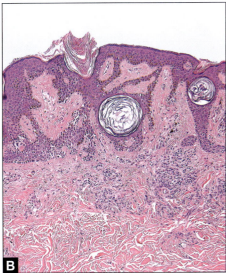
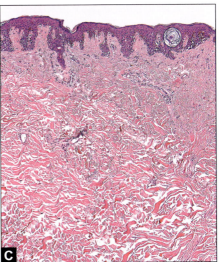

Figs 11.17A to C: Nevus spilus. (A) These are uncommon nevi with a lentiginous pattern that appears discontiguous due to "skip" areas; regions in which the nevus is either inconspicuous or altogether. In this image, note that there is a lentiginous junctional nevus on the right and a compound nevus at the left, while the central region is devoid of nevus cells. This must be differentiated from regression, which is feature common in melanomas; (B) The nevus areas within a nevus spilus may be compound as in this high power image from the right side of the lesion shown in Figure 11.17A; (C) This image (the left side of Figure 11.17A) shows the junctional component of the nevus.

Combined Nevus (Nevus with Phenotypic Heterogeneity) (Figs 11.18A to D)

■ Criteria for diagnosis

- A pigmented lesion that is clinically symmetrical and circumscribed, but varies in pigment distribution and color
- An otherwise typical nevus that contains one or more distinct cell types or architectural patterns within the dermal component.

■ Differential diagnosis

- Melanoma arising within a nevus, especially a Zitelli's or Mark's (congenital pattern) nevus
- Dermal nodule ("proliferative" nodule) within a Zitelli's or Mark's nevus
- Nevoid melanoma
- Spitz's nevus, deep penetrating nevus or blue nevus.

■ Pitfalls

- The heterogeneity may be mistaken for melanoma arising within a nevus.

■ Pearls

- Most combined nevi contain only two distinct cell populations
- The most common presentation is an otherwise typical Unna's, Miescher's or Zitelli's nevus that contains a discrete subpopulation of cells within the dermis that are more heavily pigmented and either slightly larger and more epithelioid (pigmented epithelioid cell component) or spindled (blue nevus, like component), often accompanied by melanophages
- Less common are cells similar to those of Spitz's nevi or deep penetrating nevi
- The distinctive subpopulation is almost always confined to the dermis, a feature helpful in excluding melanoma, since melanoma arising within the dermal component of a nevus is very unusual
- Overall symmetry, circumscription and maturation are maintained, cytologic atypia is not severe and mitotic figures should be absent or very rare (fewer than one per high power field).

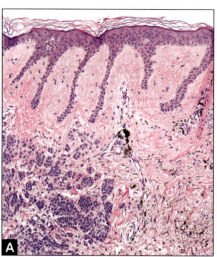

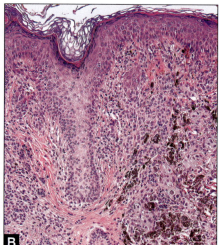

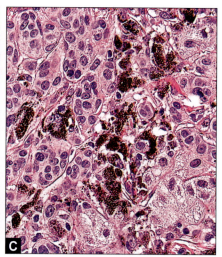

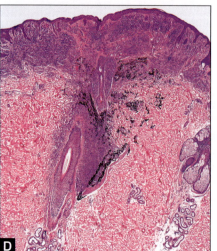

Figs 11.18A to D: (A) Combined nevus with features of a Zitelli's nevus at the left and a Tieche's (common blue) nevus. This is one of the most commonly encountered types of combined nevus; (B) Combined nevus with features of a Zitelli's pattern nevus and pigmented epithelioid cells within the dermis. This type of combined nevus may cause concern since the maturation and dispersion that characterize many benign nevi are interrupted by clusters of larger cells; (C) This image is a higher magnification of the epithelioid cells. Careful inspection for mitotic figures or a junctional component resembling melanoma may be warranted in some cases, but within the context of a nevus with otherwise benign features, it is of no concern; (D) Combined nevus with features of a Zitelli's nevus and a Seab's (deep penetrating) nevus. The upper portions of the nevus resemble a typical Zitelli's nevus, but at the base, the nevus cells become fusiform and pigmented, features of a Seab's nevus (see below for a description of Seab's nevi).

Nevi with Inflammatory Reactions, Site-Specific Features and Other Incidental Findings

The following are not specific nevus subtypes but are reaction patterns or variations that may occur within most of the subtypes described above.

Nevus with Sutton's Reaction (Halo Nevus)

- A symmetrical and circumscribed pigmented macule or papule surrounded by a symmetrical zone of depigmentation or "halo"
- Histopathologic features of a nevus (essentially any type) accompanied by a variably dense lymphohistiocytic infiltrate, that is distributed evenly and uniformly throughout the nevus (Fig. 11.19A)
- Predilection for teenagers and young adults; sometimes multiple

- Nevus cells may be obvious or may be extensively obscured by the infiltrate (Figs 11.19A and B)
- In established lesions, the nevus may be almost entirely absent, with only a few residual melanocytes and may be difficult to differentiate from a lichenoid keratosis
- The type of nevus may be difficult to discern or may be obvious
- A "halo" is a clinical description; not all nevi with Sutton's reaction exhibit a clinically evident halo
- Distinction from a regressing malignant melanoma is crucial; an inflammatory infiltrate that is uniformly distributed throughout the lesion within both the horizontal and vertical planes and is well demarcated at both the sides and base of the lesion is an important clue that the lesion is a nevus rather than a melanoma
- Marked variability within the distribution of the inflammation (i.e. asymmetry) should prompt careful examination for features of melanoma.

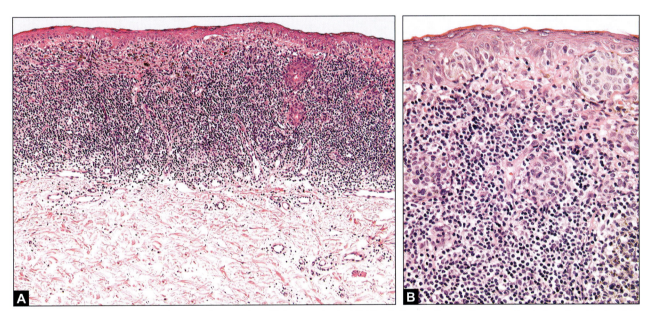

Figs 11.19A and B: (A) Nevus with Sutton's reaction (Halo reaction). (A) The infiltrate is usually comprised almost entirely of lymphocytes and these cells may partially obscure the nevus cells. Note that the infiltrate is uniform in its distribution across the base of the nevus and has a relatively distinct, even-contoured interface with the underlying dermis; (B) The infiltrating lymphocytes usually extend around and between the nevus cells. On occasion the nevus cells may appear slightly enlarge, but in general the presence of inflammation does not significantly alter the cytologic features

Nevus with Meyerson's Reaction (Eczematous Nevus)

- A nevus accompanied by epidermal spongiosis and a variable inflammatory infiltrate (Fig. 11.20)
- Inflammatory changes may obscure portions of the nevus or be accompanied by reactive changes within the nevus architecture and cytologic features that occasionally cause an otherwise banal nevus to appear atypical.

Nevi on the Breast, Genital Region and Intertriginous Areas

- Nevi on intertriginous skin and the skin of the breast and genital areas often exhibit particular features not seen when they occur at other sites ("special site nevi" or "nevi with site-specific" features) (Fig. 11.21A)
- Most are Unna's nevi, Zitelli's nevi or Clark's nevi with increased junctional architectural and cytologic heterogeneity that may prompt concern for melanoma or melanoma arising within a pre-existing nevus
- The most commonly encountered "atypical" features are: (1) increased bridging of junctional nests, (2) dyshesive nests, (3) increased lentiginous growth and (4) "skip areas" in which nevus cells are inconspicuous or absent, imparting a discontiguous pattern (Figs 11.21B and C)
- Overall symmetry, circumscription and maturation are the best evidence that the lesion is a nevus rather than a melanoma.

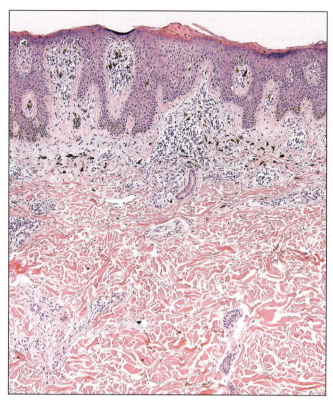

Fig. 11.20: Nevus with Meyerson's reaction/eczematous nevus. At scanning magnification, the nevus may be inconspicuous relative to the spongiotic dermatitis that accompanies it

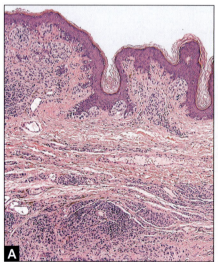
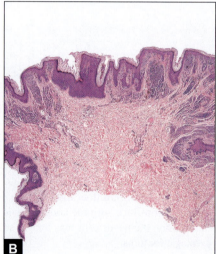
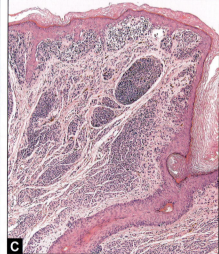

Figs 11.21A to C: Genital region nevus. (A) Lentiginous growth of the type usually seen in Clark's/dysplastic nevi is common in nevi from the genital, breast and intertriginous areas; (B) The architecture is reminiscent of an Unna's nevus but the balance and symmetry are altered by variability in the distribution of the nests. Nests predominate, but there is a zone just to the left of center in which melanocytes are inconspicuous or altogether absent (a "skip area"); (C) Two "atypical" features commonly encountered in nevi from genital and intertriginous skin are present here: (1) bridging of nests at the dermoepidermal junction and (2) dyshesion of the nested cells.

Nevi on Acral Skin (Palms and Soles, Occasionally Elbows and Knees) (Figs 11.22A to D)

- Acral nevi may have more irregular borders clinically and some exhibit atypical histopathologic features including (Fig. 11.22A): (1) ill-defined peripheral borders (Fig.11.22C), (2) increased distribution of single melanocytes above the basal layer ("pagetoid" growth pattern) (Fig.11.23D), (3) asymmetry and (4) vertically elongated spindled or dendritic cells

- The histopathologic features of acral nevi are influenced by the plane of section; the ill-defined borders and asymmetry are most prominent in sections taken parallel to dermoglyphics (fingerprint lines)
- Uniformity of the melanocytes and a lack of inflammation favor a benign acral nevus; marked cytologic atypia and dense inflammation suggest the possibility of acral melanoma
- The key pitfall is over-interpretation of these features as evidence of malignancy, but occasional examples are sufficiently atypical that definitive exclusion of melanoma is difficult or impossible.

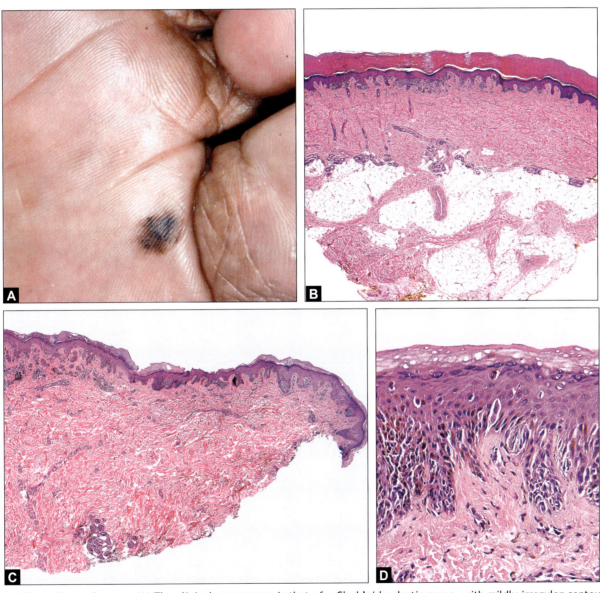

Figs 11.22A to D: Acral nevus. (A) The clinical appearance is that of a Clark's/dysplastic nevus, with mildly irregular contours and slight variability in pigmentation; (B) The appearance at scanning magnification is that of a Clark's nevus; (C) The "shoulders" of an acral nevus may be particularly broad and the peripheral border indistinct relative to nevi at other sites. Note the small nests and single cells that extend to the peripheral margin of this specimen; (D) Some acral nevi contain melanocytes within the upper epidermis. This can sometimes simulate the "pagetoid spread" of a melanoma.

Nevi on the Ear (Figs 11.23A to D)

- Nevi occurring on and around the ear exhibit certain "atypical" features that may simulate some melanomas (Fig.11.23A)

- The most common are: (1) poor circumscription (Fig.11.23B); (2) lateral extension of the junctional component beyond that within the dermis (shouldering); (3) elongated, bridging rete with horizontally oriented nests (Fig.11.23D); (4) some increased cytologic atypia.

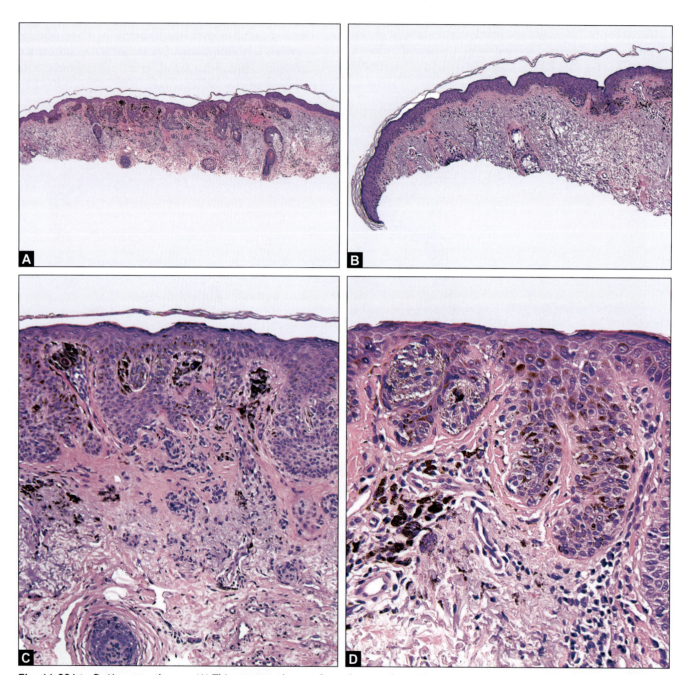

Figs 11.23A to D: Nevus on the ear. (A) This compound nevus from the ear of an older man has features of a Clark's/dysplastic nevus but also some findings that make distinction from melanoma difficult, particularly given the severe dermatoheliosis. Such lesions should be evaluated with great care; (B) Like other "special sites", nevi on the ear have a tendency to lack well-demarcated peripheral borders. Note that lesional melanocytes arranged in small groups or even as single cells extend to the margin of this biopsy; (C) Most of the melanocytes are arranged within nests in the center of the lesion, but the nests tend to be situated between individual rete rather than at their tips; (D) Elongation of the epidermal rete and lamellar fibroplasia of the dermis are common findings.

Malignant Melanoma Arising within a Compound Nevus (Figs 11.24A to D)

■ *Criteria for diagnosis*

- A pigmented lesion that exhibits features of a benign nevus, but contains a distinct region that satisfies criteria for malignant melanoma.

■ *Differential diagnosis*

- Combined nevus
- Clark's nevus with severe architectural and cytologic atypia
- Dermal nodule ('proliferative' nodule) within a Zitelli's or Mark's congenital nevus
- Nevoid melanoma.

■ *Pitfalls*

- Careful inspection of the entire dermal component is warranted to determine: (1) if the melanoma is restricted to the epidermis or involves the dermis as well (or if the entire lesion is actually a melanoma rather than melanoma arising in a nevus) and (2) the depth of the dermal melanoma component if present.

■ *Pearls*

- The most distinctive feature is a population of cells within the junctional component (with or without similar cells in the underlying dermis) that exhibit greater cytologic and architectural atypia than the surrounding nevus

- A clinical history of a pre-existing nevus that suddenly changes or enlarges should prompt careful examination for melanoma arising within a nevus
- Finding histopathologic features (e.g. a focus of inflammation or hemorrhage consistent with trauma) that might explain the changes observed clinically is often helpful in excluding melanoma and should be carefully sought
- Unlike a combined nevus, the atypical cytologic and architectural differences are almost always evident within the junctional component and the overall symmetry is disrupted
- A junctional component that becomes predominantly lentiginous rather than nested, contains atypical melanocytes within the spinous and graunular cell layers (pagetoid spread) and exhibits markedly increased cytologic atypia are the most convincing features of melanoma arising within a nevus
- The earliest manifestation is often a lentiginous growth pattern that is more pronounced at one lateral border of the nevus (i.e. a longer "shoulder" on one side).

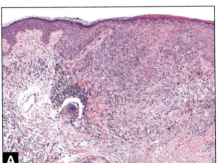
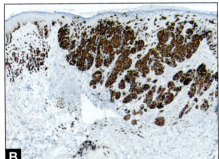
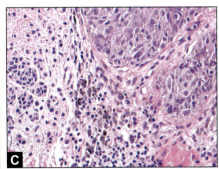
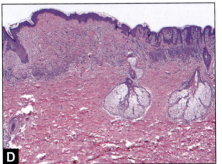

Figs 11.24A to D: Melanoma arising within a nevus. (A) Compare the left and right side of the image. At the left of the field are small nevus cells arranged in nests within the dermis, likely the remnants of a Zitelli's nevus. On the right is a melanoma characterized by markedly enlarged and atypical melanocytes; (B) The difference in cell size and architecture is highlighted by immunohistochemistry for Melan-A/Mart-1; (C) Higher magnification reveals the overt difference in size between the nevus cells and those of the melanoma; (D) In this example, melanoma (left side of field) is arising within a Clark's nevus (right).

COMPOUND OR INTRADERMAL NEO-PLASMS COMPOSED OF SPINDLED AND/OR EPITHELIOID MELANOCYTES: SPITZ'S AND REED'S NEVI

Spitz's Nevus (Nevus with Spindled and/or Epithelioid Cells) (Figs 11.25A to D)

■ *Criteria for diagnosis*

- Clinically, symmetrical papule or dome-shaped nodule (Fig. 11.25A)
- Large spindled, round or oval cells with abundant cytoplasm imparting an "epithelioid" appearance (Fig. 11.25B)
- Cells arranged in discrete nests and as single cells; nests often separated from surrounding epidermis by clefts (Fig. 11.25C)
- Epidermal hyperplasia with an acanthotic spinous layer, squamatization of the basal layer and elongated, often angular rete.

■ *Differential diagnosis*

- Melanoma with "Spitzoid" features
- Superficial spreading melanoma
- Combined nevus with "Spitzoid" component
- Reed's nevus
- Deep penetrating nevus.

■ *Pitfalls*

- Some have initial period of rapid growth that may raise clinical suspicion for melanoma
- Occasionally mistaken clinically (and rarely, histopathologically) for a pyogenic granuloma or other neoplasm, since many are red or pink in Caucasians and lack the pigmentation of other types of nevi

- Ulceration due to excoriation may occur, especially in infants and children, simulating the ulceration of melanoma
- Cytologic and architectural variability, epithelioid cells within the dermis and mitotic figures are frequent and must not be overinterpreted.

■ *Pearls*

- May occur in all races, but have been characterized predominantly in Caucasians
- Large size (> 1 cm) is not uncommon
- Pale pink globules ("Kamino bodies") are a common feature, especially in larger lesions and are a helpful clue to diagnosis, since they do not occur in melanoma
- Kamino bodies are globules of basement membrane material and stain with Periodic acid-Schiff Diastase, laminin, and type IV collagen
- Early lesions may contain only a few epithelioid cells along the dermoepidermal junction; some are multinucleated.
- Most are sharply demarcated at their peripheral borders, have a "wedge-shaped" architecture within the dermis and exhibit maturation and dispersion of cells within the dermis (progressive diminution in size of nests and individual cells, increased spacing of cells, loss of pigment) (Fig.11.25D)
- Many variants have been described, including desmoplastic (sclerotic or hyalinized dermal collagen), angiomatoid (prominent capillary sized vessels within the surrounding dermis), etc
- Lymphohistiocytic infiltrates may be dense in early lesions, but usually become inconspicuous in fully evolved nevi
- Some overlap considerably with Reed's nevi and at least some Reed's nevi share somatic genetic similarities, suggesting that the two lesions are closely-related.

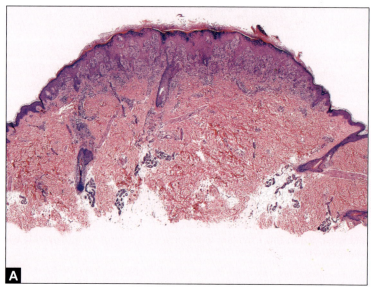

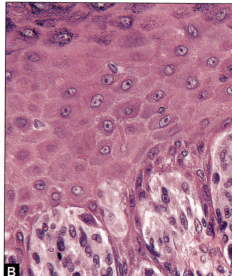

Figs 11.25A and B

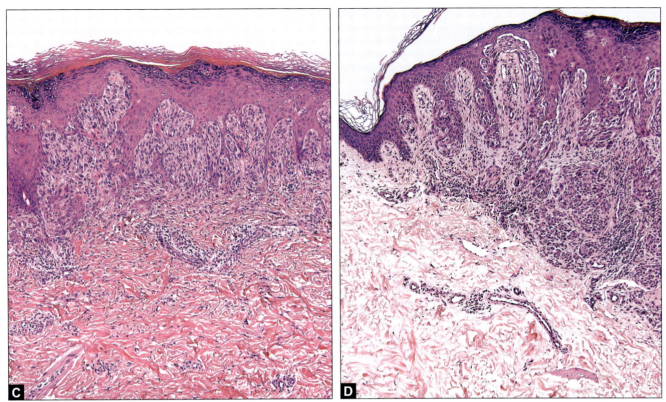

Figs 11.25A to D: Spitz's nevus. (A) A "classic" Spitz's nevus has most of the features of other benign melanocytic lesions. At scanning magnification, there is a balanced/symmetrical silhouette; (B) Spitz's nevus cells are distinct in that they are larger than most nevus cells and have an epithelioid and/or spindled shape; (C) Although nests vary in size and shape, the melanocyte nests predominate over melanocytes disposed as single cells; (D) The lesion is well demarcated at its periphery.

Reed's Nevus
(Pigmented Spindle Cell Nevus)

■ *Criteria for diagnosis*

- Dark brown or black homogeneously pigmented symmetrical macule, papule or dome-shaped nodule (Fig. 11.26A)
- Symmetrical, circumscribed collection of spindled or elongated fusiform pigmented melanocytes arranged in vertical nests at the dermoepidermal junction and within the papillary dermis (Figs 11.26B to D)
- Melanin pigment and numerous melanophages in papillary dermis.

■ *Differential diagnosis*

- Nevoid melanoma
- Congenital pattern nevus
- Compound Clark's nevus.

■ *Pitfalls*

- Malignant melanoma is often a clinical concern due to dark pigmentation and tendency for rapid initial growth

- Some cases contain several (or occasionally many) melanocytes above the dermoepidermal junction and a few mitotic figures, raising concern for melanoma.

■ *Pearls*

- Predilection for children and young adults; more common in females, especially on the thigh
- Lesions are often biopsied, since they may develop quickly and are darkly pigmented
- By dermatoscopic examination, a "starburst" pattern (pigmented streaks radiating from the center) is characteristic
- Some cases overlap considerably with pigmented variants of Spitz's nevus.

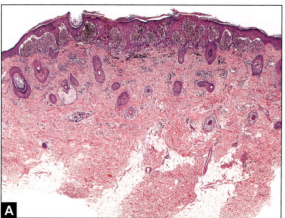
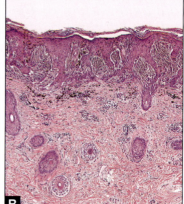
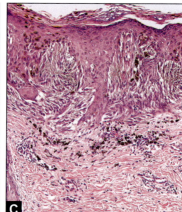
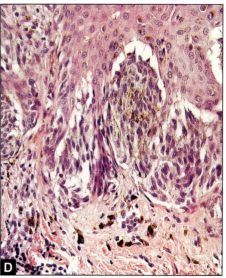

Figs 11.26A to D: Reed's nevus. (A) The silhouette is that of a benign lesion. It is balanced/symmetrical and well-demarcated at its periphery; (B) The lesional melanocytes are spindled and contain abundant cytoplasmic melanin pigment; (C) These nevi are usually confined to the epidermis or, at most, the papillary dermis. Often, however, there are numerous melanophages across the base of the lesion; (D) The prominence of the spindled shape of the cells may vary among cases and even within a given lesion, but usually spindled cells in nests such as those shown here are an obvious component.

PREDOMINANTLY DERMAL TUMORS COMPOSED OF PIGMENT SYNTHESIZING MELANOCYTES: THE "BLUE NEVUS" VARIANTS

This category represents a group of melanocytic tumors recognized by (1) a tendency to be darkly pigmented on clinical examination (often with a bluish hue, but sometimes dark brown or black); (2) localization predominantly or entirely within the dermis and (3) melanocytes with cytoplasmic melanin pigment admixed with numerous melanophages.

Beyond these commonalities, the features may vary markedly. The Tieche's variant or common blue nevus is usually a relatively superficial collection of pigmented spindled and dendritic melanocytes, while the Carney's variant (epithelioid blue nevus) is often densely cellular, involves most of the dermis and may extend into the subcutis. Spindled or fusiform cells may predominate in some types (Jadassohn's nevus), and pigmented cells and melanophages may be distributed focally in some cases (Seab's nevus).

Tieche's Nevus (Common Blue Nevus) (Figs 11.27A to D)

■ *Criteria for diagnosis*

- Blue, gray or black papule or well-demarcated macule
- Relatively circumscribed dermal collection of slender fusiform, spindled and dendritic melanocytes, some of which contain melanin pigment, admixed with a variable number of melanophages within a sclerotic dermis (Figs 11.27A and B).

■ *Differential diagnosis*

- Dermatofibroma
- Postinflammatory pigmentation (when small or paucicellular) (Fig. 11.27C)
- Combined nevus.

■ *Pitfalls*

- Some cases are extensively sclerotic and paucicellular, with only rare lesional cells
- Melanophages may be numerous and obscure the nevus cells.
- Very rarely, metastatic melanoma may simulate a Tieche's nevus
- Cells often retain HMB-45 expression (a feature uncommon in most other nevi).

■ *Pearls*

- Architectural features sometimes have a congenital pattern similar to Zitelli's nevus, with increased density of nevus cells around adnexal structures and nerves
- Dorsum of hand, foot, wrist and head are common anatomic sites
- The "Mongolian spot", Ota's nevus and Ito's nevus are large macular nevi that involve the lumbosacral region, segment of skin innervated by the first and second branch of the trigeminal nerve and the shoulder and/or upper arm respectively, that manifest in early childhood and often have cytologic features similar to Tieche's nevus
- The classical Tieche's common blue nevus does not have a junctional component; lesions with a junctional component are better classified as "combined nevus"
- When paucicellular variants are encountered, S100 immunohistochemistry may be helpful in confirming that nevus cells are present.

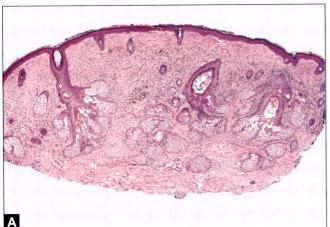 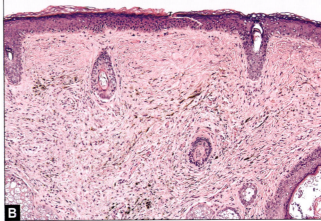

Figs 11.27A and B

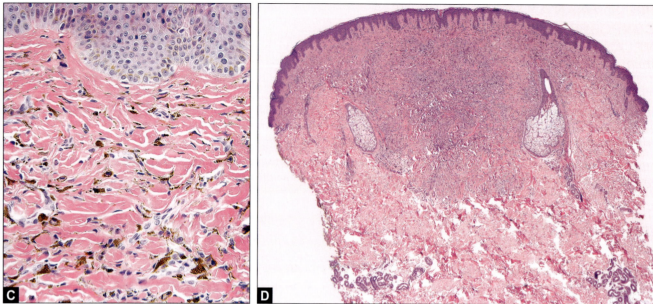

Figs 11.27A to D: Tieche's nevus (common blue nevus). (A) In its most common form, the Tieche's nevus is an entirely dermal collection of small, spindled to ovoid melanocytes with cytoplasmic melanin pigment. The edges of the nevus are usually fairly distinct; (B) The spindled and ovoid cells contain melanin pigment, but melanophages are usually numerous as well; (C) In many cases, thick, sclerotic collagen bundles surround the nevus cells and macrophages. Some may be mistaken for scars or keloids with postinflammatory hyperpigmentation; (D) Tieche's nevi vary widely in size from those that are barely perceptible (simulating postinflammatory hyperpigmentation) to lesions such as this, which extends well into the reticular dermis.

Seab's Nevus (Deep Penetrating Nevus)

■ *Criteria for diagnosis*

- A solitary, circumscribed, blue, dark brown or black papule or nodule (usually less than 1 cm in diameter)
- A "wedge-shaped" collection of relatively large fusiform to spindled melanocytes that contain varying amounts of cytoplasmic melanin pigment, along with a variable number of melanophages (Fig. 11.28A)
- A relatively inconspicuous intraepidermal component in most cases (65–80%), that is often separated from the dermal component by an uninvolved papillary dermis
- Neoplastic cells arranged in fascicles that extend along adnexal structures and neurovascular bundles into the deep dermis or superficial subcutis (Figs 11.28B and C)
- No more than one mitotic figure per 10 high power fields.

■ *Differential diagnosis*

- Other blue nevus variants
- Spitz's nevus, pigmented type, with deep dermal involvement
- Combined nevus
- Blue nevus, like melanoma.

■ *Pitfalls*

- Metastatic melanomas or heavily pigmented nodular melanomas may occasionally resemble Seab's nevus
- Some cases contain expansile nodules that may be confused with melanoma.

■ *Pearls*

- Since their original description, Seab's (deep penetrating) nevi have been shown to have features that overlap with Carney's and Tieche's nevi, supporting their inclusion within the spectrum of blue nevi
- Strong and diffuse expression of HMB45 is typical (as it is in Carney's and Tieche's nevi)
- The features overlap (extensively, in some cases) with pigmented Spitz's nevi, predilection for the face, upper trunk and proximal extremities of young adults
- The clinical features resemble those of Tieche's nevus (blue nevus)
- If the clinical impression is malignant melanoma and the lesion is in an older adult, melanoma should be suspected
- Seab's nevi are rarely seen after age of 30 years; a similar appearing lesion in an older person requires very careful exclusion of melanoma.
- May be compound or intradermal
- The term "superficial variant of deep penetrating nevus" has been used for similar lesions that are limited to the upper dermis (this confusing terminology is one reason for the eponymous designation as Seab's nevus, in our opinion)
- Expansile tumor lobules may extend into the subcutis, a feature also seen in some cellular blue nevi
- Although, patchy melanin pigmentation may also be seen in other types of nevi and in malignant melanomas, there is often a "checkerboard" distribution of the pigmented areas in Seab's nevus
- As in Spitz's tumors, mitotic figures may be apparent (but should be less than $1/mm^2$; more than 2 per 10 high power fields suggests melanoma).

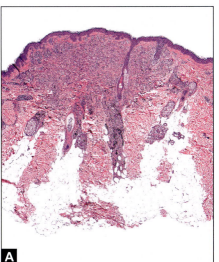 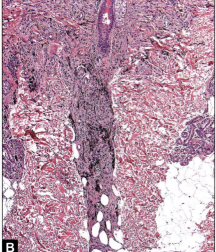 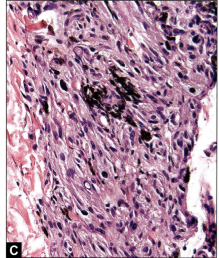

Figs 11.28A to C: Seab's nevus (deep penetrating nevus). (A) As originally described, Seab's "deep penetrating nevus" was defined as a "wedge-shaped" collection of relatively large fusiform to spindled melanocytes, some of which containedmelanin pigment, that extended into the deep dermis or even the upper subcutis; (B) The base of this lesion consists of pigmented cells and extends into the upper subcutaneous adipose tissue; (C) The cells are usually ovoid, fusiform or spindled, and by definition they must predominantly be arranged within fascicles. Haphazard distribution of the pigmented cells is characteristic.

Carney's Nevus (Epithelioid Blue Nevus, Pigmented Epithelioid Melanocytoma)

■ *Criteria for diagnosis*

- Clinically symmetrical, dark blue, brown or black, dome-shaped nodule, usually larger than 1 centimeter
- Oval or wedge-shaped dermal collection of large, round or polygonal "epithelioid" melanocytes with dense cytoplasmic melanin pigment, large vesicular nuclei and prominent nucleoli (Figs 11.29A and B)
- Dense infiltrate of heavily pigmented melanophages (Fig. 11.29C)
- Variable number of less conspicuous spindled and dendritic melanocytes, often at the periphery of the epithelioid component (Fig. 11.29D)
- No necrosis and mitotic figures absent or very rare.

■ *Differential diagnosis*

- Metastatic melanoma
- Melanoma arising within a blue nevus

- Seab's nevus
- Jadassohn's nevus.

■ *Pitfalls*

- Pigmentation of the lesional cells may obscure cytologic details
- Dense aggregates of melanophages may obscure much of the tumor in some cases
- Melanophages may be misinterpreted as lesional cells.

■ *Pearls*

- May be either sporadic or associated with Carney's complex
- Some authors advocate the term "pigmented epithelioid melanocytoma" and emphasize the tendency of the lesions to involve regional lymph nodes; this tendency clearly exists, but is not uncommon in other types of nevi.

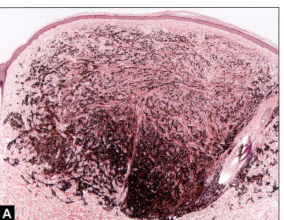
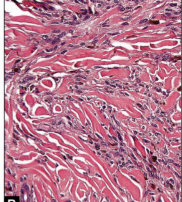
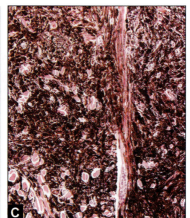
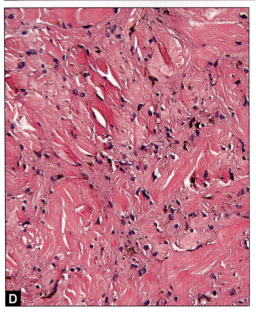

Figs 11.29A to D: Carney's nevus (epithelioid blue nevus). (A) The typical appearance at low magnification is an oval or wedge-shaped dermal collection of cells with dense cytoplasmic melanin pigment; (B) Round or polygonal "epithelioid" melanocytes make up the majority of the lesional cells; (C) Heavily pigmented melanophages may occupy large portions of the lesion. They may be difficult to differentiate from melanocytes without immunohistochemistry, and they often obscure at least some of the lesional cells; (D) In addition to the epithelioid component, at least a few areas should resemble a Tieche's nevus, with smaller spindled and ovoid melanocytes and sclerotic collagen bundles.

Jadassohn's Nevus (Cellular Blue Nevus, Blue Nevus with Spindle Cell Component) (Figs 11.30A to C)

■ Criteria for diagnosis

- Blue or black, dome-shaped papules or nodules
- Distinct nodule of fusiform or spindled cells with cytoplasm that is clear to pale pink, some with cytoplasmic melanin pigment, within an otherwise typical Tieche's or Carney's nevus (Fig. 11.30A)
- The cytologically distinct population of lesional cells may be arranged in rounded nests, surrounded by fibrous trabeculae (so-called alveolar pattern) or as fascicles of fusiform and spindled cells (fascicular pattern) or a combination of these patterns
- Less than one mitotic figure per square millimeter.

■ Differential diagnosis

- Spitz's nevus (pigmented variants)
- Other blue nevus variants, especially Tieche's and Carney's types
- Blue nevus–like melanoma
- Nodular melanoma.

■ Pitfalls

- The distinct fusiform/spindle cell population may simulate melanoma arising within a nevus
- There may be cystic degeneration, a myxoid or hyalinized stroma or hemorrhage, simulating the necrosis (necrosis en masse) of a malignant melanoma.

■ Pearls

- Usually localized to reticular dermis, often with deep extension
- Lobules that "bulge" into the subcutis (dumbbell shaped nodules) are common, but a rounded, well-demarcated, inferior margin is usually present, unlike deep nodular melanoma
- Lesional cells usually express HMB45 (like Tieche's, Carney's and Seab's nevi)
- Rare mitotic figures may be evident, but should not exceed $1/mm^2$
- Atypical mitotic figures, a mitotic index of more than $3/mm^2$ and tumor necrosis are features that favor melanoma.

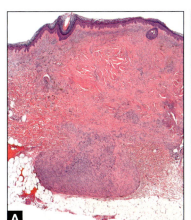 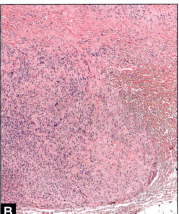 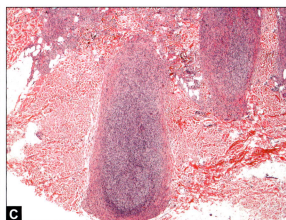

Figs 11.30A to C: Jadassohn's nevus. (A) The key feature is a well-formed nodule of fusiform or spindled cells with clear or pale pink cytoplasmic, some also containing melanin pigment, within a lesion that otherwise resembles a Tieche's or Carney's nevus; (B) The nodule has well circumscribed borders and the cells are embedded within sclerotic collagen; (C) The nodules may be solitary, but on occasion they are multiple.

Masson's Nevus (Neuronevus of Masson)

◼ *Criteria for diagnosis*

- Cytologic features of a Jadassohn's nevus along with areas of neural or "Schwannian' differentiation; absence of the well-formed nodules of a Jadassohn's nevus (Figs 11.31A and B)
- Fascicular architecture(Fig. 11.31C)
- Growth along nerves
- Areas typical of Carney's or Tieche's nevus surrounding the spindled areas or at the periphery of the tumor.

◼ *Differential diagnosis*

- Spindle cell/neurotropic melanoma
- Blue nevus–like melanoma
- Desmoplastic melanoma
- Neural tumors (especially schwannoma and malignant peripheral nerve sheath tumor)
- Other mesenchymal spindle cell tumors.

◼ *Pitfalls*

- The dense cellularity, spindled morphology and predilection for growth around nerves raises concern for malignant melanoma
- Prominent vessels with thickened hyalinized walls are sometimes present, a feature shared by schwannomas
- Degenerative change ("ancient change") is occasionally seen.

◼ *Pearls*

- Masson's nevus is essentially a rare variant of cellular blue nevus that contains spindled "Schwannian" cells arranged in fascicles and conspicuous distribution along nerves (Fig. 11.31C)
- Distinction from melanoma may be difficult, but the marked pleomorphism, high mitotic rate and necrosis usually encountered in malignant melanomas are absent
- Melanin pigment is usually present in surrounding blue nevus–like areas (unlike spindle cell /neurotropic melanoma).

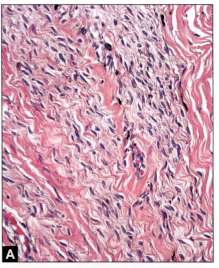
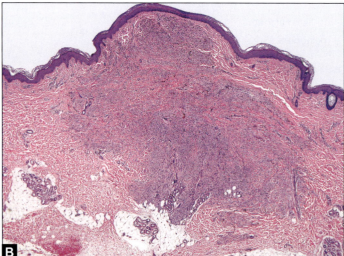
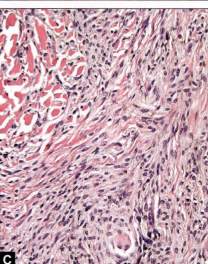

Figs 11.31A to C: Masson's nevus (neuronevus). (A) The presence of smaller spindled cells with "wavy" or "buckled" nuclei, believed to represent Schwann cell differentiation, are a defining feature; (B) The nevus is quite cellular, but well formed nodules of the type seen in a Jadassohn's nevus are absent; (C) The cells are predominantly spindled or fusiform in shape and many are arranged in long fascicles

Melanocytic Tumors of Uncertain Malignant Potential: Atypical Variants of Spitz's Nevi and the Blue Nevus Variants

Criteria for diagnosis

- A compound melanocytic tumor, with spindled, epithelioid or fusiform cells resembling a Spitz's nevus or blue nevus variant, but with one or more atypical architectural or cytologic features including:
- Ulceration (Fig.11.32A)
- Asymmetry/imbalance (Fig.11.32B)
- Poor circumscription
- Pagetoid spread (Fig. 11.32C)
- Syncytial dermal melanocytes
- Lack of maturation (Fig.11.32D)
- Necrotic melanocytes
- Marked cytologic atypia
- Increased mitotic index
- Mitotic figures near the base of the lesion
- Inflammatory reaction.

Differential diagnosis

- Malignant melanoma
- Melanocytic nevus.

Pitfalls

- Most histopathologic features useful for differentiating benign from malignant melanocytic neoplasms are not applicable to this subset of tumors.

Pearls

- In the largest study of these tumors by a panel of experts, only three histopathologic features were predictive of aggressive behavior (Fig. 11.32E):
  1. Presence of mitotic figures
  2. Mitotic figures near the base of the lesion
  3. Inflammatory reaction
- Criteria useful in the distinction of benign from malignant melanocytic tumors do not appear to apply in this group of tumors
- The tumors included in this group have features of Spitz's nevi and blue nevus variants (especially the Carney and Jadassohn types), but less important than the nevus subtype they resemble is their differentiation from conventional malignant melanoma
- More than 50% may involve regional lymph nodes, but distant metastasis and death from disease appears to be a rare event (or possibly one that occurs many years after initial diagnosis)
- It may be that these tumors represent a form of low-grade melanoma with potential for recurrence and involvement of regional lymph nodes, but a low tendency for distant metastasis.

Figure 11.32F shows atypical tumor with Spitz and Seab's patterns.

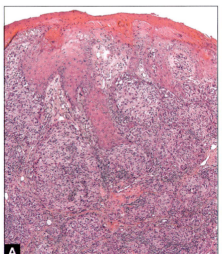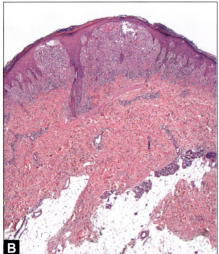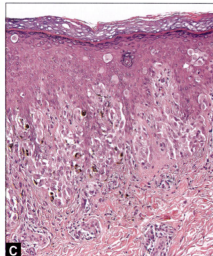

Figs 11.32A to C

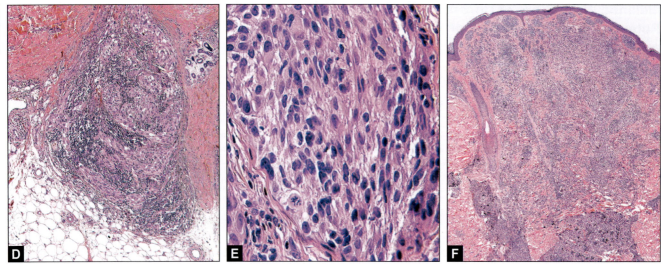

Figs 11.32A to F: Atypical Spitz tumor. (A) Ulceration is considered an atypical feature in Spitz tumors by most authorities; (B) Imbalance/asymmetry should prompt at least some concern for malignant potential; (C) Solitary melanocytes within the upper epidermis (pagetoid spread) are a feature of many atypical Spitz tumors. In an older adult, it suggests that the lesion is more likely a melanoma with "Spitzoid" features; (D) This tumor lacks maturation of the lesional melanocytes. The cells that comprise this nodule within the superficial subcutis were identical in size to those in the overlying dermis; (E) An atypical mitotic figure (bottom left) is present near the base of this tumor. In the largest study of Spitz tumors and Blue nevus variants with atypical features, only three histopathologic features were predictive of aggressive behavior: The presence of mitotic figures near the base, an increased number of mitoses and inflammation (as seen in figure 11.32D); (F) Atypical tumor with Spitz and Seab's patterns. In what could be termed an "atypical combined melanocytic tumor," this lesion resembles a Spitz tumor in the upper regions and a Seab's nevus at its base. Only one mitotic figure was evident, however, and the lesion was from a child.

COMPOUND OR INTRADERMAL NEOPLASMS COMPOSED OF MARKEDLY ATYPICAL MELANOCYTES

The major constituents of this category are melanomas. Historically, only a few major subtypes of melanoma have been recognized, including (1) Lentigo maligna melanoma; (2) Superficial spreading melanoma; (3) Nodular melanoma; (4) Acral melanoma and (5) Mucosal melanoma. These subtypes were recognized for their relatively distinct clinical, histopathologic and prognostic features. In a significant proportion of cases, however, even this basic distinction cannot be reliably made and other prognostic factors which appear are more important than histopathologic subtype. Table 11.1 shows synoptic reporting of melanoma.

Each subtype may exhibit a variety of histopathologic patterns. Until they prove to be significant prognostically, these patterns should be considered histopathologic patterns rather than clinicopathologically distinct subtypes, but they are often referred to as "histologic types". Regardless of terminology, recognizing the many patterns of melanoma may be assumed to aid in the distinction of benign from malignant lesions and in some cases, the distinction of a melanocytic neoplasm from a neoplasm of some other cell type. Table 11.2 shows staging of melanoma by pathologic characteristics.

Table 11.1: Synoptic reporting of melanoma		
Parameter	*Recommended Descriptors*	*Explanatory Notes*
Procedure type	• Biopsy, shave • Biopsy, punch • Biopsy, incisional • Excision • Re-excision	Melanomas that are transected at any margin should be noted
Tumor site	• Anatomic site (including designation as left, right or midline)	Anatomic site correlates with prognosis
Tumor size	• Greatest dimension • Additional dimensions	Required only if tumor is grossly evident
Macroscopic satellites	• Absent • Present • Indeterminate	Required only for excision specimens
Macroscopic pigmentation	• Absent • Diffuse • Patchy/Focal • Indeterminate	
Histopathologic type	• Superficial spreading melanoma • Nodular melanoma • Lentigo maligna melanoma • Acral-lentiginous melanoma • Desmoplastic and/or desmoplastic neurotropic melanoma • Melanoma arising within a blue nevus • Melanoma arising in a giant congenital nevus • Melanoma of childhood • Nevoid melanoma • Persistent melanoma • Melanoma, not otherwise classified	Current list is derived from WHO guidelines, is not exhaustive and other type of designations may be used, e.g. lentiginous melanoma If features are not characteristic of a specific type, this may simply be stated as "melanoma, type uncertain" Tumor thickness, mitotic index and ulceration usually carry greater prognostic importance than histologic subtype

Contd...

Parameter	Recommended Descriptors	Explanatory Notes
Thickness (Breslow Depth) (Fig. 11.33A)	• Maximum tumor thickness in millimeters: _____	Measure perpendicularly from the granular cell layer to deepest invasive tumor
		If tumor is ulcerated, measure from base of ulcer to deepest invasive tumor
		Avoid measuring to melanoma extending along adnexal epithelium or to any nevus cells that may be present
Anatomic Level (Clark's Level)	• I Melanoma in situ • II Melanoma in papillary dermis without filling or expanding it • III Melanoma fills and expands the papillary dermis • IV Melanoma invades reticular dermis • V Melanoma invades subcutis	Clark's level was replaced by mitotic index in the 7th edition AJCC system, but was noted that levels IV or V were retained as the criterion for classifying a tumor as T1b, if mitotic index could not be determined; many dermatopathologists have elected to continue reporting Clark's level
Ulceration (Fig. 11.33B)	• Present • Absent • Indeterminate	Ulceration is defined as: • Full-thickness epidermal defect • Fibrin deposition, neutrophilic infiltrate, necroinflammatory debris • Thinning, effacement or reactive hyperplasia of surrounding epidermis without prior trauma or surgery
		Ulceration upgrades pT substage
		A significant difference in survival has been shown for ulceration involving as little as 5% of the entire lesional diameter; as little as 2% predicts a greater likelihood of sentinel lymph node involvement
		Ulceration may be simulated by a tumor that "lifts" the overlying epidermis. Genuine ulceration is accompanied by invasion of the epidermis
Margins	• Cannot be assessed • Uninvolved by melanoma • Distance of invasive melanoma from closest peripheral margin and deep margin • Distance of in situ melanoma from closest peripheral margin and deep margin	Distance measurement are only required for excisions
		Location of involved margin or margin closest to tumor should be specified if possible
		Proximity to margins may influence additional therapy and assessment of satellitosis
Dermal Mitotic Index (Fig. 11.33C)	• Absent • $1/mm^2$ • Greater than $1mm^2$ (specify number)	Identification of even one dermal mitotic figure should be reported ($1/mm^2$), since it may prompt sentinel lymph node biopsy regardless of tumor thickness; careful inspection of three to six tissue profiles is sufficient; count should be done in "hot spot", i.e. area of tumor with highest index
Microsatellitosis	• Absent • Present • Indeterminate	Defined as tumor nests > 0.05 mm that are 0.3 mm or more from the thickest portion of the main tumor

Contd...

Parameter	Recommended Descriptors	Explanatory Notes
Lymphatic or Blood Vessel Invasion	• Absent • Present • Indeterminate	Rarely identified definitively; some authors believe tumor within the dermis directly around vessels (adventitial dermis) also confers increased risk, but further validation is pending
Perineural Invasion	• Absent • Present • Indeterminate	Common in desmoplastic melanomas and those with spindle cell morphology
Tumor Infiltrating Lymphocytes (Fig. 11.33D)	• Absent • Nonbrisk • Brisk	Absent: No lymphocytes within or around tumor Nonbrisk: Lymphocytes infiltrate dermal component only focally Brisk: Lymphocytes surround or infiltrate entire dermal component Minimal or absent lymphocytic response to melanoma is an adverse prognostic factor
Tumor Regression (Fig. 11.33E)	• Absent • Present, involving less than 75% of tumor • Present, involving more than 75% of tumor	Defined as tumor replacement by lymphohistiocytic infiltrates, but attenuation of epidermis, dermal fibrosis and melanophages are also characteristic; regression of 75% or more is an adverse prognostic factor
Growth Phase	• Horizontal/Radial • Vertical • Indeterminate	Horizontal/radial growth: Tumor is "wider than it is deep" or melanoma in situ involving three or more rete beyond the dermal component Vertical growth: Tumor is deeper than it is wide; in superficial spreading melanoma, vertical growth is signified by one or more dermal clusters larger than the largest intraepidermal cluster and/or any mitotic figures within dermal melanocytes
Nevus Remnant	• Present • Absent • Indeterminate	The significance of nevus remnants is uncertain; distinction between nevus remnant and melanoma may be difficult in some cases and "indeterminate" designation is appropriate in this situation
Sentinel Lymph Nodes	• Number of sentinel nodes examined • Number with macroscopic tumor • Number with microscopic tumor • Extranodal tumor extension • Matted nodes Location(s) of metastatic deposit(s) • Intracapsular • Subcapsular • Intramedulllary	Sentinel lymph node (SLN) status is a powerful prognostic factor in confirmed melanoma Examination of serial H and E-stained sections with intervening sections stained for S100, HMB45, and Melan-A/Mart-1 is the most sensitive method of detection Location and size of SLN tumor deposits may correlate with likelihood of tumor within additional nodes and prompt a complete lymphadenectomy SLN removal itself has not been proven to enhance survival

Contd...

Parameter	Recommended Descriptors	Explanatory Notes
Lymphadenectomy (Nonsentinel Nodes)	Metastasis size : • Size of largest metastatic deposit • Number of nodes examined • Number with macroscopic tumor • Number with microscopic tumor • Extranodal tumor extension • Matted nodes	Lymphadenectomy specimens (non-SLN) may be examined by a variety of methods, but at the very least each node should be submitted in its entirety; any node larger than 5 mm should be bisected

Source: College of American Pathologists Protocol for Melanoma of the Skin and AJCC Melanoma Staging, 7th edition; implemented 2010.

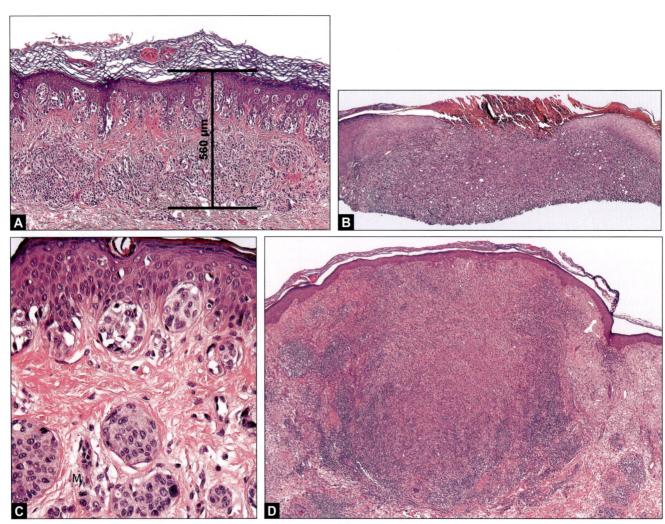

Figs 11.33A to D

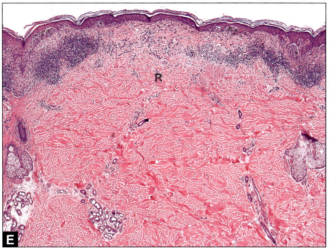

Figs 11.33A to E: (A) Melanoma thickness. Aside from sentinel node status, thickness of the primary melanoma (Breslow depth) remains the most powerful prognostic feature determined by microscopic examination. Thickness is measured from the granular layer to the deepest dermal melanoma cells, excluding those that extend along adnexal structures; (B) Ulcer in melanoma. Ulceration in a melanoma is an adverse prognostic factor that increases the substage (Table 11.1); (C) Recently, the presence of even a single mitotic figure within the dermis of a melanoma, even one with a thickness less than 1.0 mm (so-called "thin" melanomas) such as that shown here, has been shown to have prognostic significance. Note the mitotic figure within the dermis just beneath the "M" in this image; (D) Tumor infiltrating lymphocytes in melanoma. The density of tumor infiltrating lymphocytes should be reported in any melanoma with a "vertical growth phase" (i.e. mitotic figures in dermal melanocytes or nests of melanocytes larger than those in the epidermis). Tumor infiltrating lymphocytes are described rather subjectively as absent, "brisk" or "nonbrisk". If present, only an infiltrate that surrounds or infiltrates the entire dermal component are considered "brisk". This is a positive prognostic feature; (E) Regression in melanoma. Regression in its most obvious form is replacement of the melanoma by lymphohistiocytic infiltrates (the area above the "R" in this image) but attenuation of epidermis, dermal fibrosis, and melanophages are also characteristic. However, only regression of 75% or more is currently considered a significant adverse prognostic factor.

Table 11.2: Staging of melanoma by pathologic characteristics

Primary Tumor (pT)	
	pTX
	• Primary tumor cannot be assessed*
	pT0
	• No evidence of primary tumor
	pTis
	• In situ tumor only
	pT1a
	• Less than or equal to 1.0 mm thick
	• No ulceration
	• Mitotic index less than 1/mm^2
	pT1b
	• Less than or equal to 1.0 mm thick
	• Ulceration
	And/Or
	• Mitotic index more than 1/mm^2
	pT2a
	• 1.01—2.0 mm thick
	• No ulceration
	pT2b
	• 1.01—2.0 mm thick
	• Ulceration
	pT3a
	• 2.01—4.0 mm thick
	• No ulceration
	pT3b
	• 2.01—4.0 mm thick
	• Ulceration
	pT4a
	• 4.0 mm thick
	• No ulceration
	pT4b
	• More than 4.0 mm thick
	• Ulceration
	Descriptive prefixes (if applicable)
	• m (multiple tumors)
	• r (recurrent tumor)
	• y (post-treatment)

Contd...

Regional Lymph Nodes (pN)

pNX

- Regional nodes cannot be assessed

pN0

- No regional lymph node metastasis

pN1

- Metastasis in one regional lymph node

pN1a

- Clinically occult (microscopic) metastasis

pN1b

- Clinically apparent (macroscopic) metastasis

pN2

- Metastasis in two to three regional nodes

  Or

- Intralymphatic metastasis without nodal metastasis

pN2a

- Clinically occult (microscopic) metastasis

pN2b

- Clinically apparent (macroscopic) metastasis

pN2c

- Satellite or in-transit metastasis without nodal metastasis

pN3

- Metastasis in four or more regional lymph nodes

  Or

- Matted metastatic nodes

  Or

- In-transit metastasis or satellites(s) with metastasis in regional node(s)

The following should be specified for all specimens containing lymph nodes:

- Number of lymph nodes: ___
- Number with macroscopic tumor ___
- Number with microscopic tumor____
- Matted nodes: Present/Absent

Distant Metastasis (pM)

pMx

- Unknown

pM1

- Evidence of distant metastasis identified in current specimen

*The pTX designation is usually reserved for tumors that have entirely regressed

**In rare cases, where ulceration and/or mitotic index cannot be assessed or is not clear, modifiers "a" and "b" may be omitted and the tumor staged simply as pT1, pT2, etc.

Lentigo Maligna Melanoma

■ *Criteria for diagnosis*

- An in situ component typical of lentigo maligna (see lentigo maligna, above) (Fig. 11.34A)
- Dermal involvement, often focal, composed of small round or angular cells, small spindled cells (desmoplastic melanoma) or larger spindled cells.

■ *Differential diagnosis*

- Compound Clark's nevus
- Compound lentiginous melanoma
- Other compound variants of melanoma, particularly superficial spreading type.

■ *Pitfalls*

- Extension into the dermis commonly has a "desmoplastic" appearance—the neoplastic cells are spindled and the surrounding dermis is sclerotic and may be mistaken for scar (Fig. 11.34B)
- May have "skip" areas due to partial or complete regression
- Genuine dermal involvement may be difficult to differentiate from extension of atypical melanocytes along rete and adnexa

- Lesions on sun-damaged facial skin of the elderly that resemble Clark's nevi are almost always lentigo maligna melanoma.

■ *Pearls*

- Epidermal atrophy is common; solar elastosis is required by definition
- Extension of atypical cells along adnexal epithelium is common in lentigo maligna
- Cytologic atypia varies and may be mild to marked, including multinucleated giant cells
- Junctional nests, if present, usually vary markedly in size and shape and are unevenly spaced
- A dermal lymphohistiocytic infiltrate with melanophages is common
- Pagetoid spread is usually less extensive than in superficial spreading melanoma
- Dermal invasion usually occurs only in long-standing lesions
- Regression is common; its presence at an excision margin is an indication for re-excision.

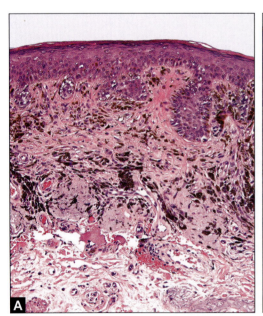 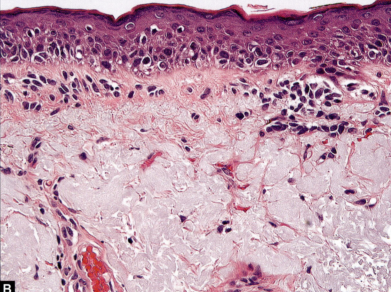

Figs 11.34A and B: Lentigo maligna melanoma. (A) The intraepidermal component is identical to that of lentigo maligna (melanoma in situ). In cases such as this, melanophages and inflammatory cells may make them difficult to detect, but close inspection reveals malignant melanocytes in the dermis that are identical to those within the epidermis; (B) In this example, the extension of malignant melanocytes into the dermis is more obvious.

Lentiginous Melanoma

■ *Criteria for diagnosis*

- A broad lesion (usually at least 6 mm) (Fig. 11.35A)
- Moderately atypical melanocytes (nuclear size usually approximates that of adjacent keratinocytes)
- Extensive lentiginous growth (melanocytes arranged predominantly as single cells) (Fig. 11.35B)
- Nests that are small, ill-defined, irregularly shaped and unevenly distributed (Fig. 11.35B)
- Intraepidermal spread (pagetoid growth) that is focal and not of the degree characteristic of superficial spreading melanoma (Fig. 11.35C)
- A lack of rete alteration, dermal lamellar fibroplasia and lymphocytic infiltration (that would suggest either a Clark's nevus or another type of melanoma) (Fig. 11.35B)
- Lack of significant solar elastosis and/or other evidence of extensive actinic damage that would qualify the tumor as lentigo maligna melanoma (Fig. 11.35C).

■ *Differential diagnosis*

- Clark's nevus
- Nevus spilus
- Lentigo maligna melanoma
- Superficial spreading melanoma
- Solar intraepidermal melanocytosis
- Junctional intraepidermal melanocytosis.

■ *Pitfalls*

- The lack of pronounced melanocyte atypia may result in under-recognition

- The lesional cells are often small, making the extensive lentiginous growth and pagetoid spread difficult to recognize without the aid of immunohistochemistry
- Partially sampled lesions are common and often preclude definitive diagnosis.

■ *Pearls*

- Lentiginous melanoma has only recently received attention in the literature
- It is slow-growing by definition
- Local persistence (recurrence) is characteristic
- Dermal involvement is minimal in most cases, is usually limited to a thickness of less than 0.7, Clark's level II, and mitotic figures and ulceration have not been described in any of the reported cases to date
- Clinical impression is often either an "atypical nevus" or melanoma
- The size of the lesion is a critical component of the diagnosis; small biopsies may not allow definitive diagnosis, since it cannot be determined whether the characteristic features involve an area of significant breadth.
- The diagnosis should be reserved for those cases that cannot be classified as one of the other major subtypes of melanoma; it could be said that it is "a melanoma of exclusion"
- May represent melanoma arising within a Clark's nevus or the evolution of a Clark's nevus into a malignant melanoma, particularly in older adults
- So-called "lentiginous junctional dysplastic nevus of the elderly" often have features that overlap with lentiginous melanoma and may be a precursor to it or identical to it.

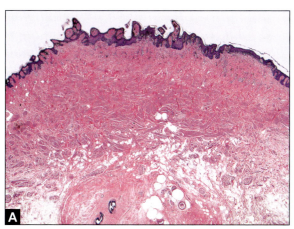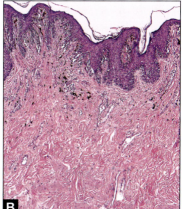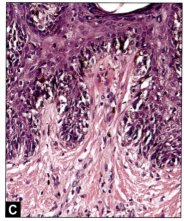

Figs 11.35A to C: Lentiginous melanoma. (A) The breadth of the lesion is a clue that it is melanoma rather than a Clark's/dysplastic nevus. The lesion occupies the junction of the entire field in this image, and was over 1.0 cm in total width; (B) Although a few nests are present, they are irregularly shaped and unevenly spaced. Lentiginous growth of single melanocytes predominates. Note the absence of lamellar fibroplasia characteristic of a Clark's nevus; (C) The atypical melanocytes have angular nuclear contours. Throughout most of the lesion, the single cells are present in contiguity. Upward "pagetoid" spread was minimal, however (differentiating it from superficial spreading melanoma) and dermatoheliosis is absent (distinguishing it from lentigo maligna melanoma).

Acral Lentiginous Melanoma

■ *Criteria for diagnosis*

- A pigmented macule, papule, ulcer or nodule (Fig. 11.36A)
- Extensive lentiginous junctional growth of atypical melanocytes (Fig. 11.36B)
- Mostly or entirely lentiginous growth in early phases; widespread dermal involvement in established lesions
- Epidermal hyperplasia and irregularly shaped nests in large, fully evolved lesions.

■ *Differential diagnosis*

- Other types of melanoma (superficial spreading, etc.)
- Acral nevi.

■ *Pitfalls*

- Lentiginous growth and melanocytes within the upper epidermis are common in acral nevi and must not be mistaken for acral lentiginous melanoma (Fig. 11.36C)
- Pagetoid spread is uncommon in early acral lentiginous melanoma and should not be relied upon as a criterion, as it is common in acral nevi.

■ *Pearls*

- Not all melanomas on acral skin are acral lentiginous type; those on the dorsal surfaces are actually more likely to be superficial spreading or nodular type.

- Acral lentiginous melanoma is usually seen on the volar skin (non hair-bearing areas)
- Other types of melanoma are very rare on volar skin
- Acral lentiginous melanoma virtually never occurs in children and is very uncommon before age of 30 years; most cases present in the seventh decade (therefore, a pigmented macule on the sole or palm of a young person is far more likely to be a nevus)
- Predilection for the feet, especially the heels
- Equal incidence in light-skinned and dark-skinned races
- Lesional cells are often vertically elongated and have thickened, elongated dendritic processes
- Lymphohistiocytic inflammation is almost always present in acral lentiginous melanoma, but is very rare in acral nevi (a very helpful feature in differentiating the two)
- Broad lesions are more likely to be evolving acral lentiginous melanoma than an acral nevus
- Cases with features that overlap with superficial spreading and nodular melanoma are not uncommon
- Nested melanocytes usually are not seen until an acral lentiginous melanoma is at least 6 mm in greatest dimension, whereas they are usually present in nevi as small as 2–3 mm
- A lesion in an adult, that is more than 6 mm in size and lacks nest formation is acral melanoma until proven otherwise.

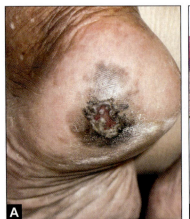 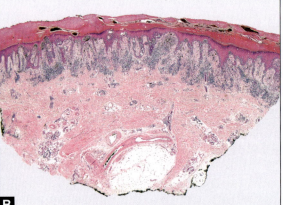 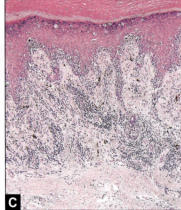

Figs 11.36A to C: Acral lentiginous melanoma. (A) This pigmented ulcerated nodule on the heel evolved rather quickly; (B) Atypical melanocytes occupy the epidermis and upper dermis; (C) The malignant cells grow in a lentiginous pattern along the junction and are distributed haphazardly throughout the full thickness of the epidermis as well.

Superficial Spreading Melanoma
(Figs 11.37A to D)

■ *Criteria for diagnosis*

- A variably pigmented macule, papule or nodule
- Atypical melanocytes within the spinous or granular layers of the epidermis in a "pagetoid" pattern (Fig. 11.37B)
- Maximum dimension of the horizontal plane greater than that of the vertical plane (a horizontally oriented, irregular, rectangular silhouette)
- One or more of the architectural criteria that favor melanoma over a benign nevus, including asymmetry/imbalance of the overall silhouette, nests that are irregularly shaped and unevenly distributed and mitotic figures within the dermis.

■ *Differential diagnosis*

- Other types of melanoma, especially lentiginous and nodular variants
- Clark's nevi with marked atypia
- Mark's nevus (deep congenital pattern nevus) with focal pagetoid growth
- Nevi of genital or acral skin with atypia
- Non-melanocytic tumors that commonly exhibit pagetoid growth, most commonly extramammary paget's disease (EPD), squamous cell carcinoma, sebaceous carcinoma, Merkel cell carcinoma (cutaneous neuroendocrine carcinoma) and epidermotropic metastatic carcinoma
- Epidermotropic metastasis from a melanoma at another site.

■ *Pitfalls*

- Extramammary Paget's disease may closely simulate the pagetoid growth of superficial spreading melanoma and pigmented variants of EPD exist, further complicating matters (Fig. 11.37C).

■ *Pearls*

- Superficial spreading melanoma usually occurs on skin that is usually covered by clothing, but intermittently exposed to sunlight
- Unlike most nevi (including Spitz's and Reed's nevi), there is often effacement of the epidermis and patchy areas in which the intraepidermal component has regressed
- There may be considerable overlap with other types of melanoma, particularly nodular type and the distinction may be artifactual
- BRAF oncogene on chromosome 7q34 is often mutated
- Other common chromosomal aberrations involve losses within chromosomes 9, 10, 6q and 8p, and gains within 1q, 6p, 7, 8q and 20
- In addition to the usually small deletions of the CDKN2A locus at 9p21, many of the other aberrations can be detected by comparative genomic hybridization.

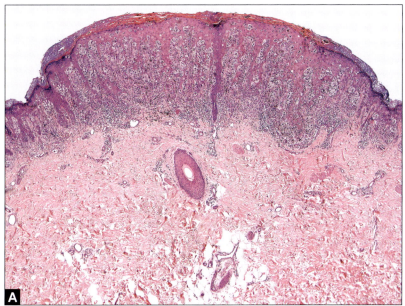 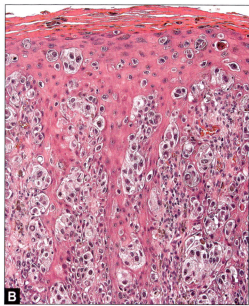

Figs 11.37A and B

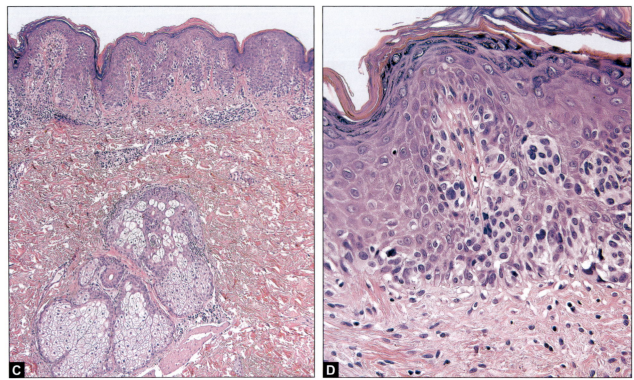

Figs 11.37A to D: Superficial spreading melanoma. (A) This lesion has a polypoid configuration due to the accumulation of malignant melanocytes within the epidermis and papillary dermis; (B) Large, atypical melanocytes distributed as solitary units throughout the full thickness of the epidermis ("pagetoid spread") is the hallmark of superficial spreading melanoma; (C) Although pagetoid spread is the most easily recognizable feature of superficial spreading melanoma, in early lesions or areas at the periphery of established lesions this may be less prominent; (D) The large, epithelioid melanocytes and the marked cytologic and architectural atypia are usually sufficient for diagnosis, however.

Nodular Melanoma (Figs 11.38A to D)

■ *Criteria for diagnosis*

- Rapidly growing tumor composed of large, atypical melanocytes
- Maximum dimension of the vertical plane greater than that of the horizontal plane (a vertically oriented, irregular, nodular silhouette) (Fig. 11.38A)
- Intraepidermal component that does not extend more than three epidermal rete beyond the dermal component
- Atypical melanocytes arranged as syncytia within the dermis with one or more mitotic figures.

■ *Differential diagnosis*

- Atypical Spitz Tumor
- Metastatic melanoma
- Melanoma arising within a pre-existing nevus
- Non-melanocytic tumors, particularly atypical fibroxanthoma (AFX), metastatic carcinoma (especially renal cell carcinoma), clear cell sarcoma, anaplastic large cell lymphoma and epithelioid sarcoma.

■ *Pitfalls*

- Extensive ulceration or regression may prevent recognition of the intraepidermal melanoma and therefore, primary nodular melanomas may be misdiagnosed as metastatic melanoma, clear cell sarcoma or other tumors

- Nodular melanomas, more than other types, tend to vary in their histopathologic appearance and may closely resemble other tumors, particularly metastatic renal cell carcinoma, various cutaneous adnexal tumors, AFX, rhabdoid tumors and sarcomas (Fig. 11.38C)
- In very rare instances, metastatic melanoma may be "epidermotropic", producing a histopathologic appearance indistinguishable from nodular melanoma.

■ *Pearls*

- A junctional component may be found with very diligent search, even if there is extensive ulceration; multiple levels may be necessary, however
- Nodular melanomas more than other types tend to have variation among the tumor cell population
- Nodular melanomas may contain nodules of large cells that compress adjacent groups of smaller cells, a feature not seen in Spitz's nevi.

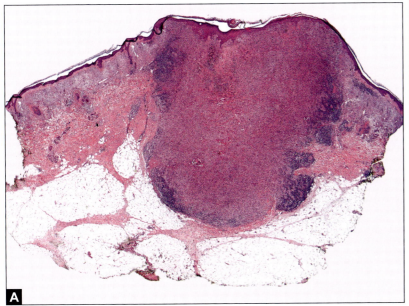
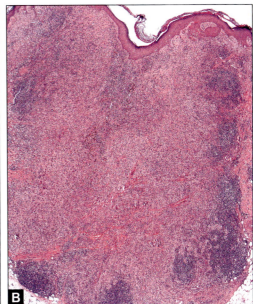

Figs 11.38A and B

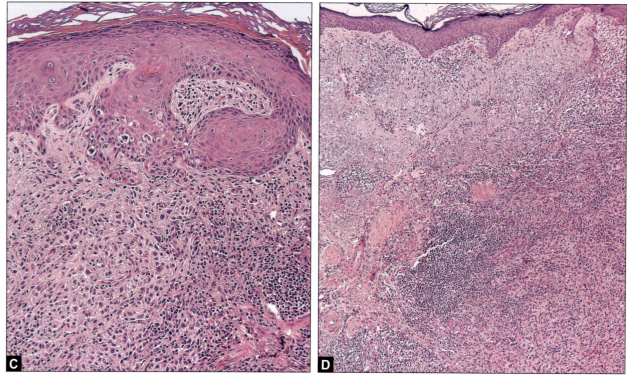

Figs 11.38A to D: Nodular melanoma. (A) A defining feature is that the tumor is greater in the "vertical" plane (from superficial to deep) than in the "horizontal" plane (from side to side); (B) The tumor appears well demarcated but the cytologic atypia is evident even at low power. The base is surrounded in most areas by lymphocytes, an example of so-called "tumor infiltrating lymphocytes," one of the histopathologic grading parameters currently used for melanomas; (C) It can be difficult to differentiate nodular melanomas from other tumors (e.g. atypical fibroxanthoma) without immunohistochemistry. In this case, however, there is an intraepidermal population of atypical melanocytes that makes the diagnosis obvious; (D) Unlike that in Figure 11.38C, some nodular melanomas lack an intraepidermal (in situ) component. Differentiating these from metastatic lesions can be challenging.

Desmoplastic Melanoma (Figs 11.39A to C)

Criteria for diagnosis

- A flesh-colored, tan or pink plaque or nodule
- Spindled melanocytes embedded within sclerotic collagen (Fig. 11.39A).

Differential diagnosis

- Scar
- Dermatofibroma
- Neurofibroma
- Morphea
- Spindled mesenchymal tumors (especially those that are fibroblastic, neural and smooth muscle)
- Desmoplatic nevus.

Pitfalls

- Most cases lack obvious melanin pigment, both clinically and histopathologically
- The vast majority of desmoplastic melanomas are negative with Fontana-Masson stains for melanin and lack expression of Melan-A/Mart-1, HMB45 and other melanocytic markers; occasionally, even S100 expression is patchy or absent (Fig. 11.39C)
- It has been estimated that, approximately 50% of desmoplastic melanomas are initially misdiagnosed
- Mistaking a desmoplastic melanoma for a benign neoplasm (e.g. neurofibroma) or a scar is a common pitfall
- Some desmoplastic nevi are over-interpreted as desmoplastic melanoma
- S100-positve Langerhans cells within the dermis may be over-interpreted as melanoma (Fig. 11.39C).

Pearls

- Features overlapping with spindle cell/neurotropic melanoma are common and the two entities may be closely-related

- Lesions that resemble neurofibromas or other neural tumors on sun-damaged skin in older patients should be carefully studied to exclude desmoplastic melanoma
- Intraepidermal melanoma may be absent in 50% (or more) of desmoplastic melanomas
- When present, lentigo maligna type melanoma is most common intraepidermal type
- The melanocytes are often arranged haphazardly among the thickened collagen bundles, but sometimes they form recognizable fascicles
- The neoplasm may extend into the subcutaneous fat producing widened septa
- Neurotropism is frequent
- Lymphoid aggregates around the periphery and base of the lesion suggest desmoplastic melanoma
- Aggregates of degenerating elastic fibers are sometimes seen, a feature not seen in most simulators of desmoplastic melanoma
- A "scar" that recurs should be carefully evaluated to exclude desmoplastic melanoma
- A polypoid "scar" that develops at the site of excision of an "atypical junctional nevus" should be carefully evaluated to exclude desmoplastic melanoma
- In adults, especially on the face and volar skin of elderly people, desmoplastic melanoma should always be considered in the differential of dermal spindle cell lesions
- Desmoplastic nevi are usually well-delineated, many contain at least a focal junctional component recognizable as nevus and most exhibit at least some degree of maturation and dispersion.

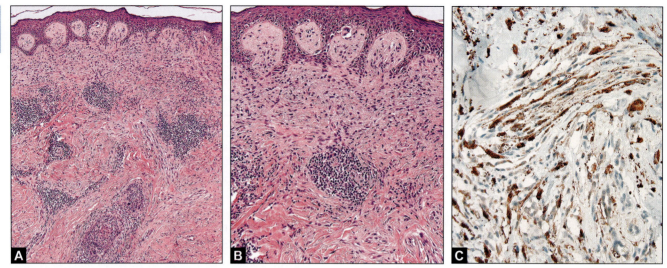

Figs 11.39A to C: Desmoplastic melanoma. (A) The epidermis contains a junctional proliferation of atypical cells. The dermis immediately beneath them is occupied by relatively small spindled melanoma cells. The lymphocytic aggregates at the periphery are a clue that desmoplastic melanoma is present; (B) The cells typically are spindled or elongated ovals. Some will invariably exhibit atypia on close examination, but many are relatively banal and may be mistaken for reactive fibroblasts (hence the notorious tendency for desmoplastic melanomas to be mistaken for scars). They generally lack the degree of atypia of the cells of a spindle cell/neurotropic melanoma; (C) By immunohistochemistry the cells of desmoplastic melanoma usually express S100 protein but are often negative for Melan-A, HMB45 and most of the other melanocyte-specific markers. The S100 stain highlights the cellular pleomorphism. Since dermal dendritic cells/Langerhans cells also express S100, care must be taken not to confuse those cells (which are present in scars) with desmoplastic melanoma cells.

Spindle Cell/Neurotropic Melanoma
(Figs 11.40A to C)

■ Criteria for diagnosis

- A melanoma composed partly or entirely of spindle-shaped melanocytes that exhibits conspicuous involvement of cutaneous nerves (Fig. 11.40A).

■ Differential diagnosis

- Neurofibroma
- Schwannoma
- Neuroma
- Spindle cell squamous carcinoma
- Scar tissue
- Masson's nevus (neuronevus).

■ Pitfalls

- Lesional cells may be cytologically banal, usually lack melanin pigment and are often few in number in early lesions
- Some cases exhibit features more typical of neural tumors than melanoma, including fascicles composed of wavy or buckled cells or verocay body-like structures that closely resemble schwannomas
- Cells usually retain S100 expression, but do not express other melanocytic markers such as HMB45 and Melan-A/ Mart-1.

■ Pearls

- Tendency to present on sun-exposed skin of the head and neck, especially the lips, cheeks and temple of older adults
- Clinically visible pigmentation is not always present; occasionally the lesion is described as occurring at or near the site of a "regressed" pigmented lesion
- Nerves that appear enlarged or are surrounded by inflammation and/or a myxoid stroma are a clue to neurotropic melanoma (Fig. 11.40C)
- Complete sampling and extensive sectioning often reveals areas of more conventional-appearing melanoma (e.g. rounded, epithelioid cells, sometimes with melanin pigment)
- A desmoplastic stroma is often present, suggesting a relationship to desmoplastic melanoma
- Neurotropic melanoma should be considered in the differential diagnosis of any lesion with a "neuroid" appearance that occurs in sun-damaged skin of the head and neck, acral skin or mucous membranes
- Like desmoplastic melanoma, lymph node metastasis is uncommon in a "pure" spindle cell/neurotropic melanoma; when found, the nodal metastasis often includes melanoma cells with a more conventional epithelioid appearance.

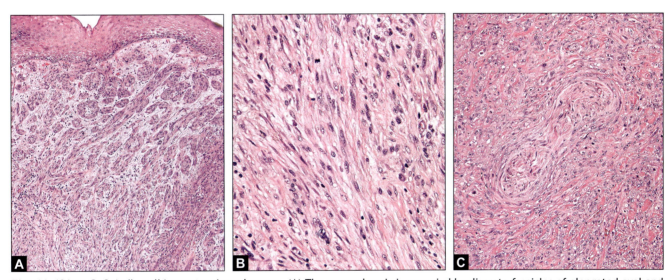

Figs 11.40A to C: Spindle cell/neurotropic melanoma. (A) The upper dermis is occupied by discrete fascicles of elongated oval and spindled cells; (B) Within the mid reticular dermis, the cells become distinctly spindled and are arranged in broad syncytial sheets. The cells are pleomorphic and have overt cytologic atypia, including cells with vesicular nuclei and prominent nucleoli; (C) As the name implies, neurotropism is a defining feature of this melanoma variant. Here, a large dermal nerve is completely ensheathed by spindled melanocytes.

Blue Nevus-Like Melanoma (Malignant Blue Nevus) (Figs 11.41A to C)

■ *Criteria for diagnosis*

- A melanoma with a dermal component that resembles a blue nevus, but has an intraepidermal component, is poorly demarcated and composed of uniformly atypical melanocytes with a mitotic index that exceeds that of a blue nevus (> 1–2 per 10 high power fields).

■ *Differential diagnosis*

- Carney's, Allen's or Masson's nevi (variants of blue nevus)
- Combined nevus
- Melanoma arising within a benign (pre-existing) blue nevus
- Metastatic melanoma.

■ *Pitfalls*

- The intraepidermal component, a key feature in differentiating blue nevus-like melanoma from benign blue nevi may be missed without sufficient sampling.

■ *Pearls*

- Features that separate a blue nevus-like melanoma from benign simulators include poor circumscription, an intraepidermal component, solid sheets of atypical melanocytes without intervening collagen bundles, nuclear hyperchromasia and pleomorphism and a mitotic index that exceeds one to two mitotic figures per 10 high power fields
- Poorly circumscribed cellular nodule occupies a variable proportion of the lesion.

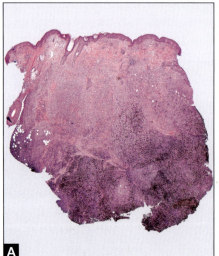
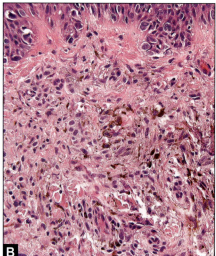
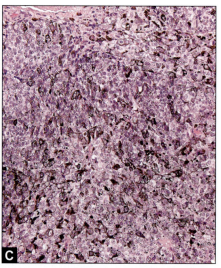

Figs 11.41A to C: Blue nevus-like melanoma. (A) At scanning magnification the lesion resembles a Carney's nevus (cellular or epithelioid blue nevus); (B) Closer inspection reveals a junctional component that is characteristic of melanoma, however; (C) The dense pigmentation obscures the cytologic detail in many of the cells, but marked atypia is evident and mitotic figures are conspicuous.

Nevoid Melanoma (Figs 11.42A to D)

Criteria for diagnosis

- A melanoma that closely resembles an "ordinary" nevus due to its silhouette (usually similar to that of an Unna's or Miescher's type) and small cell size, but with cellular density, syncytial dermal aggregates and a mitotic index that exceeds that of a nevus (Fig. 11.42A).

Differential diagnosis

- Unna's and Miescher's nevi
- Combined nevus
- Melanoma arising within a pre-existing nevus.

Pitfalls

- The silhouette and small size of the lesional melanocytes closely simulate that of a benign nevus.
- The clinical impression may be melanoma, but is often nevus or even non-melanocytic tumors such as basal cell carcinoma ("amelanotic melanoma").

Pearls

- Features that suggest nevoid melanoma include asymmetry of the silhouette of the nevus, confluence of junctional nests, more than one (and usually many) mitotic figures, necrotic dermal cells, a junctional component resembling in situ melanoma, a lack of maturation and dispersion of the nevus cells within the vertical plane, including nests within the deep dermis larger than those of the upper dermis, extensive dermal syncytial growth (solid "sheets" of tumor cells without intervening collagen bundles), irregular distribution of melanin pigment (especially pigment within the deep regions), variability in the distribution of an inflammatory infiltrate (if present) and variation in cellular density, with melanocyte nuclei that appear to overlap and lack of discernible cytoplasm ("naked nuclei") (Figs 11.42B to D).
- The prognosis is no different from that of other types of melanoma, with thickness being the primary determinant of stage.

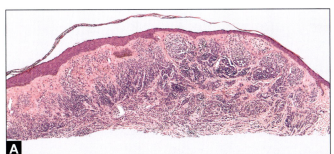
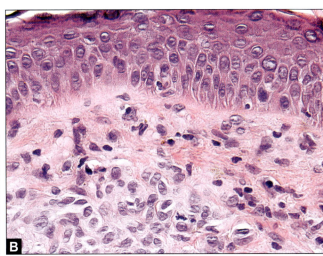

Figs 11.42A and B

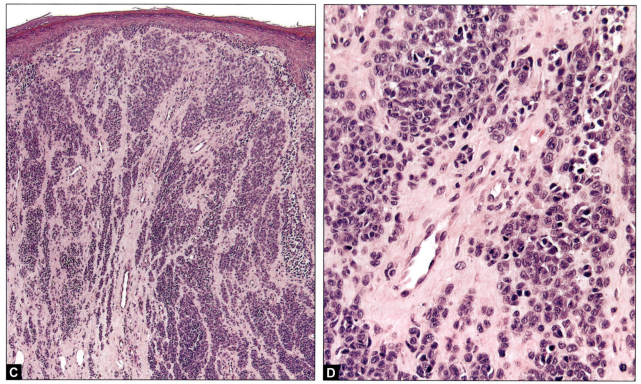

Figs 11.42A to D: Nevoid melanoma. (A) At low magnification this lesion appears similar to a common compound Miescher's pattern nevus, and there is maturation of the melanocytes at the deep aspect. However, it is imbalanced in the horizontal plane with nests of larger epithelioid cells occupying the upper dermis on the right hand side; (B) Close inspection demonstrates dermal mitotic figures and marked cytologic atypia, including large melanocytes with prominent nucleoli; (C) This case resembles a nevus since there is maturation, dispersion, and no atypical junctional component; (D) Mitotic figures are obvious within the dermal component, however; two can be seen within this single high-power field, and one has atypical features.

Spitzoid Melanoma (Figs 11.43A to G)

■ *Criteria for diagnosis*

- A tumor with cytologic and architectural features that resemble a Spitz's nevus, but with features that when considered in constellation are more characteristic of melanoma.

■ *Differential diagnosis*

- Spitz's nevus
- Seab's nevus (deep penetrating nevus)
- Other variants of melanoma.

■ *Pitfalls*

- The resemblance to a Spitz's nevus varies markedly; lesions in children may exhibit cytologic and architectural features that are more "atypical" than those in adults.

■ *Pearls*

- Features suggesting that a Spitzoid lesion is a melanoma rather than a nevus include mitotic figures, especially at the base of the lesion, an inflammatory infiltrate (sometimes including numerous plasma cells in addition to lymphocytes), greater depth than most Spitz's nevi, expansile nodules (often extending into the subcutis), extensive dermal syncytial growth (solid "sheets" of tumor cells without intervening collagen bundles), melanin pigmentation within only a subset of dermal cells (most Spitz's nevi contain little melanin pigment and if present, it is uniformly distributed), numerous melanophages, solar elastosis, striking pleomorphism and individual cell necrosis
- The patient's age should be considered; Spitz's tumors in prepubertal children are more likely to be nevi, while those in adults over age of 40 years are more likely to be Spitzoid melanomas (though, occasional Spitzoid melanomas occurring in children are well documented)
- There is some evidence that a Spitz tumor in a pre-pubertal child may behave in a more indolent manner even when many of the criteria for melanoma are present; this possibility requires further study with long-term follow-up of such cases
- Spitz's nevi, especially those with "atypical features" (i.e. some of the above criteria), have been shown to involve regional lymph nodes
- The presence of Spitz's nevus-like cells within a lymph node does "not" indicate that the primary lesion is a melanoma and the diagnostic utility of a sentinel lymph node biopsy is questionable in these lesions
- Over 60% of Spitz's tumors with features favoring nevus over melanoma may involve regional lymph nodes.

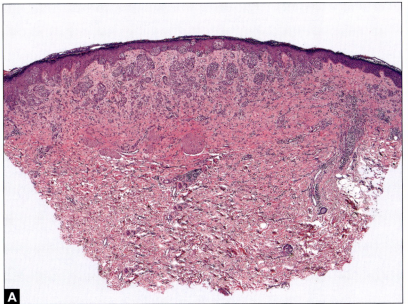 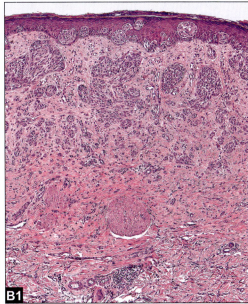

Figs 11.43A and B1

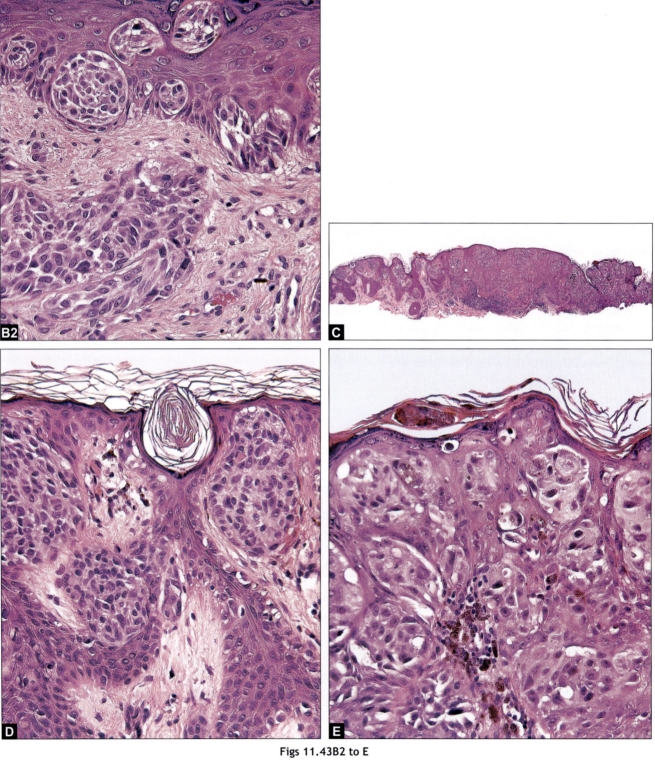

Figs 11.43B2 to E

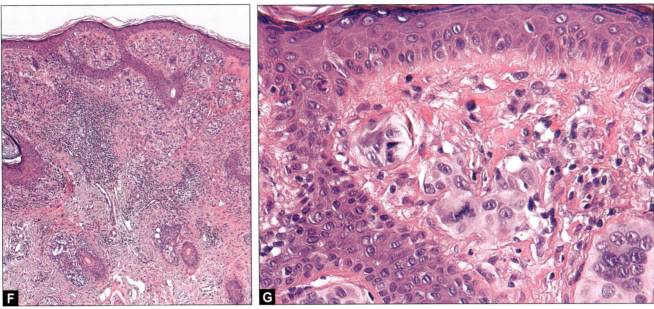

Figs 11.43A to G: (A) Spitzoid melanoma. Although some of the architectural and cytologic features resemble a Spitz nevus, note the imbalance of the lesion. The junctional component is nested at the left side of the lesion, but at the right the cells are arranged singly and irregularly; (B) Some of the large melanocytes disposed as solitary cells and even those arranged in well formed nests are arranged abnormally for a benign lesion since some are present in the upper levels of the epidermis; (C) Malignant melanoma arising within a Spitz tumor. This tumor occurred in a teenager and was reportedly present for years before it rapidly enlarged. At the left of the field the features are those of a classic Spitz tumor, but at the right there is a distinct difference in cytologic and architectural features; (D) High power examination of left hand aspect of the tumor. The features are typical of a Spitz tumor/nevus; (E) Compare the features in this field, from the right hand aspect of the tumor. There are architectural disorder and cytologic atypia that are quite obvious when compared to the remainder of the tumor; (F) Spitzoid melanoma. This lesion had recently arisen in a 53-year-old man. Although many of the cells resemble those of a Spitz nevus, the cytologic and architectural atypia are more pronounced; (G) An atypical mitotic figure is evident, and while some authors aver that these may occur in Spitz "nevi" within the context of the other features of this lesion, it strongly supports a malignant diagnosis in this case.

CHAPTER 12

Epithelial Neoplasms

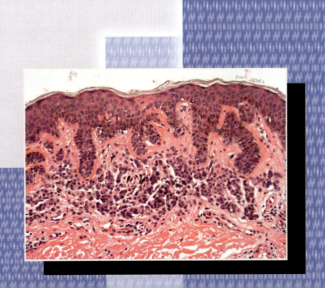

INTRODUCTION

Epithelial processes can be divided into two basic categories:
1. Neoplasms and proliferations arising from the epidermis
2. Neoplasms and proliferations arising from adnexal structures.

Both categories have benign and malignant subgroups. The neoplasms and proliferations arising from adnexae can be further subcategorized into follicular, apocrine, eccrine and sebaceous groups and are discussed in Chapter 13.

NON-NEOPLASTIC EPIDERMAL PROLIFERATIONS

- Verruca [many people classify warts as neoplasms (new growth)]
- Acanthosis nigricans
- Confluent and reticulated papillomatosis
- Prurigo nodule
- Pseudocarcinomatous epithelial hyperplasia due to infection, halogenoderma, trauma and pemphigus vegetans.

Acanthosis Nigricans/Confluent and Reticulated Papillomatosis

Acanthosis nigricans and confluent and reticulated papillomatosis demonstrate similar histopathologic findings and therefore, are grouped together here. Distinguishing the two can often be easily accomplished on clinical grounds.

■ *Criteria for diagnosis*

- Clinical history:
  - Acanthosis nigricans occurs in the axillae, nape of neck or occasionally on the palms (tripe palms) (Fig. 12.1A)
  - Confluent and reticulated papillomatosis: Occurs on trunk—seborrheic dermatitis like distribution. Lesions have reticulated appearance.
- Pathologic findings:
  - Slight papillomatous with normal thickness of the epidermis (Figs 12.1B and C)
  - Occasional pityrosporum organisms within stratum corneum in confluent and reticulated papillomatosis.

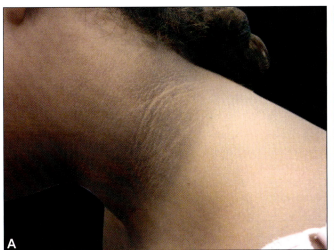

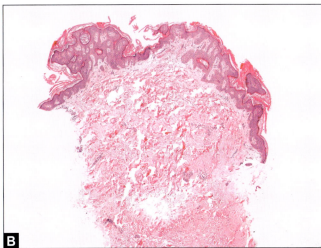

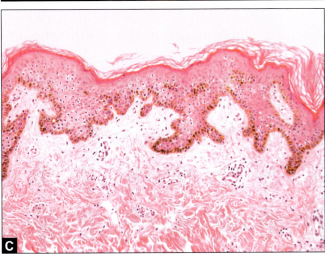

Figs 12.1A to C: Acanthosis nigricans. (A) Velvety hyperpigmented plaque on neck; (B and C) Confluent and reticulated papillomatosis: Epidermis is mamillated with overlying hyperkeratosis.

Prurigo Nodularis/Lichen Simplex Chronicus

Patients with prurigo nodularis have multiple lesions usually on the extremities that they are chronically rubbing or picking at (Fig. 12.2A) Patients with lichen simplex chronicus have a single lesion usually on the nape of the neck or ankle that they are rubbing at. Histopathologic findings in both are identical.

■ *Pathologic criteria for diagnosis*

- Epidermal acanthosis (Fig. 12.2B)
- Compact orthokeratosis
- Hypergranulosis
- Vertical streaking of collagen bundles within papillary dermis (Fig. 12.2C).

■ *Pitfalls*

- Histological features of prurigo can occur as a secondary finding in numerous dermatoses, overlying lesions and in patients with systemic diseases
- Chronic rubbing can produce epidermal papillomatosis resembling wart.

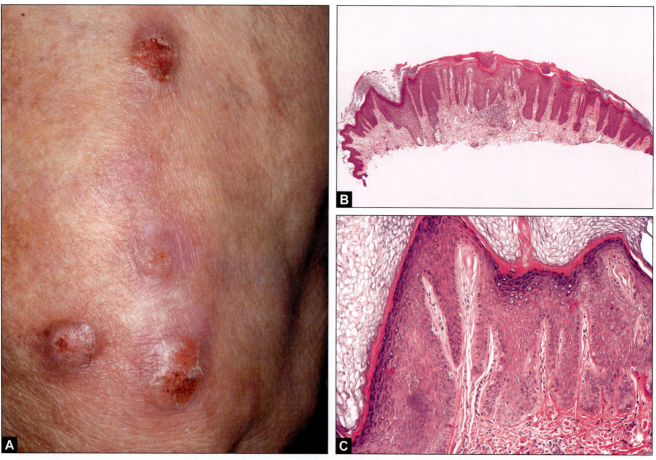

Figs 12.2A to C: Prurigo Nodule. (A) Clinical picture of prurigo nodularis; (B) Psoriasiform epidermal hyperplasia; (C) Hypergranulosis with vertical streaking of collagen bundles.

Pseudocarcinomatous Epithelial Hyperplasia

A common conundrum in dermatopathology is distinguishing pseudocarcinomatous epithelial hyperplasia and squamous cell carcinoma.

Clues to diagnosis of pseudocarcinomatous hyperplasia

- Granulomatous or suppurative inflammation due to infection (confirm with special stains and/or culture) (Fig. 12.3A)
- Hyperplastic epithelium centered on hair follicles
- Epidermal proliferation symmetric (Fig. 12.3B)
- Lack of significant solar elastosis
- Lack of significant cytologic atypia.

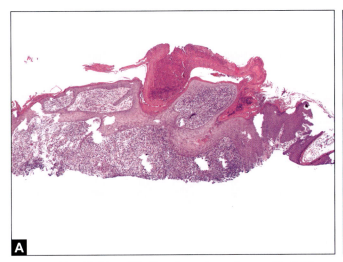 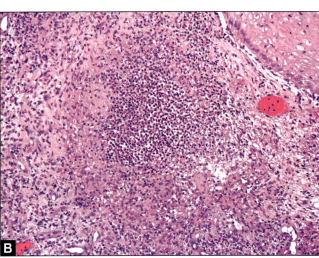

Figs 12.3A and B: Pseudocarcinomatous epithelial hyperplasia. (A) Adnexocentric centric epidermal proliferation; (B) Abscess with granulomatous inflammation clue to infectious etiology.

Verruca

▪ *Clinical criteria*

- Asymmetric papillomatous or rough papules and plaques with loss of skin lines and black puncta (Fig. 12.4A).

▪ *Pathologic criteria for diagnosis*

- Epidermal proliferation
- Inward turning rete ridges (Fig. 12.4B)
- Tortuous blood vessels within papillary dermis
- Koilocytosis (Fig. 12.4C).

▪ *Pitfalls*

- Rubbing may produce hypergranulosis simulating koilocytosis along with papillomatosis (Fig. 12.4B).

▪ *Pearls*

- Verruca in genital skin (condyloma accuminata) can histologically resemble seborrheic keratosis
- The epidermis is not papillated in flat warts.

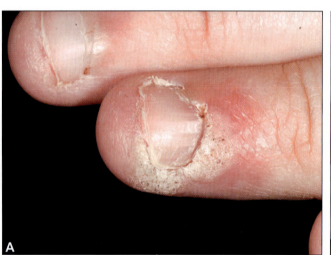

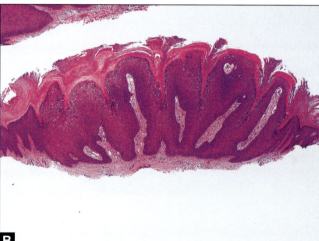

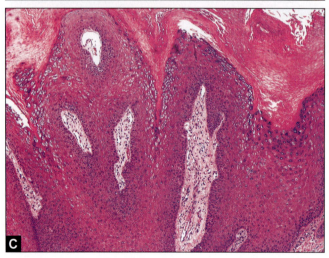

Figs 12.4A to C: Verruca. (A) Clinical picture of verruca; (B) Epidermal papillomatosis, inward turning rete ridges, parakeratosis and hypergranulosis with koilocytosis; (C) Epidermal acanthosis with koilocytosis.

BENIGN KERATINOCYTIC NEOPLASMS

- Acanthomas
  - Acantholytic
  - Epidermolytic
  - Clear cell
  - Dyskeratotic
  - Large cell
- Acrokeratosis verruciformis
- Epidermal nevus
- Flegel's disease
- Porokeratosis
- Seborrheic keratosis
- Variants of Seborrheic keratosis: Stucco keratosis, Melanoacanthoma, Dermatosis papulosa nigra
- Solar lentigo
- Warty dyskeratoma.

Acanthomas

There are a variety of benign epidermal neoplasms diagnosed as acanthomas. These neoplasms may simply be variants of seborrheic keratoses. All of them have common denominator of epidermal acanthosis and hyperkeratosis. The subtype is dependent on ancillary findings.

■ *Criteria for diagnosis*

- Epidermal acanthosis (Fig. 12.5A)
- Hyperkeratosis
- Flat base.

■ *Criteria for diagnosis of subtype*

- *Acantholytic*: Acantholysis (Fig. 12.5A)
- *Dyskeratotic*: Dyskeratotic cells with occasional Corps ronds and Corps grains (Fig. 12.5B)
- *Large cell*: A population of columnar cells at basal cell layer of epidermis (Fig. 12.5C)
- Clear cell acanthoma: See below.

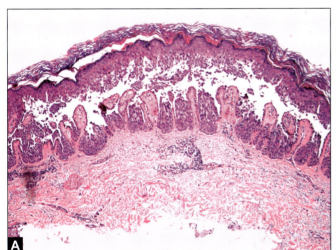

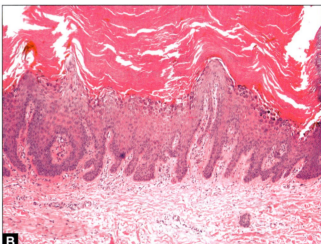

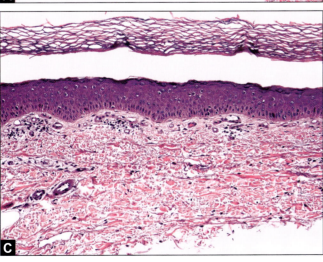

Figs 12.5A to C: Acantholytic acanthoma. (A) Epidermal acanthosis with acantholysis; (B) Dyskeratotic/Epidermolytic Acanthoma. Dyskeratotic cells are not seen in untreated wart; (C) Large cell acanthoma. Columnar shaped keratinocytes along basal layer of epidermis.

Acrokeratosis Verruciformis of Huff

Acrokeratosis verruciformis is an autosomal dominant genodermatoses linked to ATP2A2 gene defect (same gene as in Darier's disease). Patients develop warty seborrheic keratosis like lesions on dorsum hands, fingers and occasionally on feet and legs.

■ *Criteria for diagnosis*

- Clinical history:
  - Family members with similar lesions
  - Gene testing
- Pathology:
  - Papillomatous lesions resembling warts or stucco keratosis but no koilocytosis (Fig. 12.6).

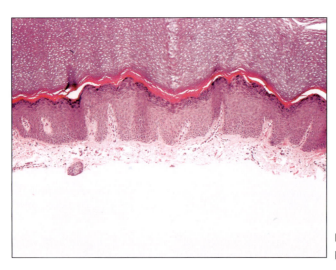

Fig. 12.6: Acrokeratosis verruciformis. Epidermal acanthosis and papillomatosis on acral skin.

Clear Cell Acanthoma

■ *Criteria for diagnosis*

- Epidermal acanthosis (Fig. 12.7A)
- Epidermal pallor
- Sharp demarcation between pale tumor cells and surrounding epidermis (Fig. 12.7B)
- Confluent parakeratosis
- Frequently neutrophils within epidermis
- Neutrophils in the keratinizing layer (Fig. 12.7C)
- Tortuous blood vessels in papillary dermis.

■ *Criteria against diagnosis*

- Clear cells with peripheral palisading: Tricholemmoma (see page 361 in Chapter 13).

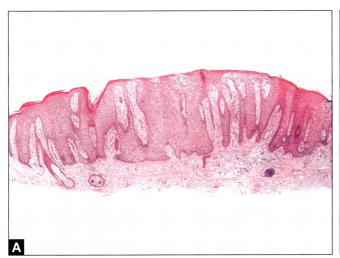

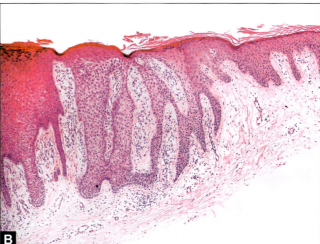

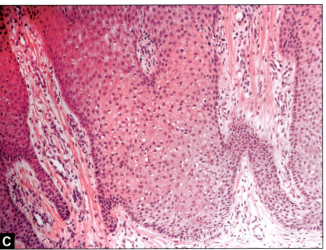

Figs 12.7A to C: Clear cell acanthoma. (A) Psoriasiform hyperplasia of pale staining epithelium; (B) Sharp demarcation between the clear cells and adjacent epidermis; (C) Neutrophils within epithelium clue to diagnosis.

Epidermal Nevus

An epidermal nevus is a type of birthmark usually presenting at birth, but occasionally delayed expression is seen (Figs 12.8A and B).

■ *Clinical criteria*

- Linear warty lesion usually following lines of Blaschko (Figs 12.8A and B).

■ *Histological criteria*

- Frequently requires clinical pathologic correlation
- Acanthotic papillomatous epidermis
- Occasional findings:
  - Psoriasiform epidermal hyperplasia
  - Warty changes
  - Epidermolytic hyperkeratosis
  - Coronoid lamella
  - Foamy cells within dermis (verruciform xanthoma)
  - Acantholysis
  - Seborrheic keratosis like changes.

■ *Pitfalls*

- Superficial biopsy of an epidermal nevus leads to fragments of skin resembling skin tags (Fig. 12.8C).

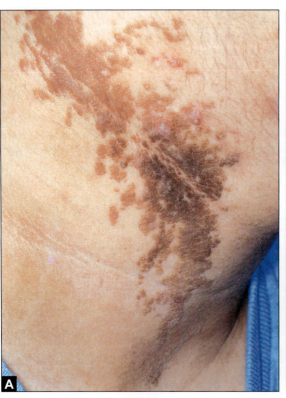

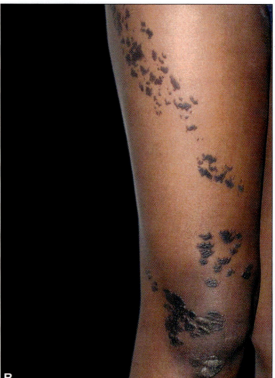

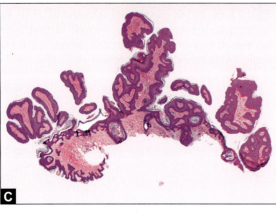

Figs 12.8A to C: Epidermal nevus. (A) Clinical picture of epidermal nevus; (B) Warty plaque in linear distribution; (C) Papillomatosis with skin tag like appearance.

Flegel's Disease (Hyperkeratosis Lenticularis Perstans)

Flegel's disease is an adult onset genodermatosis.

▪ *Clinical criteria for diagnosis*

- Family history with autosomal dominant inheritance
- Small keratotic papules on lower legs and feet.

▪ *Histologic criteria*

- Epidermal papillomatosis in periphery
- Center of the lesion often atrophic epidermis
- Lichenoid inflammation (Fig. 12.9)
- Hyperkeratosis.

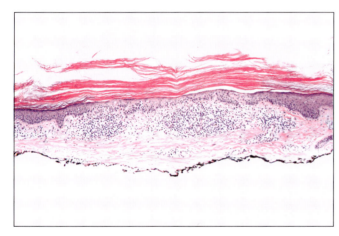

Fig. 12.9: Flegel's disease. Slight papillomatosis with central lichenoid inflammation.

Porokeratosis

Porokeratoses are a group of disorders which sometimes can be familial, but frequently idiopathic characterized by epithelial proliferation with a coronoid lamellae.

■ *Clinical criteria for diagnosis*

- Solitary (Porokeratosis of Mibelli): Plaques with a peripheral keratotic rim.
- Multiple (Disseminated actinic porokeratosis): Multiple papules with peripheral rim in sun exposed skin (Fig. 12.10A).

■ *Histological criteria (Figs 12.10B and C)*

- Coronoid lamella: Slanted parakeratotic column producing epidermal invagination with loss of granular cell layer and underlying dyskeratosis (Fig. 12.10C).

■ *Diagnostic clue*

- The central portion of disseminated superficial porokeratosis demonstrates lichenoid inflammation.

■ *Pitfalls in diagnosis*

- Coronoid lamella can be seen in other lesions besides porokeratosis, such as warts, actinic keratoses (Ackerman, AB).

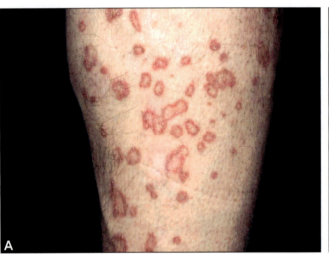

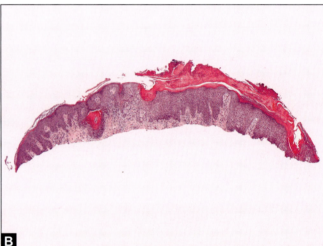

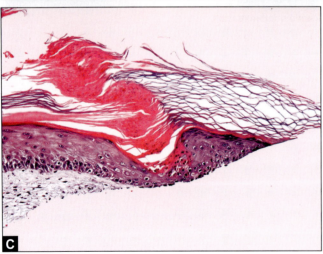

Figs 12.10A to C: (A) Disseminated superficial actinic porokeratosis—Plaques with rim in peripheryi on sun exposed skin; (B) Porokeratosis of Mibelli—Coronoid lamella at edge of specimen; (C) Coronoid lamella—Slanted parakeratotic column with epidermal invagination, loss of granular cell layer and dyskeratosis.

Seborrheic Keratosis

Seborrheic keratosis is a benign neoplasm of keratinocytes of unknown etiology developing in adults.

Criteria for diagnosis

- Epidermal acanthosis (Fig. 12.11A)
- Flat base imparting stuck on appearance (Fig. 12.11B)
- Basket weave hyperkeratosis
- Occasional horn cysts (Fig. 12.11C).

Pitfalls

- Irritated seborrheic keratosis: Numerous squamous eddies can lead to the impression of atypia and a misdiagnosis of squamous cell carcinoma
- Warts, condyloma accuminatum and epidermal nevi can resemble seborrheic keratoses (Fig. 12.11D).

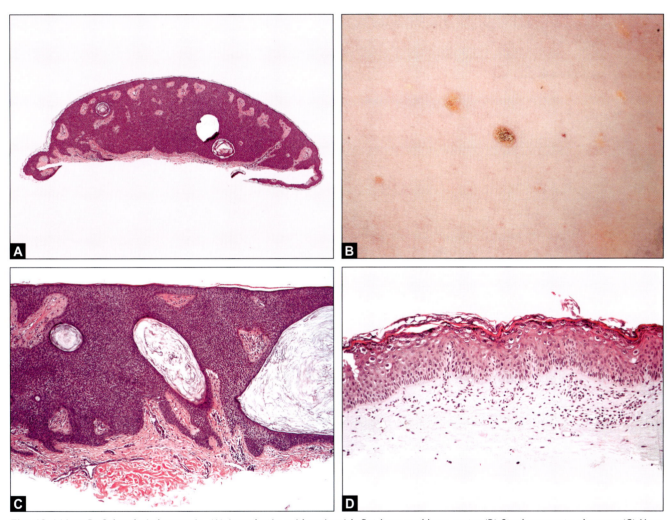

Figs 12.11A to D: Seborrheic keratosis. (A) Acanthotic epidermis with flat base and horn cysts; (B) Stuck on warty plaques; (C) Horn cysts are frequently but not always present; (D) Wart. Like a seborrheic keratosis flat base and acanthotic epidermis, but parakeratosis and koilocytosis present.

Solar Lentigo

Although a solar lentigo clinically appears to be a pigmented lesion, the pigment is within keratinocytes and therefore, solar lentigo is keratinocytic lesion. Melanocytic hyperplasia from actinic damage can be seen but the melanocytes are not atypical, relatively equally spaced, and nests of melanocytes as would be expected in a nevus are not present.

■ *Clinical criteria*

- Brown macule occurring in patients with history of sun exposure and sun damaged skin (Fig. 12.12A).

■ *Histological criteria for diagnosis*

- Uniform hyperpigmentation along the basal layers of the epidermis with elongated broad based and bulbous rete ridges (Fig. 12.12B).

■ *Pitfalls*

- Mistaking a pigmented lesion for a solar lentigo.

■ *Pearls*

- Solar lentigo can evolve into pigmented seborrheic keratosis.

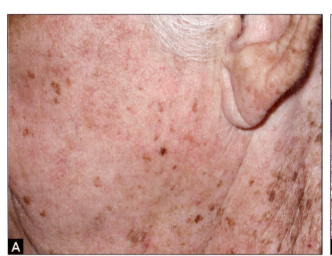
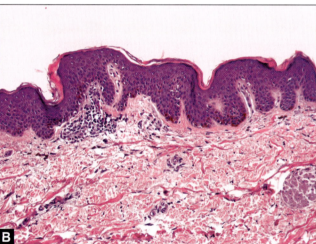

Figs 12.12A and B: Solar lentigo. (A) Brown macules on sun exposed skin; (B) Uniform pigmentation along the basal layers of elongated rete ridges in sun damaged skin.

Warty Dyskeratoma

Warty dyskeratoma is a benign keratinocytic neoplasm most frequently developing in head and neck area of adults.

▣ *Criteria for diagnosis*

- Cup shaped (Fig. 12.13A)
- Central keratin containing cavity
- Surrounding epithelium exhibiting acantholysis (Fig. 12.13B)
- Corp ronds and corps grains (Fig. 12.13B).

▣ *Pitfalls*

- An acantholytic squamous cell carcinoma also exhibits acantholysis and occasionally may have a cup shaped morphology but atypia will be present.

▣ *Criteria against diagnosis of warty dyskeratoma*

- Asymmetry
- Infiltrating base
- Epithelial atypia
- Lack of corps ronds and corps grains
- Atypical mitotic figures.

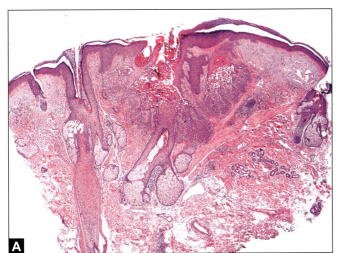 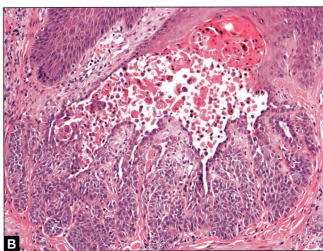

Figs 12.13A and B: Warty dyskeratoma. (A) Cup shaped, keratin filled folliculocentric neoplasm; (B) Acantholysis, dyskeratosis, Corps ronds and Corps grains.

MALIGNANT TUMORS ARISING FROM EPIDERMIS

- Actinic keratosis
- Squamous cell carcinoma
- Keratoacanthoma
- Verrucous carcinoma
- Basal cell carcinoma
- Porocarcinoma (acrosyringeal epithelium)
- Hidradenocarcinoma (acrosyringeal epithelium).

Actinic Keratosis Versus Squamous Cell Carcinoma

There is a continuum between actinic keratosis and squamous cell carcinomas and sometimes distinguishing between these two entities can seem somewhat arbitrary. Although one can argue that actinic keratoses are early squamous cell carcinomas, there is utility from clinical and treatment stand point in distinguishing between these two entities. Children grow into adults and have the same biological characteristics as adults, but as most parents will testify, should not be treated as an adult.

Actinic Keratosis

▪ *Criteria for diagnosis*

- Epithelial atypia (Fig. 12.14A)
- Solar elastosis
- Atypia spares foci where adnexal structures penetrate the epidermis (adnexae are spared from the harmful effects of ultraviolet light).

▪ *Criteria against diagnosis (Figs 12.14B and C)*

- Full thickness atypia with lack of sparing of adnexal structures (Fig. 12.14D)
- Invasion into the dermis.

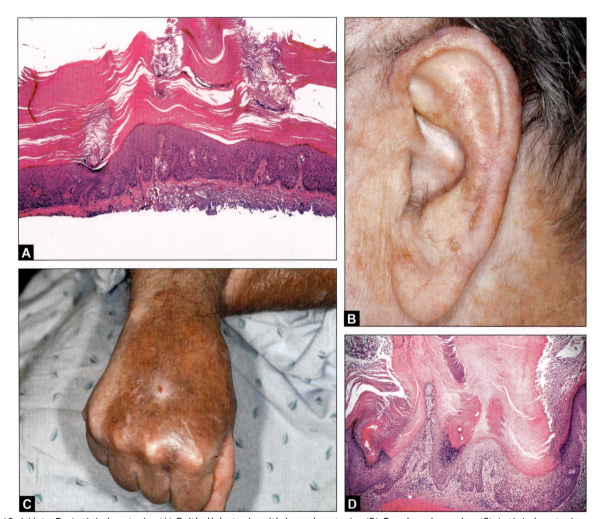

Figs 12.14A to D: Actinic keratosis. (A) Epithelial atypia with hyperkeratosis; (B) Rough red papule; (C) Actinic keratosis on dorsal hand; (D) "Flag sign" alternating foci of hyperkeratosis and parakeratosis within stratum corneum corresponding to foci of epithelial atypia that spare adnexal structures.

Squamous Cell Carcinoma

Squamous cell carcinoma is a malignant tumor arising from keratinocytes (Figs 12.15A to J). Multiple different variants of squamous cell carcinoma exist, most likely secondary to different etiologic agents. The common types of squamous cell carcinomas are listed below.

Types of Squamous Cell Carcinomas

- *Classical*: Arising from an actinic keratosis (see below) (Figs 12.15A and J).
- *Keratoacanthomatous type*: Often rapidly growing crater shaped (see below) (Figs 12.15D and I).
- *Bowenoid or squamous cell carcinoma in situ (Fig. 12.15E)*: These most likely represent a polymorphous group. Some arising from actinic damage, some may arise from human papilloma virus infection and some in the past may have arisen from carcinogen exposure, such as tars and arsenic.

- *Verrucous carcinoma (giant condyloma)*: Warty lesions arising from human papilloma virus infection most commonly seen in oral, genital and plantar skin (Figs 12.15G and H).
- *Squamous cell carcinoma in special site*: Oral, chronic wounds, chronic ulcers, and radiation.
- *Squamous cell carcinomas with special morphology*: Basaloid, acantholytic, adenoid spindle cell/desmoplastic, clear cell, etc. (Fig. 12.15F).

■ *Criteria for diagnosis*

- *In Situ*: Full thickness epithelial atypia involving adnexal structures (Fig. 12.15E)
- *Invasive*: Lobules of pleomorphic keratinocytes within the dermis (Figs 12.15B and C)
- No cause for pseudocarcinomatous epithelial hyperplasia (see above).

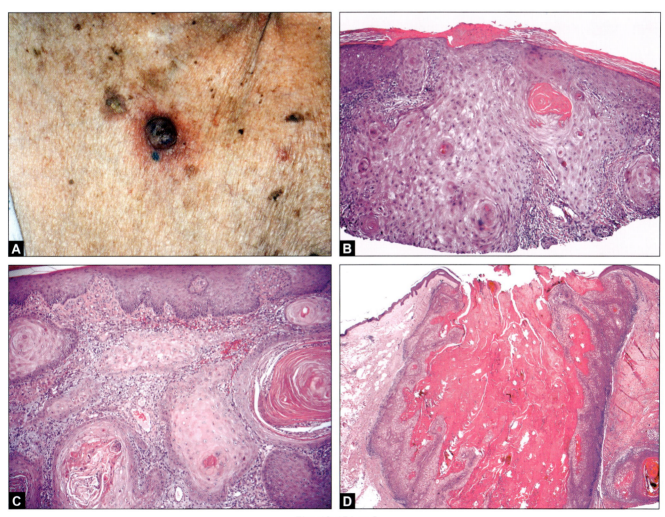

Figs 12.15A to D

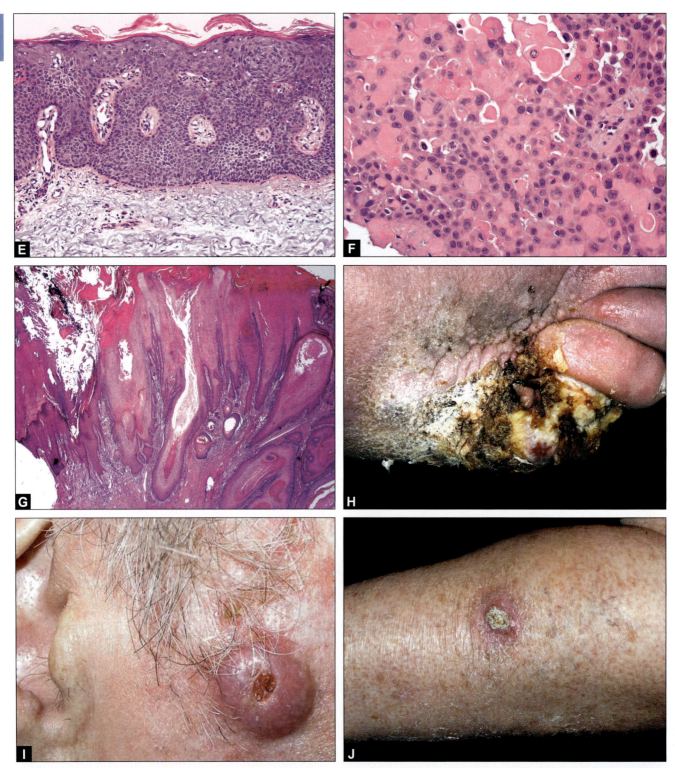

Figs 12.15A to J: Squamous cell carcinoma. (A, H, I, J) Clinical pictures of squamous cell carcinoma; (B and C) Lobules of pleomorphic keratinocytes extending into dermis; (D) Keratoacanthomatous type—Crater shaped lesion surrounded by pleomorphic epithelium; (E) Squamous cell carcinoma in situ (Bowen's disease)—Full thickness epithelial atypia; (F) Acantholytic squamous cell carcinoma; (G) Squamous cell carcinoma verrucous carcinoma type: Epidermal papillomatosis with downward extension of bulbous pushing epidermal rete ridges; (H) Clinical picture of verrucous carcinoma; (I) Squamous cell carcinoma, keratoacanthomatous type; (J) Classical actinically related squamous cell carcinoma.

Keratoacanthoma Versus Squamous Cell Carcinoma

Distinguishing between keratoacanthomas and squamous cell carcinomas remains a difficult challenge in dermatopathology (Table 12.1). Many believe that keratoacanthomas are a type of squamous cell carcinoma, and we support this opinion. The sine que non for a keratoacanthoma is the presence of involution (Fig. 12.16A). Therefore, the criteria for diagnosis of a keratoacanthoma revolve around the features that provide evidence of involution.

Table 12.1: Difference between keratoacanthoma and squamous cell carcinoma	
Keratoacanthoma	Squamous Cell Carcinoma, Keratoacanthomatous Type
• Cup shaped (Fig. 12.16B)	Cup shaped
• Epithelial atypia	Epithelial atypia haphazard throughout epithelium
(most prominent in periphery)	
• Intraepidermal microabscesses	No intraepidermal microabscesses
• Apoptosis	Apoptotic cells rare and haphazardly distributed
• Fibrosis (Fig. 12.16C)	Solar elastosis
• Eosinophils frequently	Eosinophils rare
• No precursor lesion	Precursor actinic keratosis may be present
• No atypical mitotic figures	Atypical mitotic figures

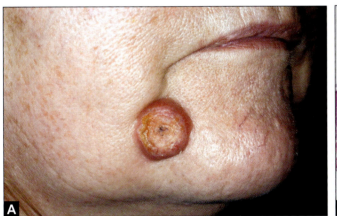

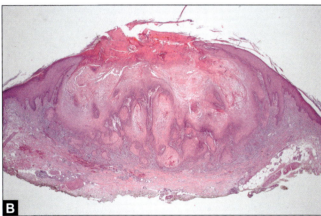

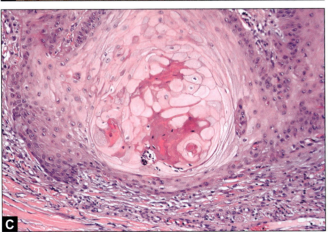

Figs 12.16A to C: Keratoacanthoma. (A) Rapidly growing nodule with central keratin filled crater; (B) Keratin filled cup shaped epidermal neoplasm; (C) Dyskeratotic cells demonstrate evidence for regression and clue for diagnosis.

Basal Cell Carcinoma

Basal cell carcinomas can frequently be diagnosed and recognized clinically. The types recognizable include:

- *Nodular* which presents as a pearly telangiectatic papule that ultimately ulcerates (Fig. 12.17A).
- *Superficial type*: Red eczematous patch with indurated border (Fig. 12.17B).
- *Morpheaform*: Scar like plaque (Fig. 12.17C).

- *Cystic*: Translucent papule or nodule
- *Fibroepitheliomatous*: Sessile nodule and plaque on trunk.

Occasionally dermatosis, lichenoid keratosis, amelanotic melanoma, seborrheic keratosis, squamous cell carcinoma, dermatofibromas, actinic keratosis and other neoplasms can be clinically mistaken for basal cell carcinomas. Inspite of the ability to clinically diagnosis basal cell carcinomas, a biopsy is required for definitive diagnosis.

■ Criteria for diagnosis

- Basophilic tumor lobules arising from the basal layer of the epidermis
- Peripheral palisading
- Clefting from the surrounding stroma
- *Germinative tumor cells*: Blue cells with indistinct nucleoli.

■ Pearls

- Basal cell carcinomas histologically can show great variability with numerous histological subtypes reported.

■ Pitfalls

- Trichoblastomas and trichoepitheliomas can be mistaken for basal cell carcinomas (see chapter 13)
- Merkel cell carcinoma can also sometimes be mistaken for a basal cell carcinoma. Unlike a basal cell carcinoma significant cytologic atypia with numerous mitotic figures are present
- Occasionally immunohistochemical studies need to be performed to confirm the diagnosis. Merkel cell carcinomas exhibit characteristic perinuclear dot staining pattern with cytokeratin 20.

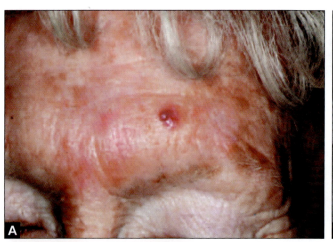

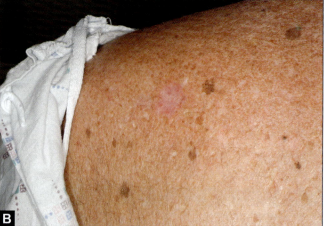

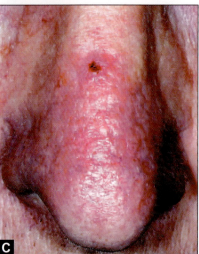

Figs 12.17A to C: Basal cell carcinomas. (A) Nodular type; (B) Superficial type; (C) Infiltrating type with poorly defined borders.

Common histological types of basal cell carcinoma (Figs 12.18A to E).

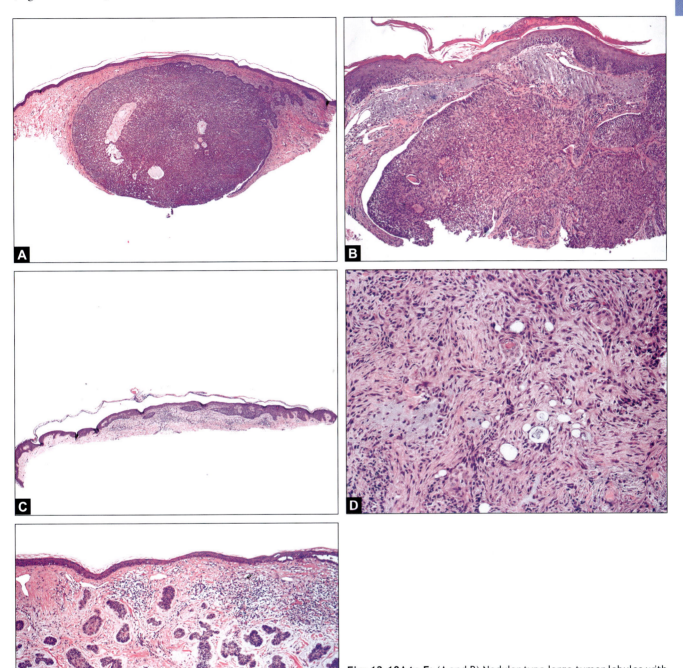

Figs 12.18A to E: (A and B) Nodular type large tumor lobules with peripheral palisading; (C) Basal cell carcinoma superficial type: Tumor lobules localized to dermal epidermal junction; (D) Basal cell carcinoma infiltrating type: Tumor lobules with jagged edges dissecting through collagen bundles (E) Basal cell carcinoma micronodular type: Tumor lobules generally sized same or smaller than hair follicles.

Color Atlas of Differential Diagnosis of Dermatopathology

BIBLIOGRAPHY

1. Billingsley EM, Davis N, Helm KF, et al. "Rapidly growing squamous cell carcinoma." J Cutan Med Surg. 1999;3(4): 193-7.

2. Deltondo JA, Helm KF. "Actinic keratosis: precancer, squamous cell carcinoma, or marker of field cancerization?" G Ital Dermatol Venereol. 2009;144(4):441-4.

3. Hashimoto T, Inamoto N, Nakamura K, et al. "Two cases of clear cell acanthoma: an immunohistochemical study." J Cutan Pathol. 1988;15(1):27-30.

4. Kaddu S, Dong H, Mayer G, et al. Warty dyskeratoma— "follicular dyskeratoma": analysis of clinicopathologic features of a distinctive follicular adnexal neoplasm." J Am Acad Dermatol. 2002;47(3):423-8.

5. Ko CJ, Barr RJ, Subtil AR, et al. "Acantholytic dyskeratotic acanthoma: a variant of a benign keratosis." J Cutan Pathol. 2008;35(3):298-301.

6. Leonardi CL, Zhu WY, Kinsey WH, et al. Seborrheic keratoses from the genital region may contain human papillomavirus DNA. Arch Dermatol. 1991;127(8):1203-6.

7. Li TH, Hsu CK, Chiu HC, et al. "Multiple asymptomatic hyperkeratotic papules on the lower part of the legs. Hyperkeratosis lenticularis perstans (HLP) (Flegel disease)." Arch Dermatol. 1997;133(7):910-1.

8. Maloney ME. (1995). "Histology of basal cell carcinoma." Clin Dermatol. 1995;13(6):545-9.

9. Megahed M, Scharffetter-Kochanek K. "Acantholytic acanthoma." Am J Dermatopathol. 1993;15(3):283-5.

10. Roewert HJ, Ackerman AB. "Large-cell acanthoma is a solar lentigo." Am J Dermatopathol. 1992;14(2):122-32.

11. Sanchez Yus E, del Rio E, Requena L. "Large-cell acanthoma is a distinctive condition." Am J Dermatopathol. 1992;14(2):140-7.

12. Sertznig P, von Felbert V, Megahed M. et al. "Porokeratosis: present concepts." J Eur Acad Dermatol Venereol. 2011;26(4):404-12.

13. Sexton M, Jones DB, Maloney ME. "Histologic pattern analysis of basal cell carcinoma. Study of a series of 1039 consecutive neoplasms." J Am Acad Dermatol. 1990;23 (6 Pt 1):1118-26.

14. Su WP. "Histopathologic varieties of epidermal nevus. A study of 160 cases." Am J Dermatopathol. 1982;4(2):161-70.

15. Toussaint S, Salcedo E, Kamino H. "Benign epidermal proliferations." Adv Dermatol. 1999;14:307-57.

16. Zayour M, Lazova R. Pseudoepitheliomatous hyperplasia: a review. Am J Dermatopathol. 2011;33(2):112-22.

CHAPTER 13

Adnexal Neoplasms

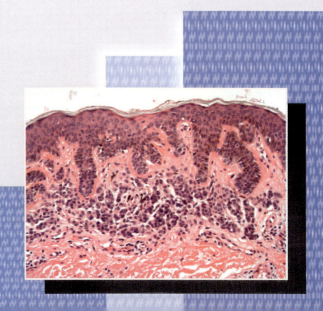

INTRODUCTION

Accurate diagnosis of adnexal neoplasms requires identification of areas of differentiation that mimic normal adnexal structures. The four major categories of adnexal tumors include: sebaceous, apocrine, eccrine, and follicular. Adnexal tumors can exhibit overlapping features, and clues to the correct diagnosis often depend on recognition of subtle areas of differentiation. For example, evidence of follicular, sebaceous and/or apocrine differentiation all provides compelling evidence against a diagnosis of an eccrine tumor because eccrine glands develop independent of the follicular-apocrine-sebaceous unit and should not exhibit areas with differentiation toward these structures.

CRITERIA FOR SEBACEOUS DIFFERENTIATION

- Vacuolated cells with scalloped nuclei
- Sebaceous ducts:
    - Duct lined by two layers of cells
    - Thin layer of orthokeratotic keratin within lumen
    - Crenulated/wavy surface.

TYPES OF SEBACEOUS NEOPLASMS

Sebaceous Hyperplasia

■ *Criteria for diagnosis*

- Clinical:
    - Yellow colored umbilicated papules on face
- Histological:
    - Lobules composed of mature sebocytes emptying into common duct (Fig. 13.1).

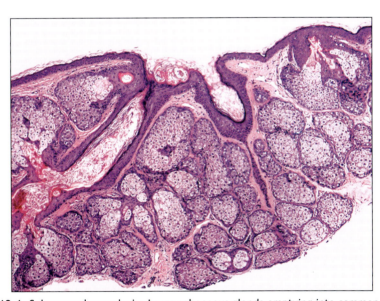

Fig. 13.1: Sebaceous hyperplasia. Large sebaceous glands emptying into common duct.

Sebaceous Adenoma

■ *Criteria for diagnosis*

- Clinical:
  - ▪ Yellow papule or plaque
- Histology:
  - ▪ Lobules composed of less than 50% immature sebocytes in the periphery with mature sebocytes and centrally located duct situated along the dermal epidermal junction (Figs 13.2A to D).

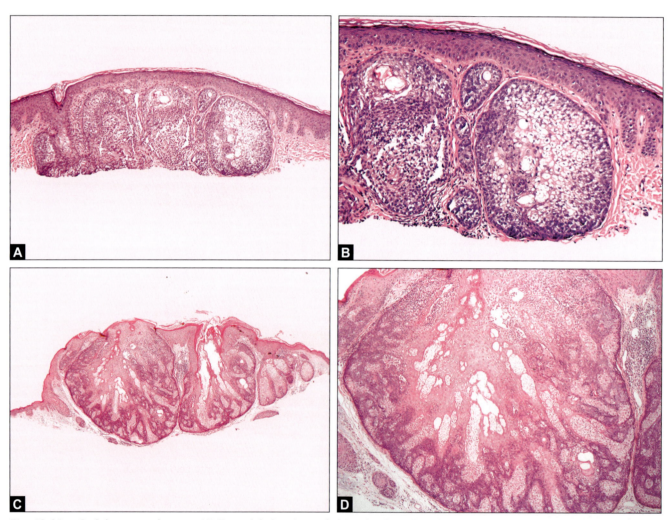

Figs 13.2A to D: Sebaceous adenoma. (A) Tumor lobules situated along the dermal epidermal junction; (B) Tumor lobules composed of predominant mature sebocytes in center with increased number of immature cells in periphery; (C and D) Normal architecture of sebaceous lobules retained.

Sebaceoma (Sebaceous Epithelioma)

■ *Criteria for diagnosis*

- *Clinical:* Yellow papule or plaque
- *Histology:* Tumor composed of lobules with predominantly immature basophilic staining sebocytes with randomly located mature sebocytes and ducts (Figs 13.3A and B).

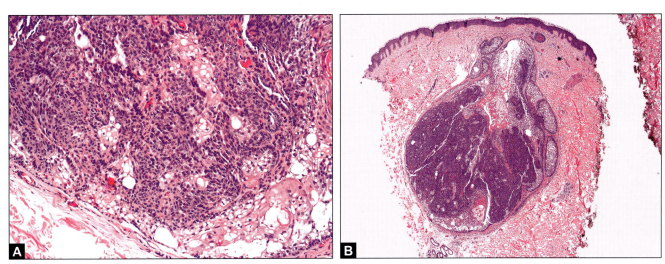

Figs 13.3A and B: Sebaceoma/sebaceous epithelioma (A and B) Tumor lobules composed of primarily immature sebocytes with sprinkling of mature clear vacuolated cells.

Sebaceous Carcinoma

- Clinical two types:
  - *Ocular*: Crusted papules on eyelids
  - *Extraocular*: Ulcerated papules, nodules, plaque

Criteria for diagnosis

- Asymmetry
- Nuclear pleomorphism
- Atypical mitotic figures (Figs 13.4A and B)
- Occasional pagetoid spread of cells within epidermis (Fig. 13.4C)
- Occasional ulceration.
- Occasional necrosis.

Pitfalls in diagnosis sebaceous carcinoma

- Squamous cell carcinoma with clear cells and tumors with areas of trichilemmal differentiation, both may exhibit clear cells with vacuolated cytoplasm resembling sebocytes.

Identifying areas with sebaceous differentiation sometimes requires immunohistochemical stains. Sebocytes express epithelial membrane antigen (EMA) and have androgen receptors, therefore, EMA and androgen receptor stains are often useful in ambiguous cases (Fig. 13.4C).

Pitfalls in diagnosis of all sebaceous neoplasms

- Distinguishing between sebaceous carcinoma, adenoma and epithelioma is difficult and not always reliable on small biopsies.

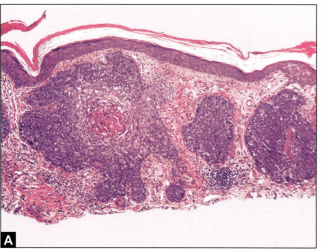

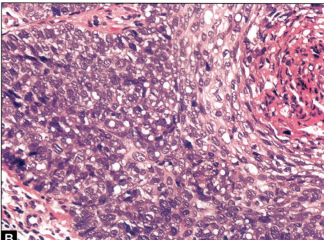

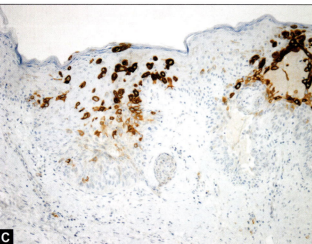

Figs 13.4A to C: Sebaceous carcinoma. (A and B) High nuclear cytoplasmic ration with atypical mitotic figures; (C) The epithelial membrane antigen stain demonstrates pagetoid spread of tumor cells within the epidermis.

Nevus Sebaceus (Organoid Nevus)

■ *Criteria for diagnosis*

Clinical

- Patch of alopecia on scalp since childhood. Often orange to yellow colored (Fig. 13.5A)
- During adolescence because warty in appearance

Histology

- Epidermal papillomatosis (Fig. 13.5B)
- Increased number of sebaceous glands (small glands in prepubertal biopsies, large glands in adolescents and adults) (Fig. 13.5C)
- Sebaceous glands connecting directly to overlying epidermis
- Loss of hair follicles (Fig. 13.5C)
- Apocrine glands in dermis

- Occasional evidence for follicular induction
- Occasional other benign and malignant adnexal tumors within (most commonly trichoblastoma).

■ *Pitfalls in diagnosis of nevus sebaceus*

- A superficial biopsy of nevus sebaceus can be confused with a seborrheic keratosis or wart
- Trichoblastomas arising within a nevus sebaceus can resemble a basal cell carcinoma.

■ *Pearls*

- Numerous other adnexal neoplasms may arise within nevus sebaceus.

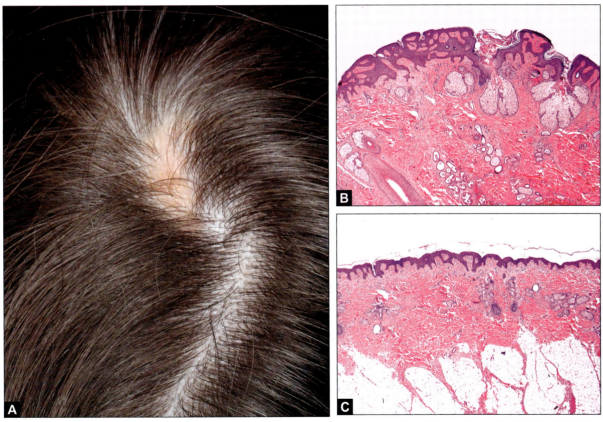

Figs 13.5A to C: Nevus sebaceus. (A) Patch of alopecia with orange color; (B) Epidermal papillomatosis with large sebaceous glands emptying directly into overlying epidermis; (C) Note absence of hair follicles. Small size sebaceous gland since excision was from prepuberal child.

Criteria for Follicular Differentiation

- Ghost cells
- Compact keratin
- Peripheral palisading
- Trichohyalin granules
- Fibroblast rich stroma
- Clear cells with peripheral palisading
- Dendritic melanocytes
- Papillary mesenchymal bodies.

Types of Benign Follicular Neoplasms

Differentiation towards follicular infundibulum and isthmus

- Dilated pore of Winer
- Nevus comedonicus
- Trichoadenoma
- Tumor of follicular infundibulum
- Trichofolliculoma (also differentiates towards entire hair follicle)
- Proliferating trichilemmal tumor.

Differentiation towards entire hair germ

- Trichoblastoma
- Trichoepithelioma

Differentiation towards hair matrix

- Pilomatricoma

Differentiation towards entire hair follicle

- Trichofolliculoma
- Hair follicle nevus

Differentiation towards outer sheath

- Tricholemmoma
- Inverted follicular keratosis

Differentiation towards follicular mesenchyme

- Fibrous papule
- Perifollicular fibroma
- Trichodiscoma
- Fibrofolliculoma

FOLLICULAR NEOPLASMS DIFFERENTIATING TOWARDS INFUNDIBULUM AND ISTHMUS

Dilated Pore of Winer

Criteria for diagnosis

- Clinical:
  - Cyst containing open pore
- Histology:
  - Cyst connecting to epidermis with dilated follicular infundibulum.

Pearls

- Dilated Pore of Winer is just an epidermal inclusion cyst with prominent opening (Fig. 13.6).

Pitfalls

- Basal cell carcinomas with pore like opening (Benedetto AV, et al).

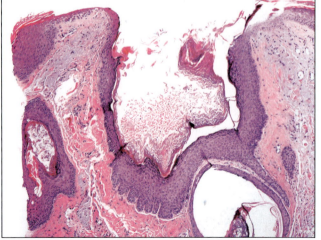

Fig. 13.6: Dilated pore of winer. Note continuity with the "pore" and milium/epidermal inclusion cyst at the base.

Pilar Sheath Acanthoma

■ *Criteria for diagnosis*

- Clinical:
  - Nodule with pore, most commonly on upper lip
- Histological:
  - Central keratin crater (Fig. 13.7A)

- Crater surrounded by lobules of epithelium exhibiting isthmus differentiation (Figs 13.7B and C).

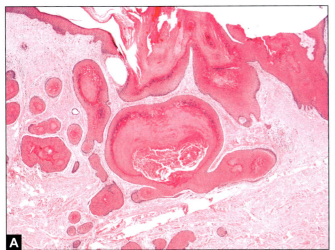

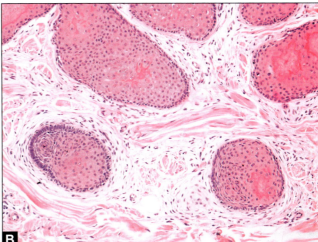

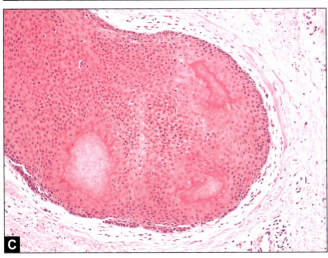

Figs 13.7A to C: Pilar Sheath acanthoma. (A) Central keratin filled cystic invagination with surrounding lobules of isthmus like follicular epithelium; (B) Lobules of follicular epithelium; (C) Note zones of compact follicular keratin within lobules.

Trichoadenoma

- Trichoadenoma clinical:
  - Nondescript papule or nodule on face or buttock.

▪ *Criteria for diagnosis*

- Numerous small milia like cysts in dermis (Figs 13.8A and B).

▪ *Pitfalls*

- Top portion of microcystic adnexal carcinoma will have horn cysts resembling trichoadenoma.

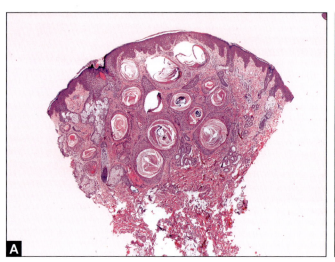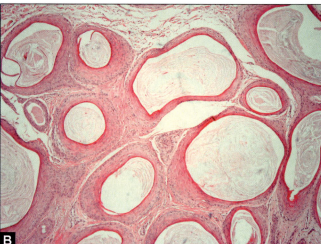

Figs 13.8A and B: Trichoadenoma. (A and B) Numerous horn cysts.

Tumor of Follicular Infundibulum

■ *Criteria for diagnosis*

- Clinical:
  - Nondescript papule
- Histologic criteria for diagnosis:
  - Elongated strands containing follicular infundibular and isthmus epithelium that anastomoses at the base (Figs 13.9A and B).

■ *Pearls*

- Tumor of follicular infundibulum frequently is found in associated with a basal cell carcinoma (Weyers W, et.al.).

■ *Pitfall in diagnosis*

- Tumor of follicular infundibulum can be mistaken for actinic keratosis, but parakeratosis is absent.

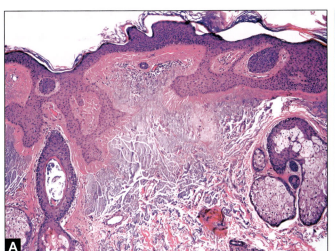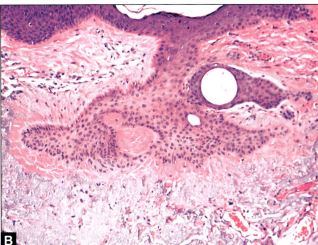

Figs 13.9A and B: Tumor of follicular infundibulum. (A and B) Plate like proliferation of follicular epithelium and horn cyst at base of follicular infundibulum.

Trichofolliculoma

■ *Criteria for diagnosis*

- Clinical:
  - Nodule with fine vellus hair protruding (Figs 13.10A and B)
- Histological:
  - Central keratin crater (Fig. 13.10C)
  - Vellus hair follicles radiate out from central crater (Figs 13.10A to C).

■ *Pitfalls*

- Peripheral portion of a trichofolliculoma can resemble a trichoepithelioma but vellus hair follicles are not seen in a trichoepithelioma.

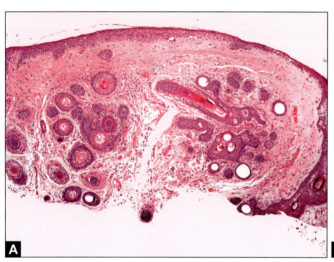

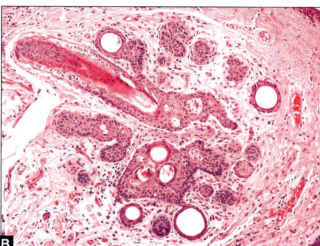

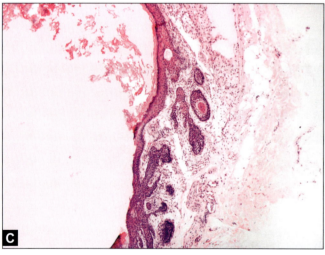

Figs 13.10A to C: Trichofolliculoma (A) Numerous small vellus hair follicles in periphery; (B) Small vellus hair follicles; (C) Central keratin filled cystic area with vellus hair follicles radiation out in periphery.

Proliferating Trichilemmal (Pilar) Tumor

■ *Criteria for diagnosis*

- Clinical:
  - Cyst on scalp in elderly female
- Histological:
  - Well circumscribed round neoplasm (Fig. 13.11A)
  - Composed of squamous epithelium with cystic and solid foci (Fig. 13.11B and C)
  - Follicular type keratinization and differentiation.

■ *Pitfalls*

- Malignant version exhibiting infiltrating borders exists.

■ *Pearls*

- "Pilar cyst" with cavity containing squamous epithelium clue to diagnosis
- AB Ackerman has hypothesized that proliferating tircholemmal tumors may represent squamous cell carcinomas arising with pilar cysts.

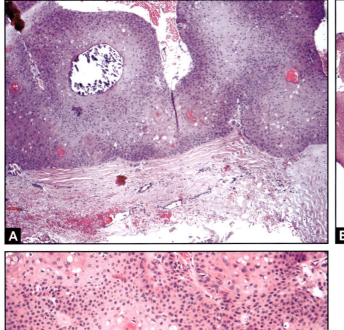

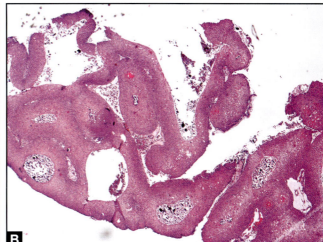

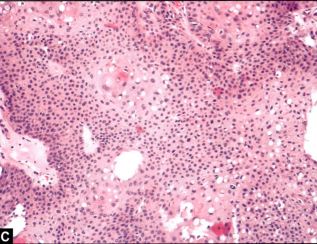

Figs 13.11A to C: Proliferating trichilemmal tumor. (A) Proliferating trichilemmal tumor: Well circumscribed border; (B) Cystic structure with solid tumor lobules in center; (C) Keratinizing epithelium can be mistaken for squamous cell carcinoma.

Pilomatricoma

Criteria for diagnosis

- Clinical:
  - Dermal or subcutaneous nodule in children and occasionally adults
  - Most commonly found in face
- Histological:
  - Ghost cells (Figs 13.12A and B)
  - Foci of calcification rarely ossification
  - Matrical cells: Blue cells with centrally located nucleoli (Fig. 13.12C).

Pearls

- Numerous mitotic figures can be seen and is not synonymous with malignancy
- May contain cystic space-matrical hair cyst.

Pitfalls

- Malignant version exists. Diagnosis is based upon infiltrating borders.

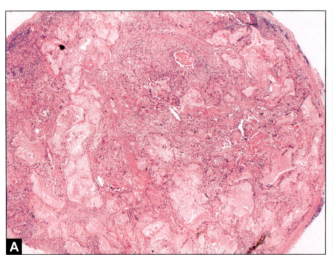

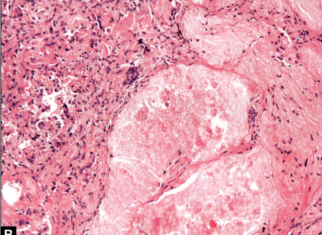

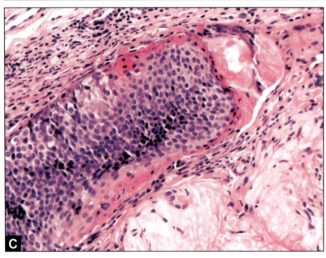

Figs 13.12A to C: Pilomatricoma. (A) Tumor composed of mixture of ghost and matrical cells; (B) Giant cells frequently surround the ghost cells; (C) Matrical cells with small centrally located nucleoli.

Tricholemmoma/Inverted Follicular Keratosis

■ *Criteria for diagnosis*

- Clinical:
  - Warty papule on face
- Histological:
  - Lobule arising from epidermis
  - Pale staining keratinocytes (Fig. 13.13A)
  - Peripheral palisading (Fig. 13.13B)
  - Thickened basement membrane zone (Fig. 13.13B)
  - Squamous eddies in inverted follicular keratosis.

■ *Pearls*

- Tricholemmomas have been associated with Cowden's syndrome (multiple hamartoma and neoplasia syndrome-tricholemmomas, and tumors, such as carcinoma of breast and thyroid)

- Tricholemmomas may be a histological expression of a type of wart (Fig. 13.13C)
- Inverted follicular keratosis are tricholemmomas with squamous eddies (Figs 13.13D and E).

■ *Pitfalls*

- A hyalinized stroma with associated reactive epithelial atypia may be seen in "desmoplastic" variant and can be misdiagnosed as squamous cell carcinoma.

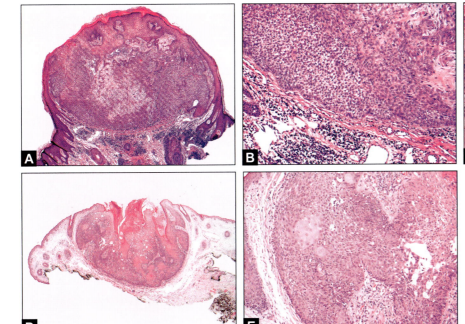

Figs 13.13A to E: Tricholemmoma. (A) Lobules composed of pale staining epithelium; (B) Peripheral palisading and thickened basement membrane zone characteristic; (C) Hypergranulosis resembling koilocytosis present. (D) Inverted follicular keratosis varient; (E) Inverted follicular keratosis variant of tricholemmoma: Notice numerous squamous eddies.

Trichofolliculoma

Discussed on page 358

Trichoepithelioma and Trichoblastoma

Trichoepitheliomas and trichoblastomas are benign adnexal tumors of the hair germ and represent a spectrum of differentiation from more differentiated (trichoepithelioma) to less (trichoblastoma). Trichoblastoma was originally described as poorly differentiated trichoepitheliomas.

■ *Criteria for diagnosis*

- Clinical:
  - Solitary papule or multiple papules inherited in autosomal dominant pattern
  - Multiple trichoepitheliomas have predilection for the nose and cheek with sparing of the upper lip.
- Histology:
  - Basophilic tumor lobules within the dermis (Figs 13.14A and B)
  - Fibroblast rich stroma (Fig. 13.15A)
  - Horn cysts in trichoepitheliomas (Fig. 13.14A)
  - Occasional calcification.

■ *Pearls*

- Familial trichoepitheliomas can be associated with other adnexal tumors, such as cylindromas and spiradenomas
- The epithelial lobules in trichoblastomas may be surrounded by lymphocytes and have been called lymphadenomas.

■ *Pitfalls*

- Trichoepitheliomas/trichoblastomas can be misdiagnosed as basal cell carcinoma (Table 13.1).

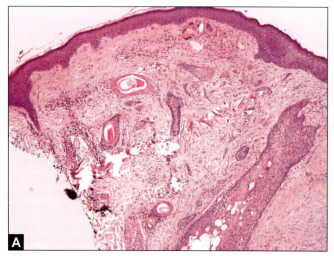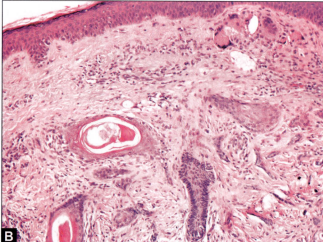

Figs 13.14A and B: Trichoepithelioma. (A) Horn cysts, basophilic tumor lobules, granulomatous inflammation and fibrotic stroma. Note no connection to epidermis unlike a basal cell carcinoma; (B) Horn cysts and basophilic staining tumor lobules. Note no clefting between tumor lobules and stroma.

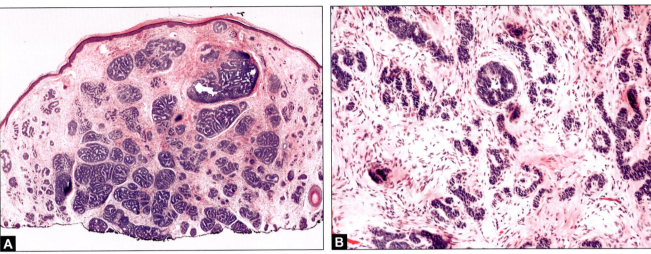

Figs 13.15A and B: Trichoblastoma. (A) Well circumscribed with fibroblast rich stroma; (B) Note that unlike a basal cell carcinoma the amount of tumor lobules and amount of stroma are approximately equivalent. In basal cell carcinoma the tumor epithelium predominates.

Table 13.1: Differentiating basal cell carcinoma from trichoblastoma/trichoepithelioma	
Basal Cell Carcinoma	*Trichoblastoma/Trichoepithelioma*
Connects to epidermis	Connection to epidermis rare
Asymmetric	Symmetric
Clefting between tumor lobules and stroma	No clefting
Mucinous stroma	Collagenous fibroblast rich stroma
Necrosis	No necrosis
Tumor epithelium predominates	Same amount of tumor epithelium and stroma (Fig. 13.15B)
Solar elastosis	Solar elastosis rare
Little evidence for follicular differentiation	Evidence for follicular differentiation
	Papillary mesenchymal bodies
	Trichohyalin granules
	Clear cells
	Rare sebocytes

Fibrous Papule

■ *Criteria for diagnosis*

Clinical

- Most commonly found as a small papule at nasolabial fold

Histological

- Dome shaped lesion
- Stellate fibroblasts
- Sclerotic collagen bundles (Figs 13.16A and B)
- Telangiectatic blood vessels.

■ *Pearls*

- Fibrous papules and angiofibromas seen in patients with tuberous sclerosis are indistinguishable
- Melanocytic hyperplasia may be present in the overlying epidermis causing confusion with a nevus.

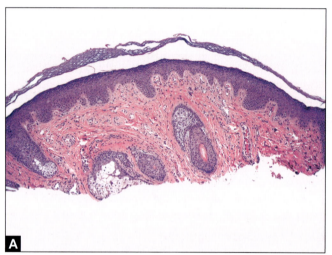 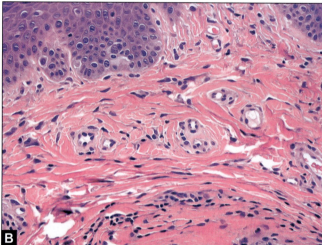

Figs 13.16A and B: Fibrous papule. (A and B) Stellate fibroblasts associated with sclerotic collagen bundles.

Trichodiscoma, Fibrofolliculoma and Neurofollicular Hamartoma

Trichodiscomas, fibrofolliculomas and neurofollicular hamartoma represent histological variation of the same neoplasm.

■ *Criteria for diagnosis*

Clinical

- Solitary or multiple lesions usually on nose or face
- Multiple lesions associated with Birt-Hogg Dube syndrome (mutation in foliculin gene leading to high risk of kidney tumors and cysts in lung).

Histologic Criteria (Figs 13.17A to E)

- Increased number of wavy spindle cells that may be S100 and/or CD34 positive.

- Slightly myxoid collagenous stoma
- Mittens of sebaceous glands in the periphery of trichodiscoma
- Proliferation of follicular infundibulum epithelium in fibrofolliculoma.

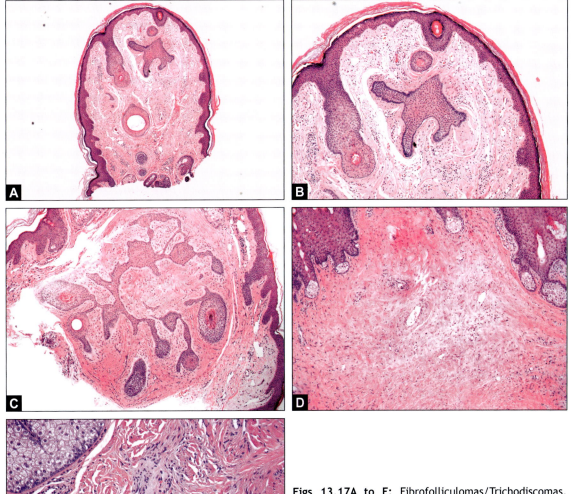

Figs 13.17A to E: Fibrofolliculomas/Trichodiscomas. (A) Lesions often have silhouette of skin tag or fibrous papule; (B) Closer inspection reveals distored follicular epithelium; (C) Anastomosing follicular epithelium with surrounding fibroblast rich stroma; (D) In Trichodiscomas only follicular stroma may be present; Sebaceous lobules in periphery are a clue to diagnosis; (E) The fibroblast rich stroma can resemble nerve bundles hence the synonym "neurofollicular hamartoma".

CRITERIA FOR APOCRINE DIFFERENTIATION

- Elongated ducts
- Ducts with columnar cells exhibiting snout like secretion
- Intraductal papillary projections
- Serous bubbly secretion
- Occasional goblet cells
- Clear cells without peripheral palisading.

NEOPLASMS EXHIBITING FOLLICULAR-SEBACEOUS APOCRINE DIFFERENTIATION

- Cylindroma
- Spiradenoma

Cylindroma

■ *Criteria for diagnosis*

Clinical

- Nodules, papules and cyst like lesions
- Frequent location on scalp (hence follicular-apocrine differentiation)
- May be inherited in AD fashion with multiple lesions (Turban tumor)

Histologic

- Lobules organized in "jig" saw puzzle configuration (Figs 13.18A and B)

- Thickened basement membrane zone around lobules
- *Two populations of cells*: Basophilic staining round cells with interspersed smaller lymphoid like cells with minimal cytoplasm
- Eosinophilic hyalinized stroma.

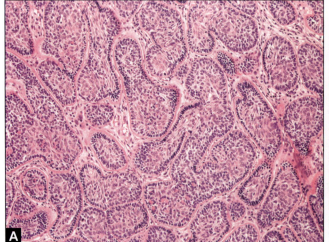 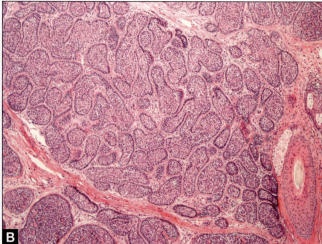

Figs 13.18A and B: Cylindroma. (A and B) Jig saw puzzled like appearance.

Spiradenoma

▪ *Criteria for diagnosis*

Clinical

- Dermal nodule which may be tender. Common location head, neck, trunk

Histological

- "Blue Balls" in the dermis (Fig. 13.19A)
- *Two populations of cells*: Basophilic staining round cells with interspersed smaller lymphoid like cells with minimal cytoplasm (Fig. 13.19B)
- Eosinophilic hyalinized stroma (Fig. 13.19C).

▪ *Pearls*

- Perivascular spaces bordered by tumor cells and lined by thickened basement membrane zone like material clue to diagnosis (van den Oord JJ, et al.) (Fig. 13.19C)
- Spiradenomas may occur in conjunction with cylindromas (cylindrospiradenoma).

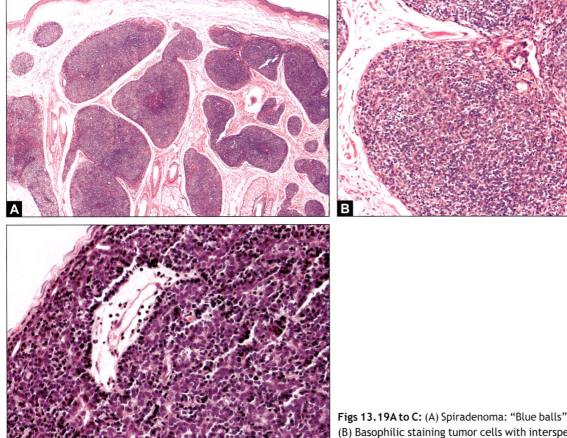

Figs 13.19A to C: (A) Spiradenoma: "Blue balls" within the dermis; (B) Basophilic staining tumor cells with interspersed lymphoid like cells; (C) Clue to diagnosis. Space containing eosinophilic hyalinized material surrounding blood vessel and tumor lobules.

TUMORS EXHIBITING BOTH ECCRINE AND APOCRINE VARIANTS

- Hidradenoma
- Poroma
- Mixed tumor (chondroid syringoma)
- Hidrocystoma.

Poroma (Figs 13.20A to C)

■ *Criteria for diagnosis*

Clinical
- Warty or pyogenic granuloma like papule plaque on plantar surface of foot, head and neck area, and occasionally elsewhere

Histological (Figs 13.20A and B)
- Composed of two cell types:
  - *Poroid*: Uniform appearing cuboidal cells (Fig. 13.20B)
  - *Cuticular*: Larger pale cells exhibiting eosinophilic keratinization

- Ducts
- Intracytoplasmic holes (attempts of forming ducts)
- Usually connection to epidermis (Fig. 13.20A)
- Hyalinized vascular stroma.

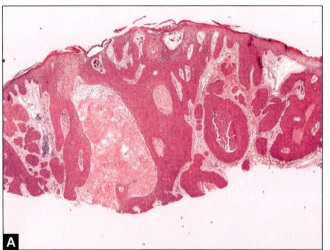

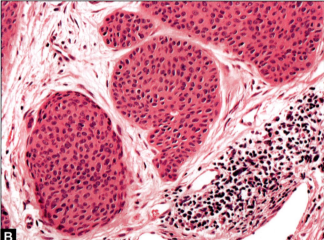

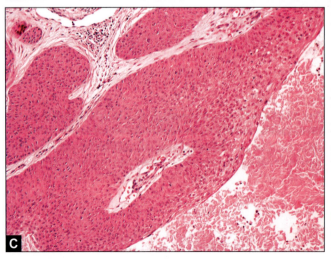

Figs 13.20A to C: Poroma. (A) Tumor connected to epidermis; (B) Uniform cuboidal (poroid) cells; (C) Solid area with adjacent area of necrosis.

Hidradenoma

■ *Criteria for diagnosis*

Clinical

- Dermal nodule with no distinguishing features

Histological

- Composed of poroid, cuticular and clear cells (Figs 13.21A and B)
- Connection to epidermis rare
- Solid and cystic areas (Fig. 13.21C)
- Ducts (more frequently found than in poroma)
- Hyalinized vascular stroma

■ *Pitfalls*

- A hidradenoma can be mistaken for a glomus tumor, but the glomus cells have indistinct cytoplasmic boundaries, surround blood vessels and are smooth muscle actin positive, and clear cells are not present (Figs 13.21D and E).

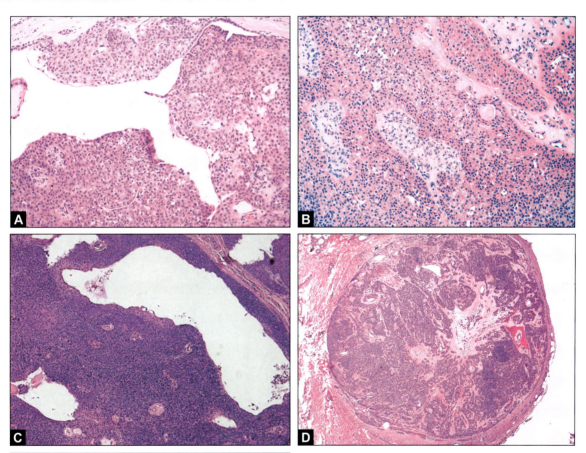

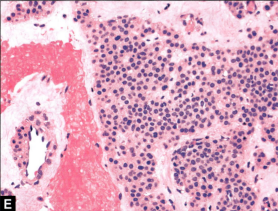

Figs 13.21A to E: (A and B) Hidradenoma: Note solid and cystic areas, and few clear cells; (C) Hidradenoma: Solid and cystic foci common; (D) Glomus tumor. Note low power resemblance to hidradenoma; (E) Glomus tumor: Uniform round glomus cells with indistinct cytoplasmic borders in perivascular distribution.

Mixed Tumor (Chrondroid Syringoma)

■ *Criteria for diagnosis*

Clinical

• Usually mistaken for an epidermal inclusion cyst

Histological

• Well circumscribed round neoplasm
• Small round ducts in syringoid (eccrine variant) (Fig. 13.22A)
• Long branching ducts and tubules (apocrine variant) (Fig. 13.22B)
• Mucinous chrondroid appearing stroma (Fig. 13.22C).

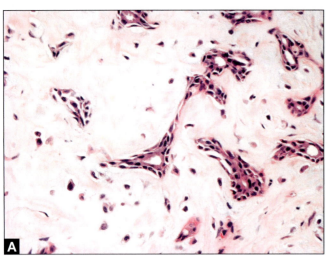

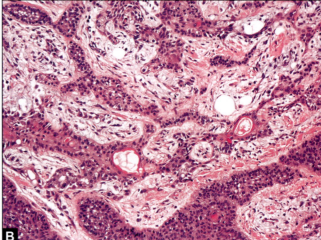

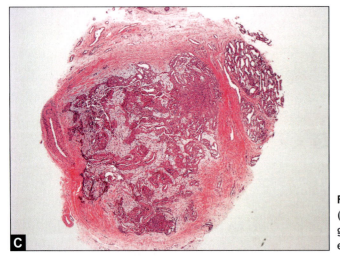

Figs 13.22A to C: Mixed tumor (Chrondroid syringoma). (A) Eccrine type of mixed tumor has small ducts resembling syringoma; (B) Apocrine type has elongated ducts; (C) Combination of epithelium and chrondroid like stroma.

PURELY APOCRINE NEOPLASMS

- Apocrine nevus
- Erosive adenomatosis of nipple
- Hidradenoma papilliferum
- Papillary tubular adenoma
- Syringocystadenoma papilliferum
- Tubular apocrine adenoma.

Hidradenoma Papilliferum, Erosive Adenomatosis of Nipple and Syringocystadenoma Papilliferum

In our opinion, these are three related apocrine neoplasms that can be primarily differentiated by their clinical location and not by histopathologic features.

■ *Criteria for diagnosis*

Clinical

- Nodules or warty plaques (Fig. 13.23A)
- Hidradenoma papilliferum: Genital skin
- Erosive adenomatosis of nipple (apocrine adenoma): On nipple
- Syringocystadenoma papilliferum: Frequently on scalp. Linear in distribution
- Occasionally arising within nevus sebaceous.

Histological

- Neoplasm composed of elongated tubules with occasional intraluminal papillary projections (Fig. 13.23B)
- Evidence for apocrine differentiation (see above) (Fig. 13.23C)
- Occasional connection to epidermis in vicinity of hair follicle/follicular infundibulum (Fig. 13.23A)
- Neoplasm entirely glandular with minimal solid areas
- Occasional plasma cells in stroma (numerous in syringocystadenoma)
- All of the above and:
  - *Location in vulva*: Hidradenoma papilliferum (Fig. 13.23D)
  - *Location on nipple*: Erosive adenomatosis of nipple.

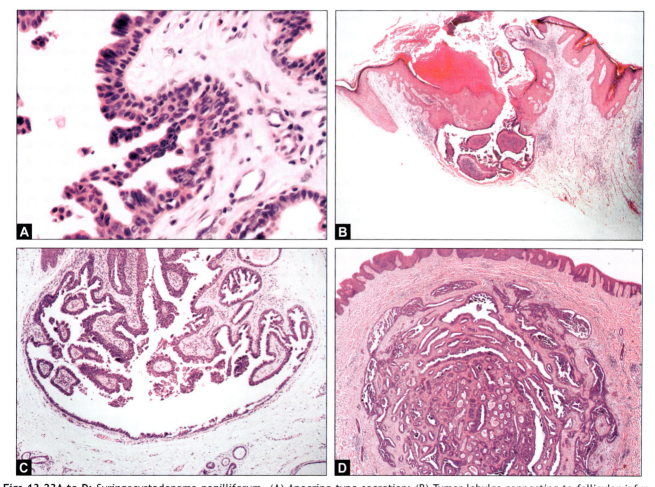

Figs 13.23A to D: Syringocystadenoma papilliferum. (A) Apocrine type secretion; (B) Tumor lobules connecting to follicular infundibulum; (C) Intraluminal papillar projections; (D) Hidradenoma papilliferum—Resembles syringocystadenoma but in contrast hidradenoma papilliferum is located in genital skin and connection to surface epithelium rare.

Tubular Apocrine Adenoma

■ *Criteria for diagnosis*

- Clinical:
  - No distinguishing features
  - Papules or nodule on scalp, axilla, face, chest or elsewhere
- Histological (Figures 13.24A and B):
  - Evidence for apocrine differentiation
  - Predominance of round apocrine glands
  - Occasional overlapping areas with syringocystadenoma papilliferum.

■ *Pearls*

- Occasionally there are tumors with overlapping features of tubular apocrine adenoma and syringocystadenoma.

■ *Pitfalls*

- The ducts may be mistaken for horn cysts and trichoadenoma but horn cysts contain keratin.

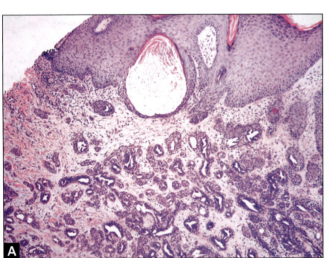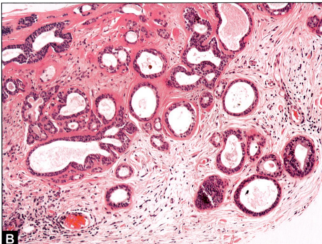

Figs 13.24A and B: Tubular apocrine adenoma. (A) Numerous tubular structures; (B) Tubules relatively round shaped.

CRITERIA FOR ECCRINE DIFFERENTIATION (DIAGNOSIS OF EXCLUSION)

- Ducts
- No evidence for apocrine/follicular/sebaceous differentiation.

ECCRINE NEOPLASMS

- Eccrine nevus
- Eccrine angiomatous nevus
- Eccrine syringofibroadenoma
- Hidrocystoma
- Syringoma

Syringoma

■ *Criteria for diagnosis*

- Clinical:
  - Usually skin colored papules around eyelids
  - Rare eruptive variant with numerous lesions on trunk or genitalia
- Histological:
  - Round small ducts in dermis
  - Ducts containing cords in periphery imparting "tadpole" or "comma" like appearance (Fig. 13.25A)
  - Hypocellular collagenous stroma (Fig. 13.25B)
  - Occasional clear cells lining ducts (Fig. 13.25C)
  - Occasional horn cysts
  - Basophilic homogenous material within lumina.

■ *Pearls*

- Clear cell syringoma is more common in patients with diabetes.

■ *Pitfalls*

- The top portion of microcystic adnexal carcinoma can resemble a syringoma (see below)

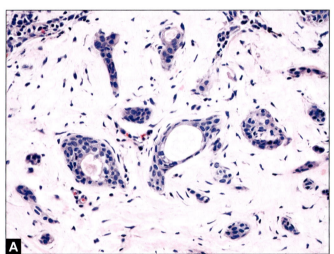

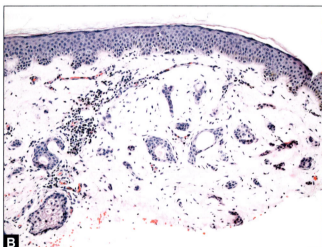

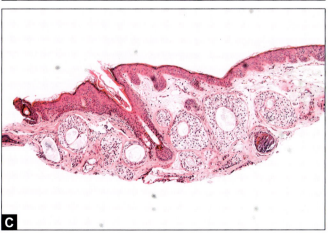

Figs 13.25A to C: Syringoma: Well circumscribed lesions with ducts, eosinophilic stroma, and cords with "tadpole" like appearance.

Malignant Adnexal Neoplasms

Malignant adnexal neoplasms can be categorized into five different pathologic types:

1. Malignant neoplasms arising within a preexisting adnexal neoplasm (Fig. 13.26)
   • Spiradenocarcinoma, porocarcinoma, hidradenocarcinoma, pilomatrical carcinoma malignant mixed tumor (usually malignant from onset), etc.
2. Adenoid-cystic carcinoma (Fig. 13.27)
   • Characteristic cribriform pattern
3. Mucinous carcinoma (Fig. 13.28)
   • Epithelial lobules embedded in lakes of mucin
4. Carcinoma with papillary configuration (Fig. 13.29)
   • Digital apocrine/eccrine adenocarcinoma

5. Carcinoma with small ducts (Fig. 13.30A to C)
   • Syringomatous carcinoma, microcystic adnexal carcinoma

◼ Pearls

• The most common malignant adnexal neoplasm is basal cell carcinoma (trichoblastic carcinoma). Basal cell carcinoma only arises from hair bearing skin and exhibits follicular differentiation.
• Basal cell carcinomas can exhibit a variety of morphological features that can be mistaken for other types of cancer. For example:
   ▪ Basal cell carcinoma with adenoid features can mimic adenoid cystic carcinoma
   ▪ Morpheaform basal cell carcinoma can mimic the pattern of metastatic adenocarcinoma.

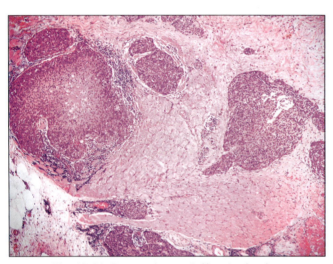

Fig. 13.26: Porocarcinoma. Infiltrating borders clue to malignancy.

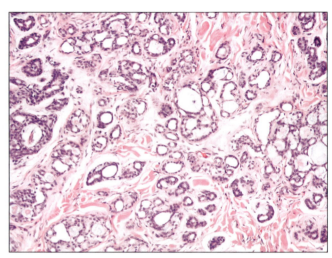

Fig. 13.27: Adenoid cystic carcinoma. Cribriform pattern is characteristic.

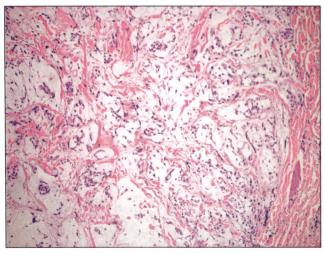

Fig. 13.28: Mucinous eccrine carcinoma. Tumor lobules swimming in lakes of mucin.

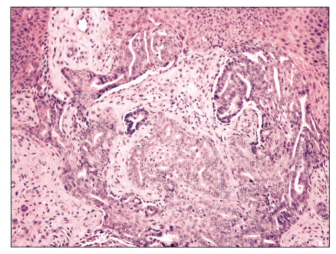

Fig. 13.29: Digital papillary adenocarcinoma. Solid foci, ducts, and papillary projections.

Differentiation between syringoma and microcystic adnexal carcinoma

- Not possible in small biopsy
- Deep dermal subcutaneous involvement not seen in syringoma
- Neurotropism in microcystic adenexal carcinoma
- Microcystic adnexal carcinoma cystic structures on surface with epithelial strands on the base
- Syringoma has cystic and tubular structures present throughout the lesion.

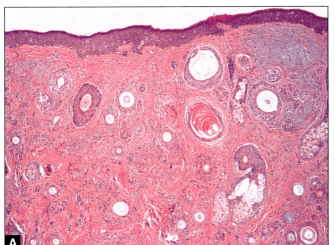

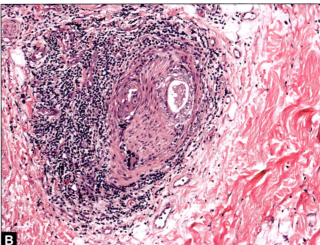

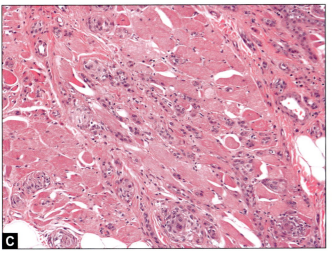

Figs 13.30A to C: Microcystic adnexal carcinoma. (A) Horn cysts that can be mistaken for trichoepithelioma/adenoma or syringoma; (B) Neurotropism characteristic finding; (C) Extention of tumor into muscle.

CYSTS

A cyst is a cavity or round space surrounded by epithelium. The name of the cyst is based either on the cyst contents or more frequently the derivation of the surrounding epithelium. Most cutaneous cysts are derived from follicular structures. Cysts present at birth or midline locations may represent embryological defects.

Follicular Cysts—Hair Follicle Related Cysts

Infundibulum Type/Epidermal Inclusion Cyst (Figs 13.31A to C)

■ *Criteria for diagnosis*

- Lining wall resembles epidermis/follicular infundibulum and contains a granular cell layer
- Cyst content looses basket-weave type keratin.

■ *Pitfalls*

- Top portion of sinus tract or fistula may resemble an epidermal inclusion cyst.

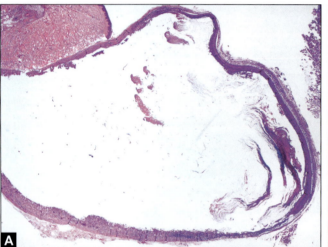

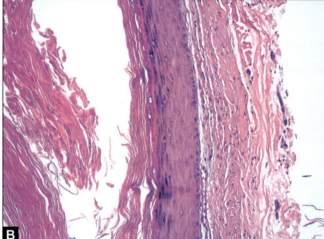

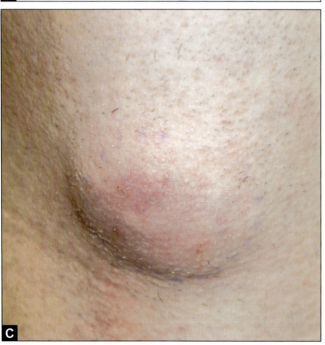

Figs 13.31A to C: Epidermal inclusion cyst. (A) Cyst with central located keratin; (B) Lining epithelium resembles epidermis; (C) Clinical picture.

Isthmus Catagen Type/Pilar/Trichilemmal Cyst

■ Criteria for diagnosis

- Clinical:
  - Most commonly located on scalp
- Lining wall resembles follicular isthmus with lack of granular cell layer (Fig. 13.32).

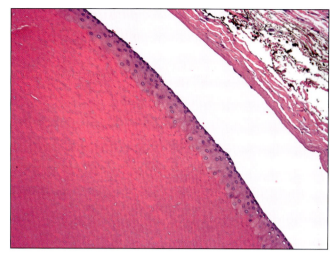

Fig. 13.32: Pilar Cyst. Compact keratin and lining epithelium lacks granular cell layer.

Steatocystoma (Cyst of Follicular-Sebaceous Duct)

■ Criteria for diagnosis

- Lining wall contains eosinophilic wavy cuticle resembling sebaceous duct (Figs 13.33A and B)
- Sebaceous gland occasionally seen in the wall.

■ Pitfalls

- Sebaceous glands can also be found in the wall of dermoid cysts, but dermoid cysts also contain hair follicles in the wall, are usually present at birth, and located around the eye/temple.

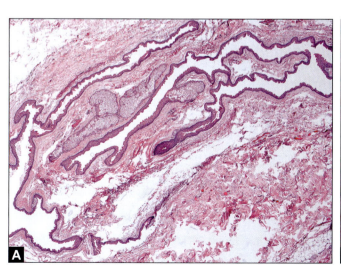 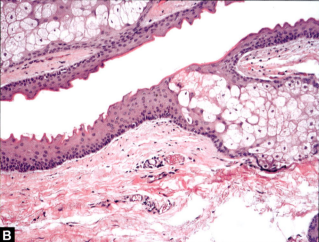

Figs 13.33A and B: Steatocystoma. (A and B) Wavy eosinophilic cuticle.

Rarer Follicular Cysts (Not Illustrated)

- *Vellus Hair cyst*: Diagnosis based upon vellus hairs in cyst cavity
- *Pigmented follicular cyst*: Diagnosis based upon pigmented hair shafts in cavity.

Apocrine/Eccrine Cysts (Hidrocystomas)

- Hidrocystomas are cysts of either the apocrine or eccrine glands (Figs 13.34A and B).

■ *Criteria for diagnosis*

Clinical
- Usually periocular location
- Translucent blue color

Histological
- Thin two-layered wall
- No cyst content visible or watery translucent material
- Lining epithelium exhibits decapitation secretion in apocrine type of hidrocystoma.

■ *Diagnostic pitfalls*

- Occasionally when a pilar cyst is excised a fragment of residual epithelium of the cyst wall can resemble a hidrocystoma
- Superficial biopsy of cystic basal cell carcinoma can also resemble hidrocystoma.

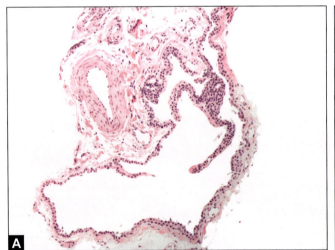 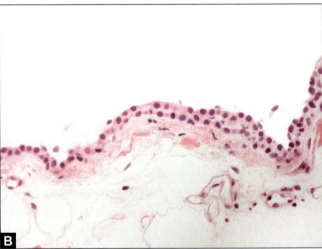

Figs 13.34A and B: Hidrocystomas. Cyst filled with clear or translucent material lined by thin one to two layered epithelium.

Embryological Cysts

- Thyroglossal duct
- Bronchogenic
- Branchial
- Cutaneous ciliated
- Dermoid
- Median Raphe cyst.

■ *Criteria for diagnosis*

Thyroglossal duct (Fig. 13.35)
- Thyroid follicles in periphery of cyst

Bronchogenic (Fig.13.36)
- Pseudostratified ciliated epithelium
- Goblet cells
- Surrounding cyst smooth muscle
- Occasional cartilage

Branchial (Fig. 13.37)
- Pseudostratified epithelium
- Surrounding lymphoid follicles

Cutaneous ciliated (Fig. 13.38)
- Location on lower extremities in females
- Cyst lined by ciliated epithelial cells

Dermoid (Fig. 13.39)
- Cyst wall or content contains hair follicles, sebaceous glands and occasional eccrine and apocrine glands.

Median Raphe Cyst
- Location on penis
- Stratified collumnar epithelium lining

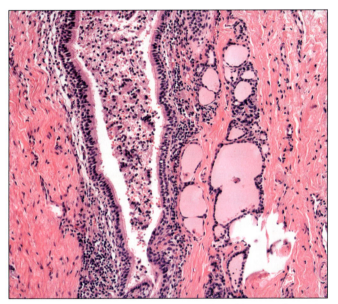

Fig. 13.35: Thyroglossal Duct cyst: Cyst lined by pseudostratified epithelium with surrounding thyroid follicles.

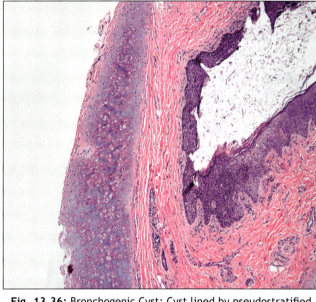

Fig. 13.36: Bronchogenic Cyst: Cyst lined by pseudostratified epithelium with surrounding cartilage.

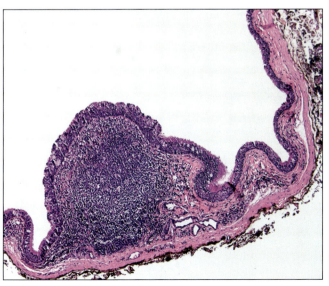

Fig. 13.37: Branchial cyst: Cyst lined by pseudostratified epithelium with surrounding lymphoid follicles.

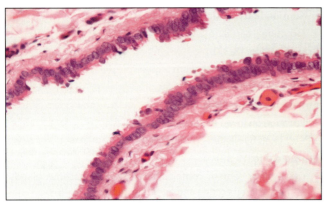

Fig. 13.38: Cutaneous Ciliated cyst: Epithelium exhibits cilia extending into lumen.

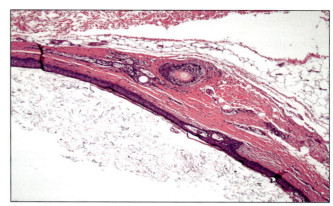

Fig. 13.39: Dermoid cyst: Keratin filled cyst with the wall and surrounding tissue contains small hair follicles and sebaceous glands extending into the cyst.

BIBLIOGRAPHY

1. Abenoza P, Ackerman AB. Neoplasms with Eccrine Differentiation. Philadelphia. Pa: Lea & Febiger; 1990. pp. 371-412.

2. Ackerman AB, De Viragh PA, Chongchitnant N. Neoplasms with Follicular Differentiation. Philadelphia: Lea and Febiger; 1993.

3. Ackerman AB, Nussen-Lee S Tan MA. Histopathologic Diagnosis of Neoplasms with Sebaceous Differentiation, Atlas and Text: Ardor Scribendi; 2009.

4. Benedetto AV, Benedetto EA, Griffin TD. Basal cell carcinoma presenting as a large pore. J Am Acad Dermatol. 2002;47(5):727-32.

5. Buckel TB, Helm, KF Ioffreda MD. Cystic basal cell carcinoma or hidrocytoma? The use of an excisional biopsy in a histopathologically challenging case. American Journal of Dermatopathology. 2004;26(1):67-9.

6. Goldstein DJ, Barr RJ, Santa Cruz DJ. Microcystic adnexal carcinoma: a distinct clinicopathologic entity. Cancer. 1982;50:566-72.

7. Helm KF, Cowen EW, Billingsley EM, et al. Trichoblastoma or trichoblastic carcinoma? J Am Acad Dermatol. 2001;44(3):547.

8. Kutzner H, Requena L, Rütten A, et al. Spindle cell predominant trichodiscoma: a fibrofolliculoma/trichodiscoma variant considered formerly to be a neurofollicular hamartoma: a clinicopathological and immunohistochemical analysis of 17 cases. Am J Dermatopathol. 2006;28(1):1-8.

9. Moore TO, Orman HL, Orman SK, Helm KF. Poromas of the head and neck. J Am Acad Dermatol. 2001;44(1):48-52.

10. Requena L, Kiryu H, Ackerman AB. Neoplasms with Apocrine Differentiation. Philadelphia, Pa: Lippincott-Raven; 1998. pp. 589-855.

11. Resnik KS, DiLeonardo M. Epithelial remnants of isthmuscatagen cysts. Am J Dermatopathol. 2004;26(3): 194-9.

12. Steffen C, Ackerman AB. Neoplasms with sebaceous differentiation. Philadelphia: Lea & Febiger; 1994.

13. Van den Oord JJ, De Wolf-Peeters C. Perivascular spaces in eccrine spiradenoma. A clue to its histological diagnosis. Am J Dermatopathol. 1995;17(3):266-70.

14. Weyers W, Hörster S, Diaz-Cascajo C. Tumor of follicular infundibulum is basal cell carcinoma. Am J Dermatopathol. 2009;31(7):634-41.

15. Wick MR, Swanson PE. Primary adenoid cystic carcinoma of the skin: a clinical, histological and immunohistochemical comparison with adenoid cystic carcinoma of salivary glands and adenoid basal cell carcinoma. Am J Dermatopathol. 1986;8:2-13.

CHAPTER 14

The Mesenchymal Tumors

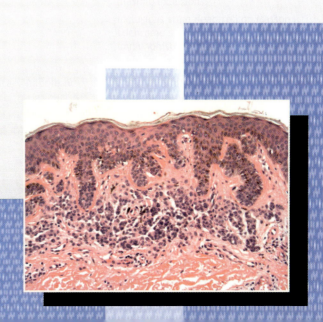

INTRODUCTION

The mesenchymal tumors are classified in most of the textbooks by their putative "cell of origin". From a practical standpoint, this is convenient when a specific lineage is immediately apparent. However, tumors that lack obvious differentiation or have features shared by two or more lineages are routinely encountered. A "spindle cell tumor", for example, may require formulation of a differential diagnosis that includes several different types of mesenchymal tumors in addition to spindle cell melanoma and spindle cell variants of squamous cell carcinoma. Therefore, approach all but the most obvious tumors with a differential diagnosis in mind. This allows judicious choice of immunohistochemical stains if they are necessary and helps prevent the occasional catastrophes that can result from misclassification.

A practical approach is to categorize the tumors by the following patterns: (1) paucicellular tumors that usually lack a specific architectural pattern; (2) cellular tumors with storiform or fascicular architecture; (3) tumors with a myxoid stroma; (4) tumors composed of epithelioid cells; (5) tumors with lipomatous differentiation; (6) tumors with vascular differentiation; (7) tumors composed of pleomorphic cells; (8) tumors composed of histiocytoid cells and; (9) tumors of round, undifferentiated-appearing cells.

PAUCICELLULAR OR PATTERNLESS TUMORS

In general, the tumors in this category are cytologically banal and have low cellularity. Most are obviously benign. Some have a definite tendency to recur, however, and a few have simulators that are aggressive. Mistaking a desmoplastic melanoma for a scar, for example, is one of the most common diagnostic disasters in all of dermatopathology. The point is that a differential diagnosis is always warranted.

Scars and Keloids

■ *Criteria for diagnosis*

- Dermis occupied by an increased number of cytologically banal fibroblasts and increased collagen fibers and prominent vessels at the site of trauma, biopsy or surgery (Fig. 14.1A)
- A scar is confined to the site of the injury.
- A keloid extends beyond the site of injury. (Fig. 14.1B).

■ *Differential diagnosis*

- Dermatofibroma
- Fibromatosis
- Desmoplastic melanoma.

■ *Pitfalls*

- Mistaking a desmoplastic melanoma for a scar is an uncommon but potentially disasterous error and represents one of the most well-known pitfalls in dermatopathology.

■ *Pearls*

- Most scars are accompanied by epidermal changes, including loss of epidermal rete
- If desmoplastic melanoma is a possibility, scrutinize the epidermis carefully for a junctional melanoma component and dermal lymphocytic aggregates. (see Chapter 11)
- Scars may have keloidal collagen bundles and thus clinical information is necessary to differentiate scars from keloids. (Figs 14.1C and D).

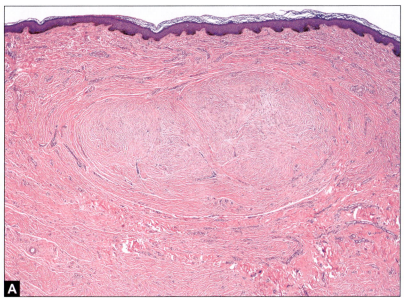

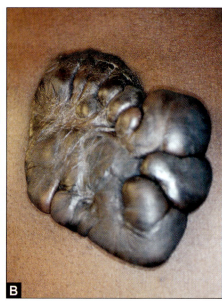

Figs 14.1A and B

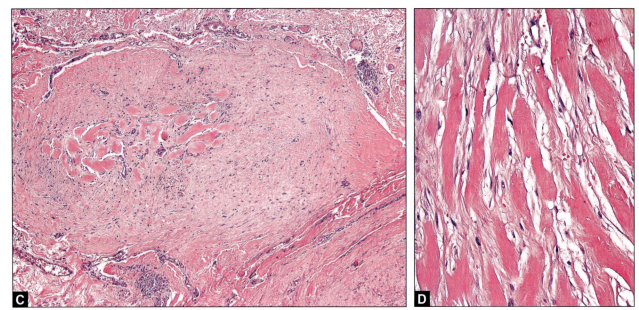

Figs 14.1A to D: (A) Hypertrophic scar. The dermis is occupied by vaguely nodular collections of collagen and an increased number of fibroblasts; (B) Keloids. This shiny, smooth plaque on the chest has extended beyond the site of the original injury; (C) This hypertrophic scar also contains keloidal collagen bundles. Unlike a true keloid, however, it did not extend beyond the area of the original injury; (D) Keloid. Thick, bright pink collagen bundles are numerous in most keloids.

Angiofibromas and Fibrous Papules

■ *Criteria for diagnosis*

- Firm, flesh-colored papule
- Ectatic vessels with a variable increase in fibroblasts, usually including some that are stellate with at least some periadnexal fibrosis in a concentric lamellar pattern (Fig. 14.2).

■ *Differential diagnosis*

- Acral fibrokeratoma
- Trichodiscoma/Fibrofolliculoma.

■ *Pitfalls*

- Superficial shave biopsies are often performed with a clinical differential stating something to the effect of "fibrous papule, rule out basal cell carcinoma." Occasionally these samples do indeed contain features of a fibrous papule but are accompanied by an underlying basal cell carcinoma not evident in the initial levels.

- Rarely, angiofibromas are composed of cells that are pleomorphic, epithelioid, have granular cytoplasm, or clear cytoplasm; these may simulate sebaceous tumors, metastatic carcinomas, granular cell tumors or melanocytic tumors.

■ *Pearls*

- If basal cell carcinoma is a possibility, additional levels should be examined since occasionally basal cell carcinoma is present in conjunction with a fibrous papule.
- Multiple angiofibromas on the face of a child or adolescent, particularly the nasolabial region, are often associated with tuberous sclerosis.
- Trichodiscomas and fibrofolliculomas are distinguished by denser periadnexal collagen and prominent folliculosebaceous elements.

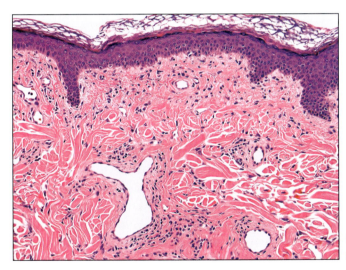

Fig. 14.2: Angiofibroma (fibrous papule). Ectatic vessels are surrounded by concentric fibrosis

Superficial Fibromatoses

■ *Criteria for diagnosis*

- A firm nodule, cord-like induration or diffuse thickening of the skin and subcutis
- A predilection for the palmar surfaces of the hands (Dupuytren's contracture) (Fig. 14.3A), plantar surfaces of the feet (Ledderhose's disease) and the penis (Peyronie's disease) (see Table 14.2).
- Banal fibroblasts and occasional multinucleated cells arranged fascicles within a collagenous stroma (Fig. 14.3B)
- Low mitotic index and absence of significant cytologic atypia.

■ *Differential diagnosis*

- Scar
- Desmoplastic fibroma/tendon sheath fibroma
- Dermatofibroma
- Myofibroma/myofibromatosis
- Calcifying aponeurotic fibroma.

■ *Pitfalls*

- Cellularity may vary markedly, ranging from paucicellular sclerotic regions (usually seen in long-standing lesions) to areas of relatively high cellularity (usually in earlier lesions); the latter may be confused with low-grade sarcomas
- Ill-defined borders are common, but some regions contain circumscribed nodules that resemble other spindle cell neoplasms.

■ *Pearls*

- In most superficial fibromatoses, the clinical presentation is characteristic
- Lesions frequently recur but never metastasize

- A family history of the disease is often discovered if sought
- Strong predilection for Caucasian males (at least three times more common in males)
- The ulnar region is favored in palmar fibromatosis and may cause contractures of the fourth and fifth digits
- Fifty percent of the cases are bilateral
- Increased frequency of all superficial fibromatoses in patients with diabetes mellitus, epileptics who take anticonvulsants, and those with alcoholic liver disease
- Lesions arise within the fascia or aponeurosis and extend upward into the subcutis
- Early lesions tend to be relatively cellular; over time cellularity diminishes and sclerotic collagen bundles become the dominant feature (Figs 14.3C and D)
- Calcifying aponeurotic fibroma is uncommon except in children, and usually contains plump epithelioid cells and calcified nodules
- Fibrosarcomas involving the superficial tissues of the hands and feet are exceedingly rare; a fibromatosis lacks the cellularity and "herringbone" fascicular architecture of a fibrosarcoma
- Palmar fibromatosis has a marked predilection for older patients (extremely rare before the age of 30)
- Plantar fibromatosis occurs across a broad age range, (onset before the age of 30 in approximately 40%)
- Penile fibromatosis (Peyronie's disease) was thought to be rare but may affect up to approximately 8% of males
- Penile fibromatosis is less frequently biopsied, but it appears to be less cellular and more sclerotic than the other types and have a higher incidence of metaplastic ossification.

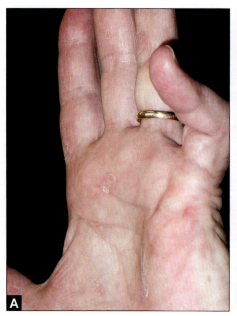
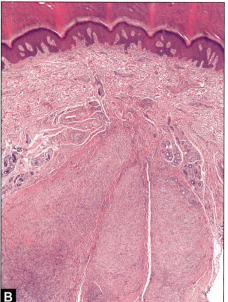

Figs 14.3A and B

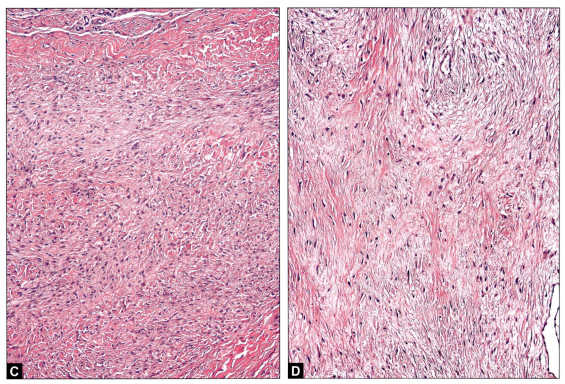

Figs 14.3A to D: Superficial fibromatosis. (A) There is contracture of the fifth digit on the hand of this elderly man(Dupuytren's contracture); (B) The lesional borders are often ill-defined, but as illustrated here, well demarcated nodules may also be present; (C) Early lesions are usually relatively cellular and may form vague fascicles; (D) In long standing tumors, the cellularity decreases and irregular collagen bundles predominate.

Deep Fibromatosis (Desmoid tumor, Desmoid fibromatosis)

Criteria for diagnosis

- Indurated plaques or nodules that arise from aponeuroses, fascia or intramuscular fibrous tissue
- Infiltrative, ill-defined nodules of cytologically banal spindled cells arranged in fascicles or haphazardly within a collagenous to myxoid stroma (Fig. 14.4A)
- Vimentin positive; variably positive for smooth muscle actin (SMA) and beta-catenin; negative for desmin.

Differential diagnosis

- Scar
- Dermatofibroma/dermatomyofibroma
- Superficial fibromatosis
- Fibrosing dermatitis.

Pitfalls

- Beta-catenin is positive only in 60–70% of cases
- The low cellularity and haphazard architecture make margin assessment difficult in re-excisions of desmoid tumors (Fig. 14.4B)
- Diffuse infiltration makes excision and assessment of margins very difficult in many cases.

Pearls

- The term "deep" fibromatosis is misleading since these tumors occasionally involve skin and even appear largely confined to the dermis and subcutis in some sections
- Marked tendency for repeated local recurrence that may be locally destructive; no metastatic potential
- Immunohistochemistry for beta-catenin is helpful in excluding other fibroblastic tumors but keep in mind that it is expressed in only 60–70% of desmoids tumors (Fig. 14.4C).

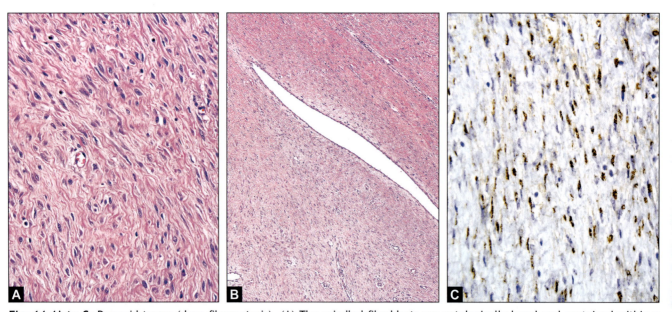

Figs 14.4A to C: Desmoid tumor (deep fibromatosis). (A) The spindled fibroblasts are cytologically banal and contained within a fibrous stroma; (B) Cellularity is relatively low and there is often no discernible pattern. Elongated, ectatic vessels are common in established tumors; (C) Nuclear and cytoplasmic reactivity for antibodies directed against beta-catenin is characteristic, but sensitivity has been estimated at only 60–70%.

Multinucleate Giant Cell Angiohistiocytoma

Criteria for diagnosis

- One or more papules on the distal extremities
- Increased number of small vessels in the superficial dermis with cytologically banal stellate and multinucleated cells within a fibrous stroma (Figs 14.5A and B).

Differential diagnosis

- Acroangiodermatitis
- Chronic dermatitis with multinucleate cells
- Angiomas/hemangiomas.

Pitfalls

- The number of supposedly characteristic multinucleate cells varies.

Pearls

- Since similar features are often seen in long-standing chronic dermatitis with lichen simplex chronicus/prurigo change, multinucleate giant cell angiohistiocytoma may be a reactionary phenomenon rather than a "true" neoplasm.

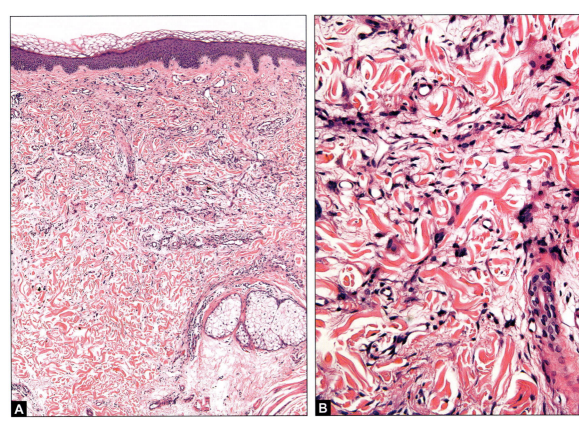

Figs 14.5A and B: Multinucleate cell angiohistiocytoma. (A) The papillary dermis contains an increased number of spindled and stellate cells, as well as numerous capillary-sized vessels; (B) Stellate and multinucleated cells are conspicuous.

Tendon Sheath Fibroma

■ *Criteria for diagnosis*

- A slowly enlarging nodule attached to a tendon sheath (Fig. 14.6A)
- Early cellular tumors are cellular and have a fasciitis-like appearance; later tumors are paucicellular and sclerotic or hyalinized (Fig. 14.6B).

■ *Differential diagnosis*

- Nodular fasciitis
- Giant cell tumor of the tendon sheath.

■ *Pitfalls*

- Early lesions may contain areas indistinguishable from nodular fasciitis
- In some cases, a definite connection to the tendon sheath is not evident.

■ *Pearls*

- Hands and feet are most common site (see Table 14.2)
- Ages 20–50 with male predominance
- A t(2;11)(q31-32;q12) translocation has been identified (Ide F et al. 1999)
- May recur but does not metastasize.

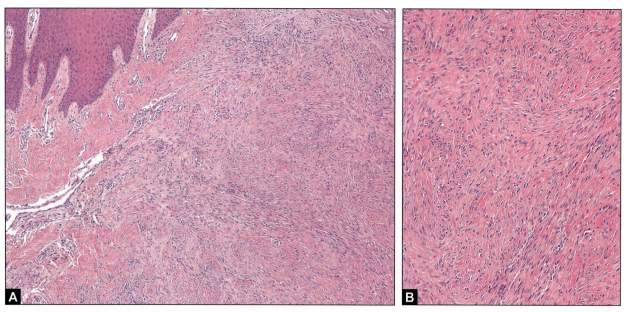

Figs 14.6A and B: Tendon sheath fibroma. (A) An early tendon sheath fibroma. Extension into the upper dermis is somewhat uncommon but may be seen depending on the site; (B) Some lesions are cellular and closely resemble a fibromatosis, but tendon sheath fibromas are usually more circumscribed and may have a "capsule" of compressed collagen bundles. In this case, the surgeon reported an obvious contiguity with a tendon.

Desmoplastic Fibroblastoma

Criteria for diagnosis

- A slowly enlarging nodule within the subcutis or deeper soft tissue
- Early cellular tumors are cellular and have a fasciitis-like appearance; later tumors have low cellularity and haphazardly arranged small fibrocytes (Figs 14.7A and B).

Differential diagnosis

- Tendon sheath fibroma
- Superficial fibromatosis
- Nodular fasciitis
- Neurofibroma.

Pitfalls

- The histopathologic features may be virtually identical to those of a tendon sheath fibroma
- Occasionally, neurofibromas have a very similar architecture.

Pearls

- Hands and feet are the most common site (see Table 14.2)
- Ages 20–50 with male predominance
- Desmoplastic fibromas rarely recur, unlike fibromatoses and tendon sheath fibromas
- Very few cases have been studied cytogenetically, but they have shown the same translocation as tendon sheath fibroma t(2;11)(q31-32;q12) (Ide et al, 1999).

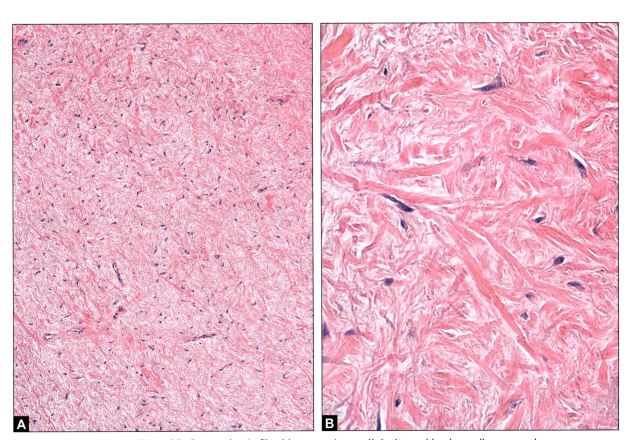

Figs 14.7A and B: Desmoplastic fibroblastoma. Low cellularity and haphazardly arranged small fibrocytes are characteristic of established tumors.

Neurofibroma and Variants

■ *Criteria for diagnosis*

- Dermis and/or subcutis occupied by small, cytologically banal cells that may be ovoid, fusiform, spindled, or "buckled" in a homogenous eosinophilic stroma or a loose collagenous stroma (Figs 14.8A and B)
- Stroma may be one or more of the following types:
  - Pale eosinophilic and homogenous ('neuropil-like') (Fig. 14.8B)
  - Thin collagen fibers arranged haphazardly or in vague fascicles
  - Myxoid (see Myxoid Tumors) (Fig. 14.8C)
- Immunohistochemistry:
  - S100   + in approximately 50–70% of lesional cells
  - CD34   + in variable number of cells
  - EMA   + in scattered cells

■ *Differential diagnosis*

- The diffuse variant of neurofibroma may closely simulate dermatofibrosarcoma protuberans (DFSP) (see below)
- The plexiform variant of neurofibroma may be difficult to distinguish from schwannoma (see below) (Fig. 14.8D)
- Rarely, "ancient change" (or degenerative atypia) is present and may be confused with desmoplastic melanoma (or rarely, a malignant peripheral nerve sheath tumor).

■ *Pitfalls*

- Some cases are predominantly myxoid and may be mistaken for other myxoid tumors (see Myxoid Tumors, below)
- Rarely, desmoplastic melanoma may simulate neurofibroma
- Occasional cases contain degenerative atypia ('ancient change') which results in pleomorphic cells that may be mistaken for evidence of malignancy.

■ *Pearls*

- Sporadic neurofibromas have a very low risk of malignant transformation and simple excision is adequate therapy
- Before making a diagnosis of a neurofibroma in sun-damaged skin, be certain to exclude desmoplastic melanoma

- Remember that S100 is expressed by only about half the cells in a typical neurofibroma (useful for differentiation from a schwannomas, which are almost entirely S100+)
- Myxoid variant is uncommon and has a predilection for the extremities and may simulate nerve sheath myxomas or dermal mucinosis.

■ *Diffuse neurofibroma*

- An uncommon variant of neurofibroma notable for its tendency to simulate the superficial portions of (DFSP)
- Ill-defined plaque-like elevations of the skin with a predilection for the head and neck region of children and young adults (Fig. 14.8E)
- Lesional cells are similar to those of conventional neurofibroma but growth is more diffuse and infiltrative, involving the entire dermis and usually the subcutis with permeation around adnexal structures and extension into fat
- Wagner-Meissner bodies are a characteristic feature that aids in distinguishing diffuse NF from DFSPs (Fig. 14.8F)
- Although S100+ cells usually predominate, a subset of the cells express CD34, and careful distinction from DFSP is essential.

■ *Plexiform neurofibroma*

- Cutaneous neurofibromas may have a plexiform pattern, but plexiform neurofibroma is a term reserved for tumors that involve large segments of deep nerves, since genuine plexiform neurofibromas are considered pathognomonic of neurofibromatosis.
- Plexiform pattern neurofibromas are characterized by marked enlargement of nerves by spindled and ovoid cells
- The expanded nerve bundles surrounded by intact perineurium and epineurium may simulate the encapsulated appearance typical of schwannomas, and distinction between the two may be difficult
- Some claim that neurofilament protein (NFP) positivity within scattered cells differentiates neurofibromas from schwannomas, but this has been disputed; we do not recommend relying on NFP alone to make this distinction.

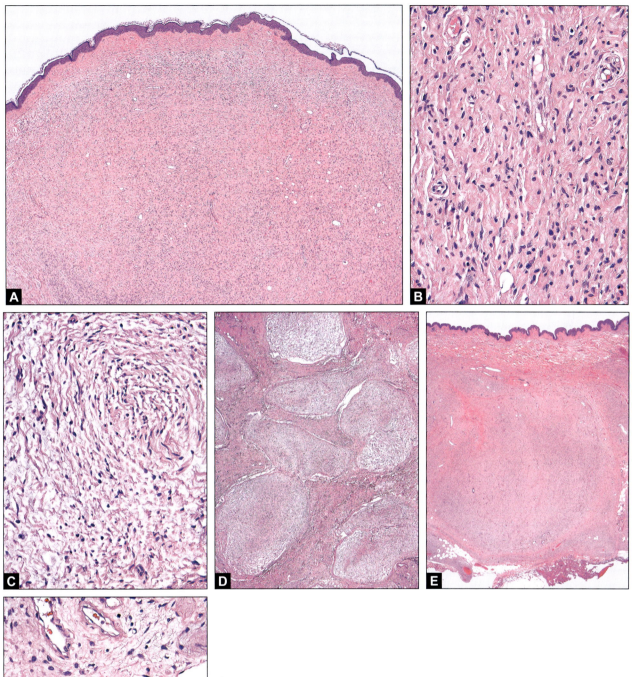

Figs 14.8A to F: Neurofibroma. (A) Typical lesions are dome shaped nodules with a dermis occupied by a diffuse collection of randomly oriented small spindled and ovoid cells; (B) Cytologically banal spindled and ovoid cells within a pale collagenous stroma; (C) Neurofibroma, myxoid type. Occasionally the stroma is distinctly myxoid; (D) Neurofibroma with a plexiform pattern. Discrete nodules are present; (E) Neurofibroma, diffuse type. This variant is sometimes referred to as the "plaque variant", and may be confused with a dermatofibrosarcoma protuberans because of its diffuse involvement of the dermis and extension into the subcutis; (F) Meissner bodies, if present, are helpful in distinguishing a neurofibroma from simulators. They resemble the Meissner bodies of normal skin.

Sclerotic Fibroma (Storiform Collagenoma)

■ *Criteria for diagnosis*

- Solitary flesh colored papule or nodule (may be multiple in Cowden's disease)
- Well demarcated nodule of dense collagenous matrix with collagen bundles separated by clefts populated by cytologically banal spindled and stellate cells (Figs 14.9A and B)

■ *Differential diagnosis*

- Old scar/keloid
- Fibrosing dermopathies
- Sclerotic variant of perineurioma
- Desmoplastic nevus.

■ *Pitfalls*

- Occasional multinucleated cells may be seen, sometimes causing confusion with pleomorphic fibroma.

■ *Pearls*

- Benign tumors that are cured by simple excision
- Particularly when multiple lesions are detected, there is an association with Cowden's disease.

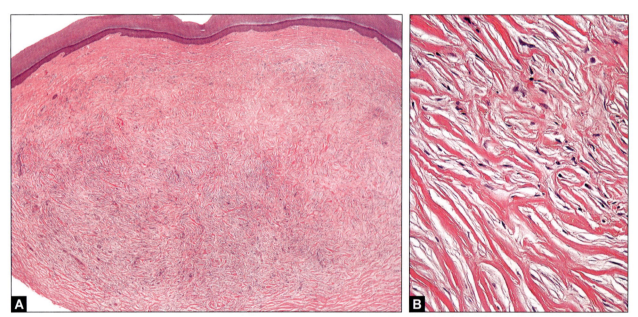

Figs 14.9A and B: Sclerotic fibroma. (A) Wavy collagen bundles predominate; (B) The collagen bundles are thick and separated by clefts. Fibroblasts are reduced in number and in some areas they may be absent altogether.

Perineurioma

■ *Criteria for diagnosis*

- Ill-defined dermal nodules of epithelial membrane antigen+ (EMA+)/glucose transporter 1(GLUT 1+)/S100–spindled or ovoid cells with a haphazard, vaguely whorled or fascicular arrangement (Fig. 14.10A)
- Neoplastic cells have thin, elongated cytoplasmic processes.

■ *Differential diagnosis*

- Neurofibroma
- Dermatofibroma
- Dermatofibrosarcoma protuberans
- Desmoplastic melanomas
- Low-grade fibromyxoid sarcomas
- Superficial acral fibromyxoma.

■ *Pitfalls*

- Perineuriomas may occasionaly resemble the superficial portions of a DFSP; positivity of both for CD34 compounds this problem (see below)
- The neoplastic cells of perineurioma by definition must express EMA, but the staining is often subtle or faint, and requires examination on high power
- Up to 20% of the cases may exhibit one or more "atypical" features, including significant mitotic activity, scattered pleomorphic cells, focal hypercellularity or diffuse infiltrative growth (but these features do not appear or imply malignancy).
- Rare malignant peripheral nerve sheath tumors (MPNSTs) resemble perineuriomas (but have overt malignant features, including marked pleomorphism and mitotic activity).

■ *Pearls*

- Uncommon; primarily affects adults, most often the extremities and trunk
- Benign tumors that only rarely recur locally, even when "atypical" features are presents
- Superficial portions of DFSP may occasionally very closely resemble perineuriomas — but perineuriomas usually entrap dermal collagen bundles, express EMA, exhibit clefting and express CD34 only weakly (Fig. 14.10B).
- GLUT-1 staining may be more robust than EMA; may be useful in cases in which EMA is difficult to assess, but GLUT-1 is not specific.
- Nerve sheath myxoma
- Dermatofibroma
- Absence of S100 expression helps exclude desmoplastic melanomas.
- Lack of a capsule helps to exclude schwannoma.

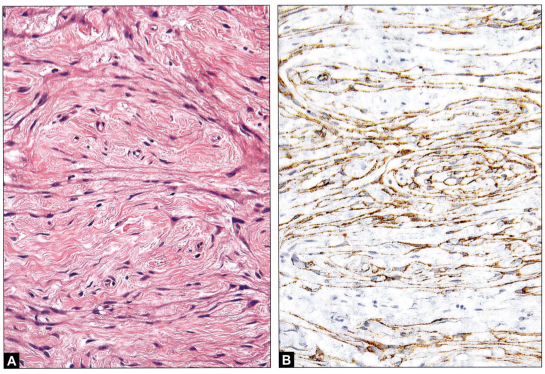

Figs 14.10A and B: Perineurioma. (A) The lesional cells are spindled or stellate and have long dendritic processes; (B) The cells express epithelial membrane antigen, which highlights their elongated dendritic processes.

Acral Fibrokeratoma

■ *Criteria for diagnosis*

- A polypoid projection on acral skin (Fig. 14.11A) (see Table 14.2)
- An expanded dermis composed of vertically oriented elongated collagen bundles (Fig. 14.11B).

■ *Differential diagnosis*

- Supernummary digit/rudimentary digit (Fig. 14.11C)
- Verruca vulgaris.

■ *Pitfalls*

- Superficial biopsies may often be nonspecific and may not include the subtle neural vestiges of supernummary digit

- Features similar to those of acral fibrokeratoma may be a nonspecific finding overlying tumors located in the deep dermal or subcutis (Fig. 14.11C).

■ *Pearls*

- Considered a type of angiofibroma by some
- Considered a regressing wart by some.

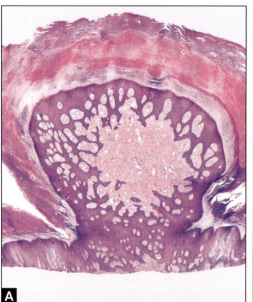

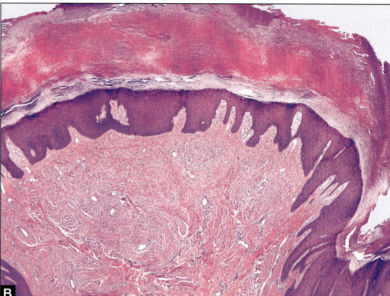

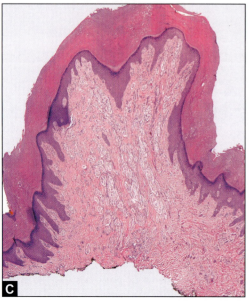

Figs 14.11A to C: Acral fibrokeratoma. (A) A polypoid projection on acral skin is the most common presentation; (B) The polypoid configuration is imparted by an expanded dermis; (C) Rudimentary digit (accessory digit). These are sometimes confused with acral fibrokeratomas histopathologically, but can be distinguished by the large nerve bundles within the central dermis. The clinical presentation is quite different from acral fibrokeratoma as well.

Elastofibroma

Criteria for diagnosis

- Slow-growing tumor, almost exclusively occuring in the subcutis/fascia of the subscapular area of elderly people
- Haphazardly arranged, pale pink collagen bundles and amorphous pale material representing degenerated elastic fibers (Fig. 14.12A)
- Elastic fibers, seen best with elastin stains, such as Verhoeff-Van Gieson, that are clumped and form thin cords with serrated edges and small rounded globules (Figs 14.12B and C).

Differential diagnosis

- Various depositional disorders
- Fibrolipoma

Pitfalls

- Definitive diagnosis may require elastic stains to demonstrate that the amorphous material is degenerating elastic tissue.

Pearls

- Elastic tissue stains highlight the globular, serrated or beaded appearing degenerating elastic fibers
- The subscapular location and presentation in an older or elderly adult are highly characteristic
- The "tumor" is likely a degenerative process caused by repetitive stress or manual labor.

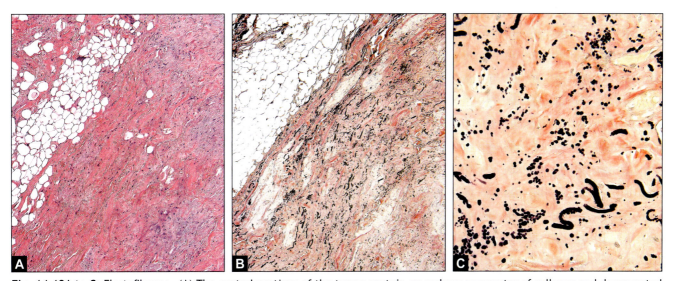

Figs 14.12A to C: Elastofibroma. (A) The central portions of the tumor contain amorphous aggregates of collagen and degenerated elastin fibers; (B) Elastic fibers, seen best with elastin stains, such as Verhoeff-Van Gieson, are fragmented, clumped, and form thin cords and round globules with serrated edges and small rounded globules; (C) Thick cords of elastin with serrated edges are characteristic.

Pleomorphic Fibroma

■ *Criteria for diagnosis*

- Slow-growing, dome shaped or polypoid papule
- Well circumscribed paucicellular tumors composed of widely scattered cells within a sclerotic dermis (or rarely, a variably myxoid stroma)
- CD34+ pleomorphic, multinucleated cells are present, but spindled, stellate and rounded cells are also evident (Fig. 14.13A).

■ *Differential diagnosis*

- Angiofibroma
- Desmoplastic nevus (with degenerative atypia)
- Myxoid tumors (in cases where myxoid stroma predominates)

■ *Pitfalls*

- The cellular pleomorphism may be overinterpreted as evidence of malignancy
- Isolated case reports describe "transformation" of pleomorphic fibromas into myxofibrosarcoma; in case where a myxoid stroma predominates, deep extension of the tumor must be excluded, and there should be continued clinical surveillance.

■ *Pearls*

- Despite the pleomorphism, these are benign tumors that only rarely recur (Fig. 14.13B)
- Conservative excision is recommended to prevent recurrence
- In cases with predominantly myxoid stroma, excision is warranted to exclude the possibility of a deeper myxoid tumor.

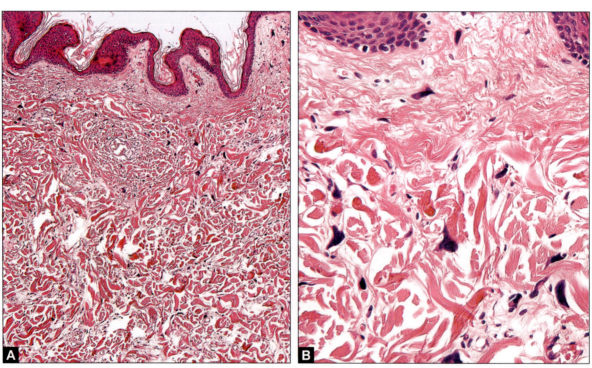

Figs 14.13A and B: Pleomorphic fibroma. (A) Cellularity is generally low, but even at low power the pleomorphic cells are conspicuous; (B) The pleomorphic cells are alarming at first glance, but the low cellularity and absence of mitotic figures are reassuring features.

THE FASCICULAR AND STORIFORM TUMORS

Nodular Fasciitis (and Other Fasciitis Variants)

■ *Criteria for diagnosis*

- A rapidly growing nodule composed of plump, immature-appearing but monomorphic myofibroblasts with conspicuous nucleoli arranged in short fascicles or haphazardly within a myxoid to collagenous stroma that does not contain thin, branching curvilinear vessels (Figs 14.14A and B).

■ *Differential diagnosis*

- Myxomas
- Myxofibrosarcoma
- Dermatofibroma/fibrous histiocytoma
- Fibromatosis
- Fibrosarcoma.

■ *Pitfalls*

- Appearance may vary greatly among lesions and within a given lesion, and inadequate sampling may prevent definitive diagnosis.

■ *Pearls*

- Most cases contain extravasted erythrocytes and lymphocytes in a patchy distribution, an important clue to the diagnosis
- Myxomas are far less cellular.

- Fibromatoses contain more elongated fascicular growth
- Fibrosarcomas are generally more densely cellular and elongated fascicles usually predomiante.
- Myxofibrosarcomas exhibit cellular pleomorphism and a characteristic thin, branching curvilinear vessels
- Central collections of multinucleated giant cells may be present
- Most common benign lesion to be misdiagnosed as a sarcoma
- Stroma varies from myxoid and edematous-appearing in early lesions to dense and collagenous in long-standing lesions
- Lesions can occur virtually at any anatomic site and although they grow rapidly, they are generally self-limited and rarely exceed 3 cm in maximum dimension
- Nodular fasciitis almost never recurs even if incompletely excised; recurrence should prompt consideration of another diagnosis.

Proliferative Fasciitis

- A subcutaneous lesion that contains large ganglion-like cells, some of which are multinucleated, but otherwise is very similar to nodular fasciitis (Fig. 14.14C)
- The differential diagnosis may include ganglioneuroma due to the presence of ganglion-like cells.

Proliferative Myositis

- An intramuscular lesion that is similar to proliferative fasciitis and also contains large ganglion-like cells
- Often produces secondary atrophy of skeletal muscle fibers.

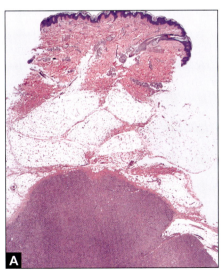 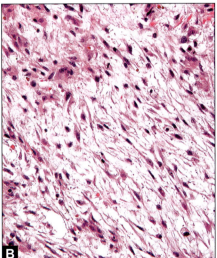 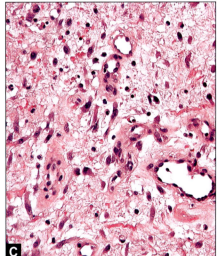

Figs 14.14A to C: Nodular fasciitis. (A) A densely cellular nodule occupies the subcutis. The tumors often have infiltrative borders, but some, like this example, are well demarcated in some areas; (B) Areas with haphazardly arranged plump spindled cells within a loose collagenous stroma (the so-called "tissue culture" appearance) are characteristic; (C) Proliferative fasciitis. The architecture is similar to nodular fasciitis, but large "ganglion-like" cells are present.

Dermatofibroma and Variants

Figures 14.15A to C show dermatofibroma.

Criteria for diagnosis

- Firm, slowly growing papule
- Flesh-colored, white or brown-red color
- Cytologically banal spindled to ovoid cells arranged haphazardly and/or in fascicles of varying length
- Factor 13a expressed by many cells in most cases.

Differential diagnosis

- Scar
- Collagenous neurofibroma
- Dermatomyofibroma
- Granuloma annulare
- Blue nevus
- Desmoplastic nevus
- Dermatofibrosarcoma protuberans
- Atypical fibrous histiocytoma (AFH).

Pitfalls

- Superficial biopsies may simulate scars and other fibrosing processes
- "Follicular induction" within the overlying hyperplastic epidermis may closely simulate basal cell carcinoma in some cases
- A minority have epidermal atrophy instead of hyperplasia (possibly due to trauma)
- Minimal extension into the subcutis is not uncommon and depending on its degree, may cause confusion with DFSP
- Many variants of dermatofibroma exist, cellularity may vary dramatically in some cases, and therefore the differential diagnosis may be very broad in some situations.

Pearls

- Benign lesions with minimal tendency to recurrence
- Predilection for the extremities of adults, but may occur at virtually any site and within any age group
- Most cases exhibit characteristic epidermal hyperplasia directly over the neoplasm
- Many cases contain scattered cells with foamy cytoplasm (usually absent in DFSP)
- Spindled cells that encircle rounded collagen fibers (collagen balls) are characteristic (but not entirely specific) features
- A wide variety of histopathologic patterns results in a broad differential diagnosis
- Most diagnostic challenges are caused by the following subtypes:

    - *Epithelioid cell type*: Round cells with vesicular nuclei, visible nucleoli and multinucleated cells may cause confusion with Spitz's nevi and other tumors (Fig. 14.15D).
    - *Granular cell type*: The features may be virtually identical to those of a granular cell tumor, but they express factor 13a and are S100 negative; often there are other areas that are typical of an "ordinary" dermatofibroma (Fig. 14.15E).
    - *Clear cell type*: The cells have clear cytoplasm and can be mistaken for a variety of other tumors, including nevi, melanomas and carcinomas.
    - *Lipidized type*: Abundant foamy cytoplasm simulates xanthomas or xanthogranulomas (Fig. 14.15F).
    - *Sclerosing hemangioma type*: Hemorrhage and hemosiderin are present; the latter is sometimes mistaken for the melanin pigment of a nevus or melanoma; multinucleated cells are often numerous (Fig. 14.15G).
    - *Cellular type*: The dense cellularity can be misinterpreted as a sarcoma (Fig. 14.15H).
    - Atypical dermatofibroma
- Factor 13a is usually positive; occasional cases express CD68 and smooth muscle actin.
- CD34 expression is very uncommon, and its expression may cause confusion with DFSP.
- S100 is negative.

Cellular Dermatofibroma

- A variant of dermatofibroma in which there is markedly increased cellularity, mitotic figures and often of a larger size
- Approximately 25% of cellular dermatofibromas recur, and conservative but complete excision is recommended if possible since recurrences may be more diffuse and further excisions may produce suboptimal cosmetic results.

Atypical Dermatofibroma (Dermatofibroma with Monster Cells)

- A variant of dermatofibroma that contains some cells that are markedly enlarged, cytologically atypical, and have an increased mitotic index.
- Complete excision is prudent since there is a higher likelihood of recurrence.

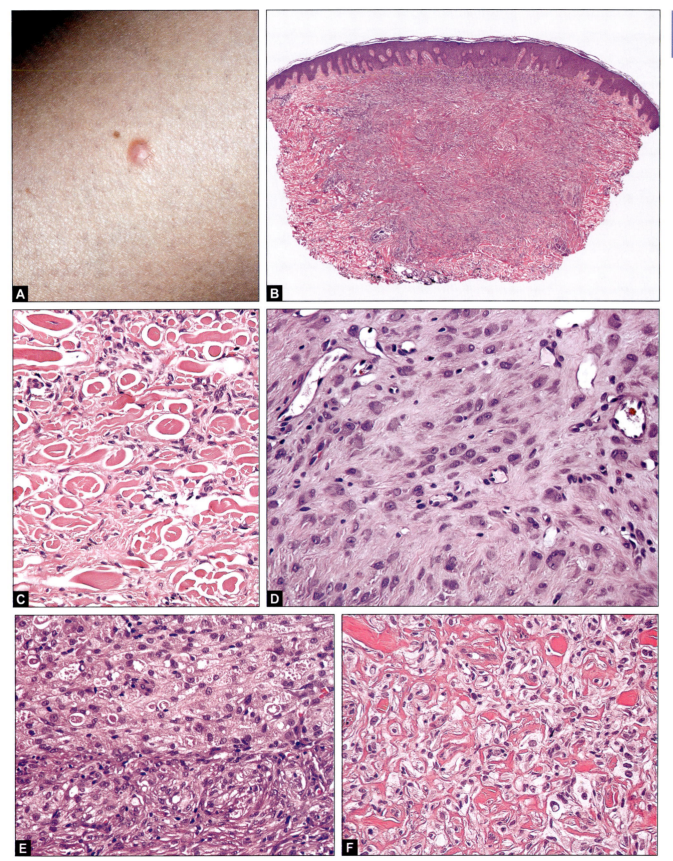

Figs 14.15A to F

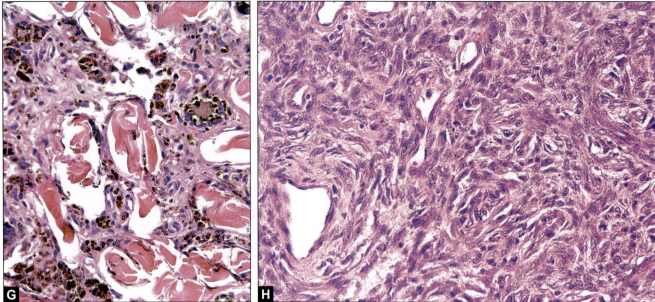

Figs 14.15A to H: Dermatofibroma. (A) A pink, shiny papule is a typical presentation; (B) Most cases are relatively well-demarcated nodules that occupy the dermis; (C) The tumor cells surround rounded collagen 'balls' at the periphery; (D) Dermatofibroma, epithelioid cell variant. The cells are round rather than spindled, and some contain vesicular nuclei and conspicuous nucleoli. Binucleated and multinucleated cells; (E) Rarely, granular cells (upper half of the field) may compose part or all of the neoplasm. Unlike a genuine granular cell tumor, the cells express factor 13a but not S100; (F) Dermatofibroma, lipidized variant. Cells containing intracytoplasmic lipid resemble those of histiocytomas. There is a predilection for the ankle; (G) Dermatofibroma, hemosiderotic variant. The extensive hemosiderin deposition often causes these tumors to appear dark brown clinically and may be mistaken for a melanoma. This variant is sometimes mistaken for a Spitz's nevus or an epithelioid perineurioma, but the cells are S100 and epithelial membrane antigen negative; (H) Dermatofibroma, cellular variant. The dense cellularity can be overinterpreted as evidence of malignancy, especially when mitotic figures are conspicuous.

Dermatomyofibroma

■ *Criteria for diagnosis*

- A flesh colored or hypopigmented plaque
- Cytologically banal spindled cells arranged in fascicles that run parallel to the overlying epidermis (Fig. 14.16A)
- Centered within dermis with limited extension into the subcutis (Fig. 14.16B)
- Positive expression of SMA and/or muscle specific actin; negative for CD34 and usually negative for factor 13a.

■ *Differential diagnosis*

- Dermatofibroma
- Leiomyoma
- Dermatofibrosarcoma protuberans
- Fibromatoses
- Scar

■ *Pitfalls*

- Features may overlap with those of cutaneous leiomyoma in some cases.
- Factor 13a, CD34 and S100 may label dermal dendrocytes scattered among or at the periphery of the neoplastic cells.

■ *Pearls*

- Uncommon relative to dermatofibromas
- The long fascicles arranged parallel to the epidermis are a helpful clue since they are usually not seen in either dermatofibromas or leiomyomas
- Unlike fibromatoses, beta-catenin is not expressed.

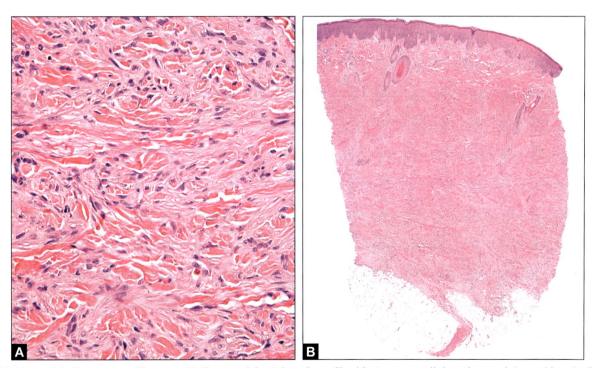

Figs 14.16A and B: Dermatomyofibroma. (A) Elongated fascicles of myofibroblasts run parallel to the overlying epidermis. Dermal collagen bundles are present between the fascicles; (B) The tumor often appears poorly demarcated at its periphery, by comparison to a dermatofibroma.

Dermatofibrosarcoma Protuberans

■ *Criteria for diagnosis*

- Indurated plaque, nodule, or multinodular mass (Fig. 14.17A)
- Monomorphic slender spindled cells that diffusely permeate the dermis and subcutis, often with a prominent storiform architecture in the mid to deep dermis (Figs 14.17B and C)

■ *Differential diagnosis*

- Dermatofibroma
- Neurofibroma, diffuse type
- Perineurioma
- Giant cell fibroblastoma (see below)
- Fibrosarcoma.

■ *Pitfalls*

- Samples that do not include the subcutis may preclude definitive diagnosis since the pattern of subcutaneous infiltration is a defining feature of DFSP (Figs 14.17D and E)
- The superficial portions may closely simulate the diffuse variant of neurofibroma and other benign tumors
- The myxoid variant is difficult to differentiate from other myxoid tumors (see section on "myxoid tumors").

■ *Pearls*

- Predilection for the trunk and proximal extremities of young to middle-aged adults, but any site and age group may be affected.
- S100 (positive in neurofibromas) is helpful in excluding diffuse neurofibromas

- CD34 expression is typically strong and diffuse in DFSP
- Even with wide local excision, recurrence develops in 20% of the cases, usually when margins are narrow
- Most DFSPs appear to be driven by overexpression of platelet derived growth factor β-chain (PDGFβ) and activation of its receptor (PDGFR)
- A translocation, t(17;22)(q22;q13), fuses exon 2 of the PDGFβ gene to exons of the collagen type 1 α1 gene (COL1A1)
- The fusion places the PDGFβ gene under control of the highly active COL1A1 promotor, leading PDGFβ overexpression
- Imatinib mesylate (Gleevec) blocks PDGFR signaling, and imatinib therapy can produce shrinkage or regression in some tumors
- Rare cases metastasize, but usually only after multiple local recurrences
- Rare cases contain areas identical to conventional fibrosarcoma; the prognostic significance of this remains unclear, but some data suggest that there is no difference if complete wide local excision with negative margins is achieved
- Criteria for the diagnosis of fibrosarcoma arising within a DFSP:
  - Fascicular rather than storiform growth pattern
  - Plump spindle cells with more vesicular nuclei
  - CD34 expression diminished or absent
  - Increased mitotic rate 7–15/10 high power field (HPF) (versus 1–3 per 10 HPF in conventional DFSP).

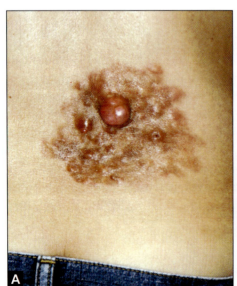
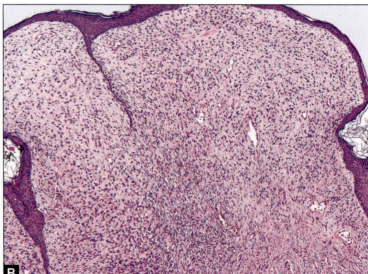

Figs 14.17A and B

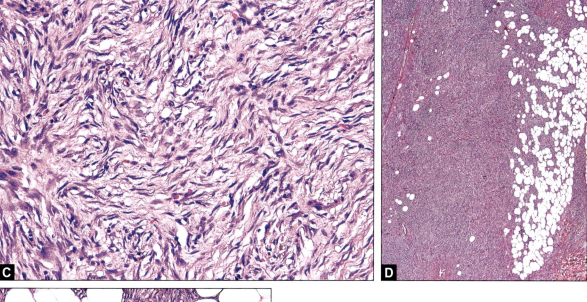

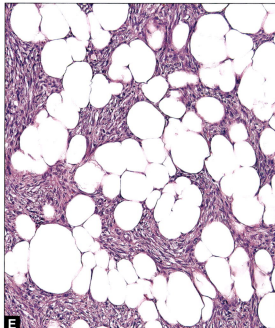

Figs 14.17A to E: Dermatofibrosarcoma protuberans (DFSP). (A) A red-brown plaque studded with papules and nodules on the lower back of a middle aged male; (B) The papillary dermis is occupied by a diffuse collection of spindled cells. The characteristic storiform pattern is often absent in the most superficial portions; (C) Slender spindled cells are arranged in a distinctive storiform pattern within most of the tumor; (D) Replacement of the reticular dermis and portions of the subcutis is characteristic; (E) Infiltration around small groups of adipocytes (imparting a 'lace-like' pattern) is a key feature.

Solitary Fibrous Tumor

■ *Criteria for diagnosis*

- Well demarcated or partially encapsulated dermal or subcutaneous tumors composed of monomorphic but plump CD34+ spindled and ovoid cells arranged haphazardly or in short fascicles within a fibrous stroma containing ectatic blood vessels with angular and branching contours.

■ *Differential diagnosis*

- DFSP
- Dermatofibroma
- Spindle cell lipoma.

■ *Pitfalls*

- Partially sampled lesions may closely simulate DFSP or intradermal spindle cell lipoma, since both express CD34.

■ *Pearls*

- Uncommon tumors that usually present in adults with a median age of 50 years.

- The vast majority of solitary fibrous tumors are benign
- Rare cases may recur or metastasize
- The arrangement of the cells is often referred to as "patternless" (Fig. 14.18A)
- Alternating cellular and hypocellular zones, angular ectatic vessels with thickened, hyalinized walls are common features (Fig. 14.18B)
- The relationship between atypical histopathologic features (e.g. cytologic atypia, mitotic index, necrosis) and prognosis is not entirely clear
- CD34 expression allows distinction from dermatofibromas
- Unlike DFSP and intradermal spindle cell lipomas, solitary fibrous tumors are well demarcated and/or partially encapsulated
- Subcutaneous spindle cell lipomas may be well demarcated and/or encapsulated, but typically contain more adipocytes that solitary fibrous tumors
- Many cases express CD99 and Bcl2 in addition to CD34.

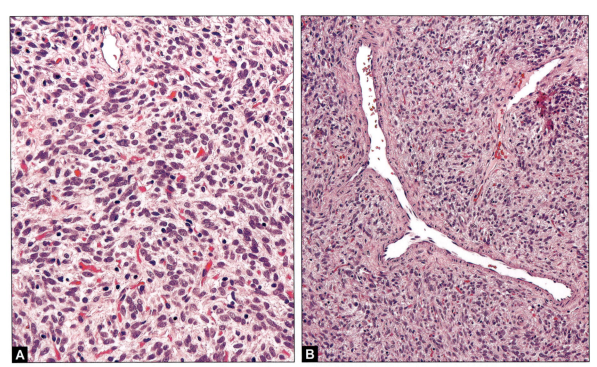

Figs 14.18A and B: Solitary fibrous tumor. (A) The architecture is often described as "patternless." The tumors may be relatively cellular and cells may be plump, but the nuclear features are banal; (B) Vessels are often prominent many are ectatic and branched, the so-called "staghorn" pattern originally associated with hemangiopericytomas. Unlike dermatofibrosarcoma protuberans, the cells are plump and often ovoid, and the tumor lacks the storiform architecture of a dermatofibrosarcoma protuberans.

Traumatic Neuroma

■ *Criteria for diagnosis*

- Small, firm nodule at the site of prior trauma
- Fibrous tissue containing a haphazard proliferation of small nerve bundles that emanate from the end of an intact nerve (Fig. 14.19A).

■ *Differential diagnosis*

- Localized interdigital neuritis (Morton's neuroma)
- Solitary neuroma
- Schwannoma
- Neurofibroma.

■ *Pitfalls*

- If the "parent" nerve is not sampled, distinction from peripheral nerve sheath tumors may be difficult, particularly if a history of prior trauma is not provided (Fig. 14.19B).

■ *Pearls*

- Most cases involve the distal extremities, especially the digits (see Table 14.2)
- The small bundles are composed of varying proportions of schwann cells and axons
- If there is a history of trauma, the presence of haphazardly arranged small nerve bundles within the vicinity of an intact normal appearing nerve is virtually diagnostic.

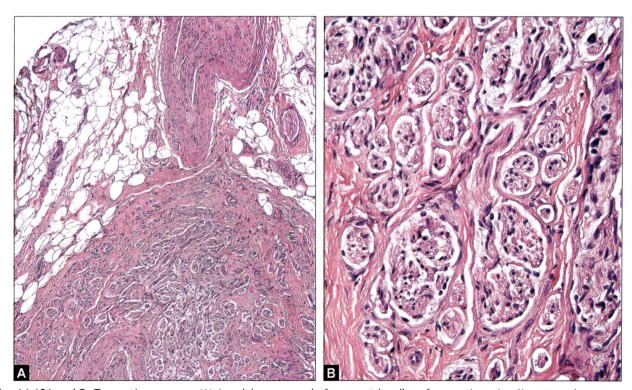

Figs 14.19A and B: Traumatic neuroma. (A) A nodule composed of compact bundles of nerve tissue is adjacent to the transected "parent nerve" at the right of the field; (B) The proliferation of small nerve bundles can be mistaken for neural neoplasms if the parent nerve is not seen or if the clinical scenario is unknown.

Localized Interdigital Neuritis (Morton's Neuroma)

■ *Criteria for diagnosis*

- A firm, fusiform enlargement of the plantar digital nerve at its bifurcation point
- Edema and fibrosis within the nerve and concentric fibrosis that envelops the epineurium and perineurium (Fig. 14.20)
- No proliferation of nerve bundles (Fig. 14.20) (see Table 14.2).

■ *Differential diagnosis*

- Traumatic neuroma
- Solitary neuroma
- Schwannoma
- Neurofibroma

■ *Pitfalls*

- If the fibrosis is extensive, there is potential for confusion with superficial fibromatosis or a fibroma of the tendon sheath.

■ *Pearls*

- The condition is actually a fibrosing inflammatory reaction, not a genuine neuroma
- The clinical history is very characteristic; the vast majority of cases present with paroxysmal pain in the sole of the foot and involve the plantar digital nerve between the heads of the third and fourth metatarsals, and less often between the second and third
- Predilection for women (possibly caused by high-heeled shoes)
- The extensive fibrosis and lack of numerous small nerve bundles differentiate it from traumatic neuroma and the peripheral nerve sheath tumors.

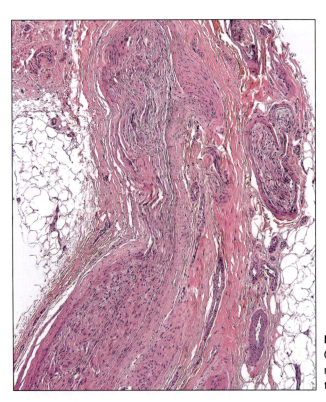

Fig. 14.20: Localized interdigital neuritis (Morton's neuroma). Concentric fibrosis surrounds the epineurium and perineurium of nerves. There is no proliferation of small nerve bundles as in a traumatic neuroma.

Palisaded and Encapsulated Neuroma/Solitary Neuroma

■ *Criteria for diagnosis*

- Dermal nodule composed of short cellular fascicles of cytologically banal spindled cells separated by small clefts and surrounded by rim of compact fibrous tissue (Fig. 14.21A).

■ *Differential diagnosis*

- Schwannoma
- Neurofibroma

■ *Pitfalls*

- Partially sampled lesions can be difficult to distinguish from schwannomas and some types of fibrous tumors
- "Palisading" and "encapsulation" are misleading since palisading is rarely seen and the tumors, while sharply demarcated are not surrounded by distinct capsule in many cases (Fig. 14.21B).

■ *Pearls*

- Vast majority occur in the head and neck region, particularly on the face
- Benign tumors that almost never recur even with incomplete excision
- Schwannomas may have many overlapping features but typically have a prominent collagenous capsule, lack distinct clefting, usually vary in cellular density and architecture, and are often adjacent to normal appearing nerves.

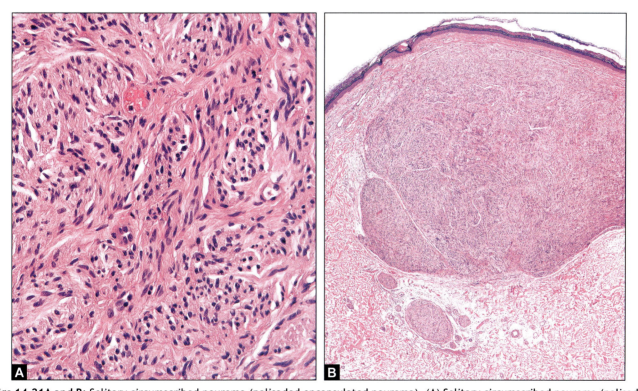

Figs 14.21A and B: Solitary circumscribed neuroma (palisaded encapsulated neuroma). (A) Solitary circumscribed neuroma (palisaded encapsulated neuroma). Rounded, compact fascicles are separated by clefts; (B) A sharply demarcated tumor occupies the dermis.

Schwannoma

■ *Criteria for diagnosis*

- An encapsulated nodule centered within the dermis or subcutis composed of wavy S100+ spindled cells arranged in densely cellular nodules (Antoni A areas) in some regions but diffusely in others (Antoni B areas) (Figs 14.22A to C).

■ *Differential diagnosis*

- Neurofibroma
- Cellular schwannoma (Table 14.1)
- Malignant peripheral nerve sheath tumor (Table 14.1).

■ *Pitfalls*

- Some cases exhibit nuclear pleomorphism that may cause confusion with malignant tumors (Fig. 14.22D).

■ *Pearls*

- The sharp circumscription and fibrous capsule help to differentiate schwannomas (including cellular schwannomas) from other nerve sheath tumors, including MPNST (Fig. 14.22E)

- Helpful clues to diagnosis are vessels with thick, hyalinized walls and often portions of a normal appearing nerve adjacent to the tumor (Fig. 14.22F)
- In rare cases, multiple nodules may be present (schwannomatosis)
- Rarely, a schwannoma is composed almost entirely of round or ovoid epithelioid cells
- All are strongly and diffusely S100+ but negative for melanocytic markers
- Neurofibromas lack the well-developed capsule of a schwannoma
- Malignant peripheral nerve sheath tumors lack a capsule, are more pleomorphic, have a higher mitotic index, and express S100 only focally.

Table 14.1: Cellular schwannoma versus malignant peripheral nerve sheath tumor		
Feature	Cellular Schwannoma	MPNST
Common in skin	Yes	No
Capsule	Yes	No
Necrosis	Rare	Common
Pleomorphism	Mild to moderate	Marked
Mitotic index	< 4 per 10 HPF	> 4 per 10 HPF
Erosion of underlying bone	Uncommon	Common
S100 expression	Diffuse and strong	Focal and weak
Recurrence	Less than 5%	Frequent
Metastasis	Never	Common

(MPNST: Malignant peripheral nerve sheath tumors; HPF: High-power field).

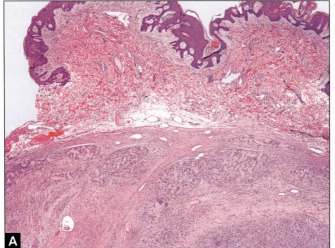
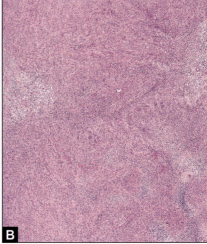

Figs 14.22A and B

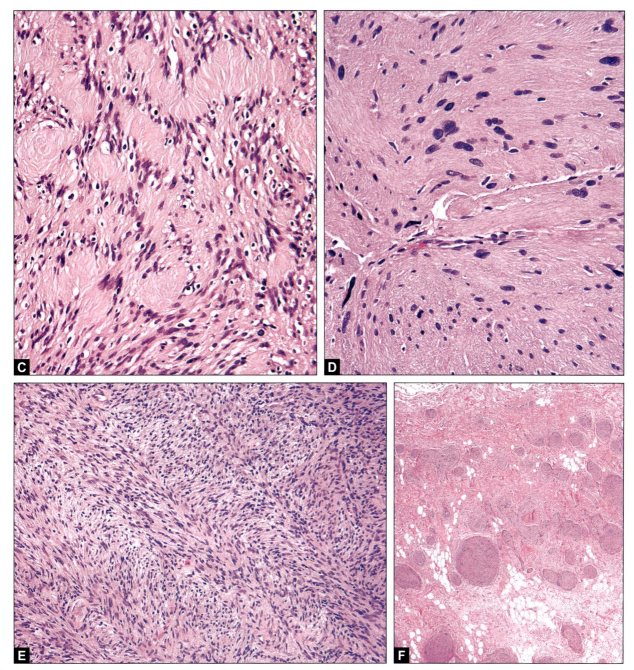

Figs 14.22A to F: Schwannoma. (A) Even at low power, the typical "organized" lobules (Antoni A areas) and patternless diffuse regions (Antoni B areas) are evident; (B) Some areas lack a distinct architectural pattern; (C) Nuclear palisades and Verocay bodies are formed from rows of nuclei separated by cytoplasmic processes. These are often seen within the nodular Antoni A regions; (D) Schwannoma with degenerative change (ancient change). There is marked nuclear plemorphism but mitotic figures are usually few or altogether absent; (E) Cellular schwannoma. Many of the features resemble a malignant spindle cell tumor, particularly a malignant peripheral nerve sheath tumor, fibrosarcoma or synovial sarcoma. However, mitotic figures number fewer than 4 per 10 high-power fields, the cells are less pleomorphic, and the tumors are usually encapsulated. Unlike a malignant peripheral nerve sheath tumor, S100 expression is usually strong and diffuse; (F) Plexiform variants are composed of discrete nodules of neoplastic cells.

Low Grade Fibromyxoid Sarcoma

■ *Criteria for diagnosis*

- A tumor of low to moderate cellularity with fibrous zones alternating with myxoid areas populated by evenly distributed cytologically banal spindled and stellate cells that express vimentin and sometimes SMA but not CD34, S100, desmin or beta-catenin (Fig. 14.23).

■ *Differential diagnosis*

- Low grade myxofibrosarcoma
- Myxoid neurofibroma
- Myxoid DFSP
- Desmoid fibromatosis.

■ *Pitfalls*

- The tumors may appear well-circumscribed grossly but microscopic examination usually shows infiltrative growth
- Since the characteristic architectural features (alternating fibrous regions and myxoid regions, collagen "rosettes") are often necessary for differentiating it from other tumors, low grade fibromyxoid sarcomas (LGFMS) may be very difficult to diagnose without an excision or a large excisional biopsy (Fig. 14.23).

■ *Pearls*

- Affects a wide age range but favors young to middle-aged adults
- Recurrence and metastasis is well-documented in cases that are incompletely excised
- Metastases often occur several years or even decades after presentation
- Relative to other fibrous and myxoid tumors, LGFMS are uncommon in the skin; most arise deep to the fascia
- Lower extremities are the most common site, followed by the chest wall or axilla, buttock and head neck
- Characteristically contains a translocation t(7;16), which results in fusion of the *FUS* gene on chromosome 7 and the CREB3L2 gene on chromosome 16
- The *FUS/CREB3L2* fusion transcript may be detected by reverse transcription-polymerase chain reaction or a break-apart probe for the FUS gene.

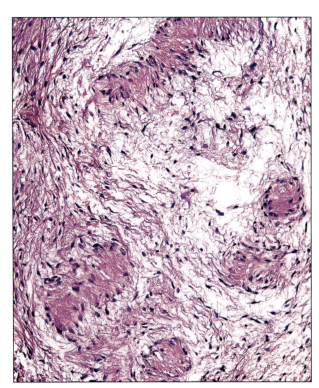

Fig. 14.23: Low-grade fibromyxoid sarcoma. These tumors are uncommon in the skin. There is usually an abrupt transition from myxoid to fibrous areas. "Rosettes" composed of cells in a vaguely palisaded arrangement are characteristic (but must be differentiated from the Meissner bodies of neurofibromas or Verocay bodies of schwannomas).

Leiomyoma

■ *Criteria for diagnosis*

- Solitary or multiple flesh colored or pale pink dermal nodules
- Fascicles of plump but cytologically banal spindled cells, usually well demarcated at the periphery (Fig. 14.24A).

■ *Differential diagnosis*

- Leiomyosarcoma
- Smooth muscle hamartoma (Fig. 14.24B).

■ *Pitfalls*

- Occasionally there is some variability in cytolomorphology that could be overinterpreted as evidence of malignancy.

■ *Pearls*

- More than one or two mitotic figures suggest the possibility of leiomyosarcoma, particularly when there is some cellular pleomorphism.

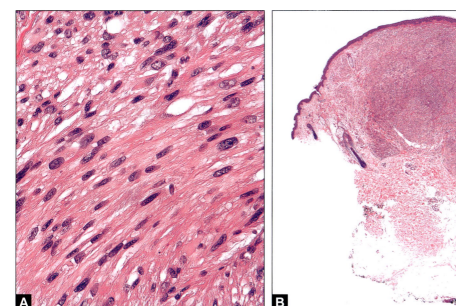
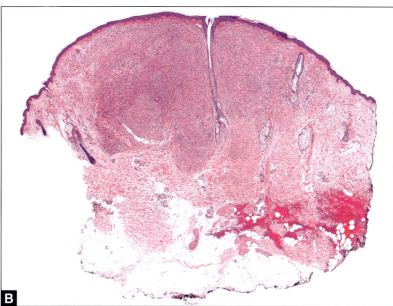

Figs 14.24A and B: Leiomyoma. (A) Fascicles of plump but cytologically banal cells with cylindrical (cigar shaped) nuclei compose most of the tumor. There may be mild variability in nuclear size and shape but mitotic activity is low by comparison to leiomyosarcomas; (B) Many dermal leiomyomas are referred to as "pilar leiomyomas" since, as in this case, the fascicles of neoplastic smooth muscle cells appear to emerge from the arrector pili.

Cutaneous Leiomyosarcoma

■ *Criteria for diagnosis*

- A solitary dermal nodule
- A dermis occupied by a poorly circumscribed nodule of plump spindled cells that are pleomorphic, contain at least some mitotic figures and express SMA (Fig. 14.25A)
- Absent or minimal extension into the subcutis (Fig. 14.25B).

■ *Differential diagnosis*

- Atypical fibroxanthoma (AFX)
- Spindle cell variant of squamous cell carcinoma
- Spindle cell melanoma
- Spindle cell angiosarcoma
- Cutaneous metastasis from leiomyosarcomas arising at other sites.

■ *Pitfalls*

- Rarely there may be expression of cytokeratin within a few tumor cells
- Cutaneous metastases from leiomyosarcomas at other sites must be excluded for definitive diagnosis
- Definitive diagnosis can only be made on biopsies/excisions that allow evaluation of the subcutis.

■ *Pearls*

- The term cutaneous leiomyosarcoma should be reserved for those tumors that can be shown to be centered within the dermis, with only minimal extension into the subcutis
- Recurrence develops in approximately 50%
- Cases with significant extension into the subcutis may metastasize, but cutaneous leiomyosarcoma confined predominantly to the dermis are nonmetastasizing tumors.
- The presence of multiple lesions suggests the possibility of cutaneous metastases from a leiomyosarcoma arising at another site
- The vast majority are relatively well differentiated; occasional multinucleated cells may be present, but the pleomorphism is generally far less than that of an AFX
- Prognosis is dependent solely on the depth of the tumor; mitotic index, grade and other features do not predict metastasis if the strict definition of confinement to the dermis is used
- Every effort should be made to completely excise these tumors (e.g. wide local excision) since complete excision is curative.
- Recurrences tend to exhibit more involvement of the subcutis and therefore metastatic potential.

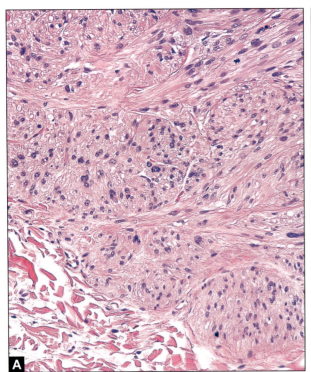 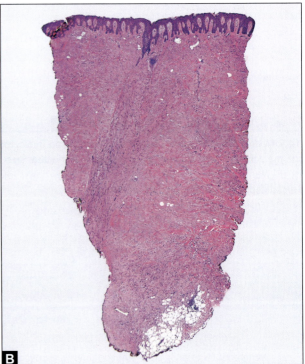

Figs 14.25A and B: Leiomyosarcoma. (A) The cells exhibit greater pleomorphism and there is an increased mitotic index by comparison to leiomyoma; (B) The tumor is based within the dermis, but there is extension into the subcutis. While those contained within the dermis never metastasize, when the subcutis is involved, there is at least some potential for local recurrence or rarely, metastasis.

Myofibroma (and Myofibromatosis)

Criteria for diagnosis

- *Myofibroma*: A solitary flesh colored or violaceous nodule
- *Myofibromatosis*: A condition in which multiple myofibromas present at birth or in infancy
- Well demarcated nodular or multinodular tumor composed of two cell populations:
  - Spindled cells arranged in fascicles plus oval or round undifferentiated appearing cells
  - A "zonal" appearance with rounded hypocellular sclerotic regions and cellular regions surrounding angular ectatic vesses (Fig. 14.26A).

Differential diagnosis

- Nodular fasciitis (when spindled cell component predominates)
- Cellular dermatofibroma
- Leiomyoma
- Myopericytoma

Pitfalls

- Lobules of tumor cells may extend into vessels; this "vascular invasion" appearance is not evidence of malignancy (Fig. 14.26B)
- Tumor necrosis and occasional mitoses may be seen, and are not evidence of malignancy
- Solitary myofibromas may lack a distinct zonal pattern.

Pearls

- Head, neck and trunk are favored sites for myofibromas
- Solitary myofibromas may recur locally but do not metastasize; conservative complete excision is recommended treatment
- Myofibromatosis does not metastasize but may involve underlying viscera, making complete excision difficult, and recurrence/persistence is not uncommon.

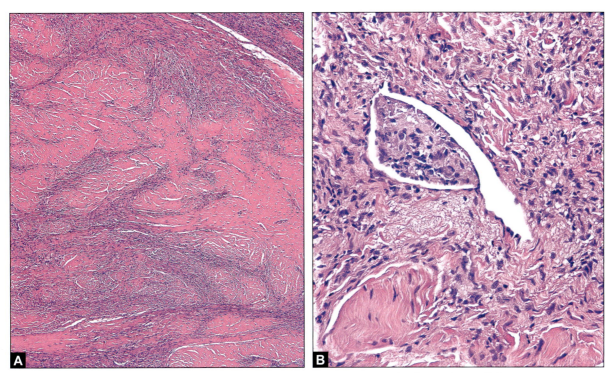

Figs 14.26A and B: Myofibroma. (A) A "biphasic" appearance is characteristic, with sclerotic hypocellular zones alternating with cellular areas; (B) Within the cellular regions, there is often vascular "pseudoinvasion." This does not imply a risk of metastasis.

Infantile Digital Fibromatosis (Inclusion Body Fibromatosis)

Criteria for diagnosis

- Solitary or multiple firm nodules on the fingers or toes of an infant or child (Fig. 14.27A) (see Table 14.2)
- Collagneous stroma containing cytologically banal spindled myofibroblasts, some of which contain small, round eosinophilic cytoplasmic inclusions that are deep red on Masson trichrome stain and express actin by immunohistochemistry but do not stain with periodic acid-Schiff, Alcian blue or colloidal iron stains (Figs 14.27B to D).

Differential diagnosis

- Nodular fasciitis
- Superficial fibromatosis.

Pitfalls

- Inclusions may be few in some cases and difficult to detect on H & E

- In some cases, actin positivity may only be detectable in alcohol fixed tissue or after treatment with KOH or trypsin preteated formalin-fixed tissue

Pearls

- Sixty percent of the cases recur locally, but none metastasize and many regress spontaneously over a period of months to years
- Predilection for third, fourth and fifth digits; thumb involved rarely, but no case has occurred on the great toe
- Functional impairment or persistent joint deformity in some cases
- Inclusions appear to be derived from actin filaments.

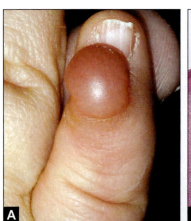
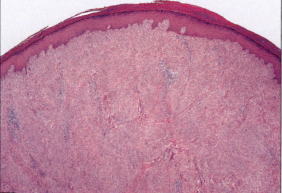
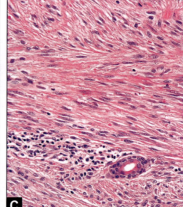

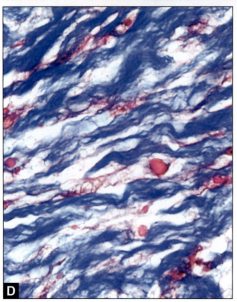

Figs 14.27A to D: Inclusion body fibromatosis. (A) This firm nodule developed on the fifth toe of a 2-year-old child; (B) The nodule is composed of spindled cells that occupy the entire dermis; (C) The tumor is composed of plump spindle cells, some of which contain characteristic cytoplasmic inclusions adjacent to their nuclei; (D) The inclusion bodies are bright pink with Masson's trichrome stain.

Tumor	Clinical Features	Histopathologic Features
Traumatic neuroma	Small, firm nodule at site of prior trauma	Fibrous tissue containing haphazard proliferation of small nerve bundles that emanate from the end of an intact ('parent') nerve; (parent nerve not always present in sampled sections)
Morton's neuroma	Presents with paroxysmal pain in the sole of the foot between heads of 3rd and 4th metatarsals, less often between 2nd and 3rd	Fusiform enlargement of plantar digital nerve Edema and fibrosis within the nerve and concentric fibrosis that envelops the epineurium and perineurium No proliferation of nerve bundles
Digital myxoid pseudocyst	Solitary papule on the distal digit, often periungual	Amorphous basophilic myxoid material within a cystic space and/or within the surrounding fibrous tissue
Ganglion cyst	Solitary nodule on the wrist or hand	Same as digital myxoid pseudocyst
Acral fibrokeratoma	Polypoid projection on acral skin	Expanded dermis that contains vertically-oriented, elongated collagen bundles
Rudimentary/accessory digit	Polypoid projection on acral skin	Similar to acral fibrokeratoma, but central dermis occupied by large nerve bundles
Tendon sheath fibroma	Deep, slowly enlarging nodule attached to a tendon sheath	Circumscribed nodule of spindled cells with variable cellularity ranging from fasciitis-like appearance to paucicellular and sclerotic or hyalinized
Acral/digital fibromyxoma	Solitary, slow-growing, nontender papule or nodule on the fingers and toes; frequently involves the nailbed	Myxoid to fibrous stroma populated by cytologically banal CD34+ spindled cells
Superficial fibromatosis	Firm, cord-like induration or diffuse thickening of the skin and subcutis in adult Caucasian males	*Early*: nodules of fibroblasts that occupy the dermis with relatively high cellularity, may form vague fascicles *Late*: Decreased cellularity with increased irregular, sclerotic collagen bundles
Infantile digital fibromatosis	Solitary or multiple firm nodules on the fingers or toes of an infant or child	Collagenous stroma containing banal spindled myofibroblasts, some of which contain small round eosinophilic cytoplasmic inclusions Inclusions stain deep red on Masson trichrome stain and express actin by immunohistochemistry
Nerve sheath myxoma	Slowly growing, solitary papule or nodule	Nodules of round, spindled, and ovoid cells surrounded by fibrous trabeculae; cells express S100
Giant cell tumor of the tendon sheath (Tenosynovial giant cell tumor)	Nodule overlying the interphalangeal joint of a finger	Nodules with even, rounded contours composed of various proportions of mononuclear cells, xanthoma cells, and multinucleated giant cells

Contd...

Tumor	Clinical Features	Histopathologic Features
Epithelioid sarcoma	Slow-growing dermal or subcutaneous tumor on the hand or wrist of a young adult; frequently with overlying ulceration	Nodules of round, ovoid, or polygonal cells with abundant cytoplasm and large, vesicular nuclei (i.e. 'epithelioid'), occasionally with spindled cells as well; central necrosis within nodules
		Tumor extends into skin from deep soft tissue
		Neoplastic cells express vimentin and focally cytokeratins; variable expression of CD34 in at least 50% of cases
Acral lentiginous melanoma	Expanding brown-black macule, patch or plaque on acral surface;	Pleomorphic melanocytes, often spindled, which in rare cases may simulate sarcoma (since intraepidermal component may be inconspicuous or absent due to ulceration and necrosis)

Fibrous Hamartoma of Infancy

■ Criteria for diagnosis

- Rapidly growing mass in the deep dermis or subcutis that almost always develops within the first 2 years of life but may continue to grow (Fig. 14.28A)
- Presence of three distinct components: (1) intersecting fibrous trabeculae containing spindled cells; (2) small round to stellate immature cells within a myxoid Alcian blue-positive matrix; (3) interspersed mature adipocytes (Fig. 14.28B).

■ Differential diagnosis

- Infantile fibromatosis (Fig. 14.28C)
- Myofibromatosis
- Calcifying aponeurotic fibroma.

■ Pitfalls

- In some cases, the undifferentiated spindled cell component may be inconspicuous
- Mature adipose tissue may predominate in some cases, resembling nevus lipomatosus superficialis or lipoma.

■ Pearls

- Benign, but recurrence develops in approximately 16%
- Usually cured by local excision and re-excision if recurrent
- Predilection for males
- Up to 20% present at birth
- Axillae, groin, proximal extremities, shoulders, back and forearm are the most common sites
- Actin positivity may be present within the mature appearing fibroblasts; CD34 positivity in some cases.

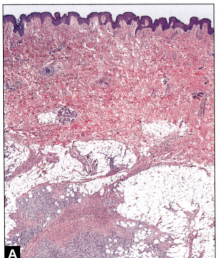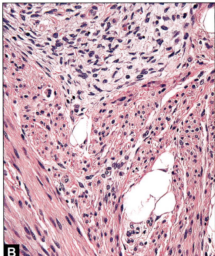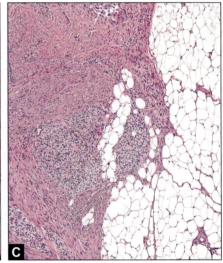

Figs 14.28A to C: Fibrous hamartoma of infancy. (A) The deep dermis and subcutis contain elongated fascicles of spindled cells with eosinophilic cytoplasm admixed with nodules of ovoid cells arranged in nodules; (B) In this field, all three components are present: undifferentiated mesenchymal cells (top of the field), fibroblastic/myofibroblastic elements (lower half of field) and mature adipocytes; (C) There is an abrupt transition between the different cell types.

Plexiform Fibrohistiocytic Tumor

Criteria for diagnosis

- Slowly growing nodule centered within the subcutis (Fig. 14.29A)
- Two components: (1) spindled cells (that express smooth muscle actin) in intersecting fascicles; (2) small rounded nodules of histiocytoid cells that express CD68, some of which may be multinucleated (Figs 14.29B and C)
- Variable expression of SMA within the spindled cells and CD68 within the histiocytoid cells
- Absence of S100, factor 13a, lysozyme, keratin and desmin expression.

Differential diagnosis

- Fibromatosis
- Granulomatous procceses including infections
- Neurothekeomas

Pitfalls

- The two components may not be equally represented, and in some cases the fascicles of spindled cells predominate, simulating a fibromatosis.

Pearls

- Predilection for proximal extremities
- Almost exclusively in children and adults younger than age 30
- Classic cases exhibit a characteristic biphasic appearance in which the histiocytoid cells are surrounded by the intersecting spindle cell fascicles
- Recurrence is common but metastasis is uncommon; lymph nodes and pulmonary metastases have been described but death from disease is extremely uncommon
- Imaging of the lungs should be performed since in rare cases pulmonary involvement is present at the time of initial diagnosis
- No histologic features have been shown to be predictive of metastatic potential
- Plexiform fibrohistiocytic tumor is probably closely related to (or possibly synonymous with) neurothekeomas.

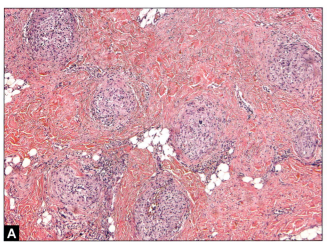

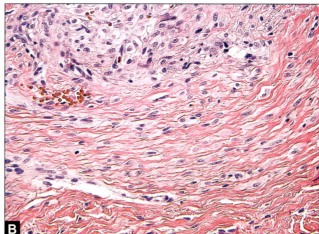

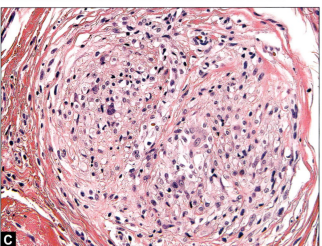

Figs 14.29A to C: Plexiform fibrohistiocytic tumor. (A) The most striking feature at low power is usually the small rounded nodules of histiocytoid cells (resembling granulomas) within the deep dermis and subcutis; (B) There is a biphasic architecture with long fascicles of plump spindled cells in addition to the histiocyte-like nodules; (C) The nodules are typically compact and in addition to the histiocyte like cells they tend to contain multinucleated cells as well.

Neurothekeoma

■ *Criteria for diagnosis*

- Firm, solitary, slowly growing nodule in the skin or superficial subcutis (Fig. 14.30A)
- Multilobulated collections of spindled and ovoid cells arranged in densely cellular bundles and whorled fascicles
- Tumor cells express smooth muscle actin, CD10, factor 13a, protein gene product 9.5 and microphthalmia transcription factor (MiTF)
- Negative for S100, glial fibrillary acidic protein (GFAP) and Melan-A/Mart-1.

■ *Differential diagnosis*

- Nerve sheath myxoma
- Plexiform fibrohistiocytic tumor
- Perivascular epithelioid cell tumor
- Melanocytic tumors.

■ *Pitfalls*

- Occasional examples are paucicellular, and some have a myxoid stroma leading to potential confusion with nerve sheath myxoma (Fig. 14.30B)

- Some cases exhibit conspicuous mitotic activity and some degree of pleomorphism, causing confusion with a malignant neoplasm.

■ *Pearls*

- Peak incidence in the second decade; slight predilection for females
- Favored sites are the head (particularly nose, cheeks and periorbital region), the upper extremities and shoulder girdle (Fig. 14.30A)
- Most are benign, but recurrence occurs in some cases
- Origin is unclear, but neurothekomas share more features with fibrohistiocytic and pericytic tumors and are not derived from schwann cells and the peripheral nerve sheath (Table 14.3).
- Absence of S100 and GFAP expression helps exclude nerve sheath myxoma; lack of Melan-A/Mart-1 excludes melanocytic tumors
- Morphologic and immunohistochemical features overlap with those of plexiform fibrohistiocytic tumor, and the two may represent variants of a single entity
- Plexiform fibrohistiocytic tumor typically occurs in the deeper soft tissue and has a predilection for the extremities.

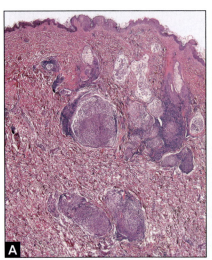 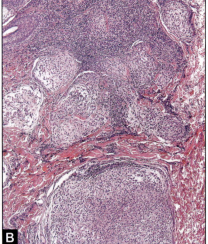

Figs 14.30A and B: Neurothekeoma. (A) This case was located on the cheek. Discrete lobules of tumor cells occupy the dermis; (B) The nodules are separated by intervening collagen bundles and are composed of ovoid cells within an eosinophilic to myxoid cytoplasm. The myxoid component is usually less than that of a nerve sheath myxoma.

Table 14.3: Comparison of nerve sheath myxoma and neurothekeoma		
Feature	*Nerve Sheath Myxoma*	*Neurothekeoma*
Anatomic site	Distal extremities (fingers and hand), head and neck	Head (nose, cheeks, and periorbital region), upper extremities, and shoulder girdle
Depth	Usually limited to the dermis	Dermis and /or superficial subcutis
Histopathologic features	Myxoid lobules centered within the dermis surrounded by fibrous septa	Multilobulated collections of spindled and ovoid cells arranged in densely cellular bundles and whorled fascicles
		Nodules separated by intervening collagen bundles
Immunohistochemical features	Tumor cells express S100 and often GFAP, CD57, and neuron specific enolase; cells at periphery often EMA positive	Tumor cells express smooth muscle actin, CD10, factor 13a, PGP 9.5, and MITF;
		Negative for S100, GFAP, and Melan-A/ Mart-1

Malignant Peripheral Nerve Sheath Tumor, Spindle Cell Pattern

■ *Criteria for diagnosis*

- Subcutaneous nodules, often large
- A collection of spindled to epithelioid cells within a collagenous to myxoid stroma with cytologic atypia and a high mitotic index.

■ *Differential diagnosis*

- Cellular schwannoma
- Spindle cell melanoma
- Synovial sarcoma
- Fibrosarcoma

■ *Pitfalls*

- Loss of S100 expression is common (except in epithelioid variants, which may retain significant expression) and other features must be used to differentiate MPNST from other spindle cell tumors (Fig. 14.31A)
- Distinction from spindle cell variant of melanoma may be difficult if S100 expression is retained (since spindle cell melanomas will also usually lack Melan-A and HMB-45 expression) (Fig. 14.31B)

- Differentiation from synovial sarcoma is often difficult and may require molecular analysis to exclude synovial sarcoma (Table 14.4 and 14.5).

■ *Pearls*

- Lesions should be extensively sampled, including their periphery, since this occasionally reveals an adjacent neurofibroma, which virtually confirms the diagnosis
- Unlike cellular schwannomas, MPNSTs lack a capsule
- The weak and patchy positivity for S100 helps exclude cellular schwannoma and spindle cell melanoma
- Histologic features have been shown to be predictive of metastatic potential.

Spindle Cell/Neurotropic Melanoma

- Spindle cell melanoma is easily confused with some spindle cell tumors and its early form may appear as a relatively subtle expansion of dermal nerve bundles (see Chapter 11).

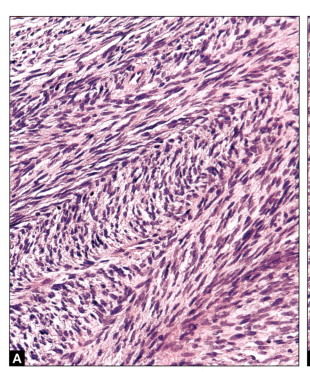 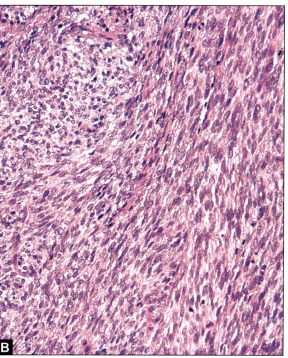

Figs 14.31A and B: Malignant peripheral nerve sheath tumor, spindle cell pattern. (A) Malignant peripheral nerve sheath tumor, spindle cell pattern. In some cases, spindled malignant peripheral nerve sheath tumors are indistinguishable from fibrosarcomas and other tumors that may exhibit the so-called "herringbone" architecture (tightly formed fascicles of spindled cells); (B) These rarely arise within the skin, but deep-seated tumors may extend upward into the subcutis and dermis occasionally. Differentiation from spindle cell melanomas can be difficult in some cases.

Table 14.4: Common genetic abnormalities of cutaneous mesenchymal tumors

Tumor	Cytogenetic Abnormality	Molecular Event
Lipoma	t with 12q15;	HGMA2 fusions
	t with 6p21	HGMA1 rearrangements
Atypical lipoma/Well differentiated liposarcoma	Amplified 12q13—15	Amplification of MDM2 (and CDK4, GLL, and SAS)
Pleomorphic lipoma	Deletion of 16q or	Unknown
Spindle cell lipoma	(less commonly) 13q	
Myxoid lipoma		
Desmoplastic fibroblastoma, tendon sheath fibroma	t(2;11)(q31—32;q12)	Unknown
Epithelioid hemangioendothelioma	t(1;3)(p36.3;q25)	Unknown
Giant cell tumor of the tendon sheath	t(1;2)(p13;q37)	Fusion of CSF1 and COL6A3 genes
Low-grade fibromyxoid sarcoma	t(7;16)(q33;p11.2) in >95%	Fusion of FUS and CREB3L2 genes (>95%) and FUS and CREB3L1 genes (<5%)
	t(11;16)(p13;p11.2) in <5%	
Myxoid/round cell liposarcoma	t(12;16)(q13;p11)	Fusion of FUS and CHOP genes
Pericytoma	t(7;12)(p2;q13)	ACTB-GL
Synovial sarcoma	t(X;18)(p11.2;q11.2)	Fusion of SYT with SSX1
		SSX2, or SSX4
Clear cell sarcoma	t(12;22)(q13;q12)	Fusion of EWS-ATF1

Table 14.5: Comparison of benign and malignant granular cell tumors

Feature	Benign	Malignant
Size	Usually < 2 cm	Often > 2 cm
Borders	Circumscribed	Infiltrative growth
Mitotic index	Usually < 1/10 HPF	≥ 2/10 HPF
Cytologic features	Round or oval cells in nests	Spindled cells in fascicles
Ulceration	Rare	Sometimes
Necrosis	Rare	Sometimes
Lymphovascular invasion	Never	Sometimes
Cytologic atypia	Mild	Marked

HPF: High-power field.

THE MYXOID TUMORS

Cutaneous Focal Mucinosis

■ *Criteria for diagnosis*

- A dome shaped flesh colored or white dermal papule, usually solitary and painless
- Basophilic amorphous myxoid material or mucinous "pool" containing scattered fibroblasts those are spindled, stellate and/or triangular but cytologically banal (Figs 14.32A and B)
- Focal, but not necessarily well-demarcated.

■ *Differential diagnosis*

- Ganglion cyst/digital mucous pseudocyst (histopathologically)
- Various cutaneous mucinoses (see Chapter 10)
- Cutaneous angiomyxoma, other myxoid neoplasms.

■ *Pitfalls*

- Cutaneous angiomyxomas may have some overlapping features; they are benign tumors but have a tendency to recur
- Without clinical correlation, the histopathologic features could be confused with papular mucinosis.

■ *Pearls*

- May be a depositional condition rather than a neoplasm
- Neutrophils and prominent vascularity are absent, unlike cutaneous myxoma/superficial angiomyxoma
- Common anatomic sites are the extremities, face, neck or trunk but not the hands or digits, unlike myxoid pseudocysts and ganglion cysts
- Cellularity varies but is usually less than that of most myxoid tumors
- Intracytoplasmic vacuoles are common.

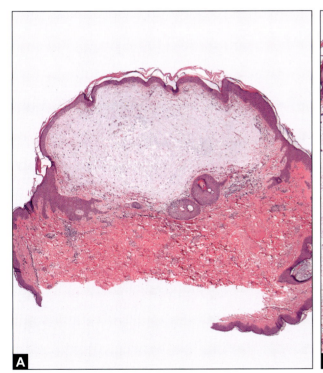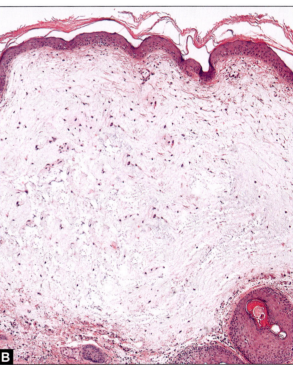

Figs 14.32A and B: Cutaneous focal mucinosis. (A) A diffuse collection of mucin occupies the papillary dermis; (B) Stellate and spindled fibroblasts are present, but they are fewer in number than in most myxoid neoplasms.

The Acral Myxoid Pseudocysts

Ganglion Cyst/Digital Myxoid Pseudocyst/ Cutaneous Myxoid Cyst

■ *Criteria for diagnosis*

- Clinical presentation as a solitary papule or nodule on the wrist, hand or digits; mildly painful in about half of cases (see Table 14.2)
- Thick bands of fibrous tissue surrounding a cystic space that may or may not have a synovial lining (Fig. 14.33A)
- Amorphous basophilic "mucin" within the cystic space and/or within the surrounding fibrous tissue (Fig. 14.33A).

■ *Differential diagnosis*

- Cutaneous focal mucinosis
- Superficial angiomyxoma
- Nerve sheath myxoma.

■ *Pitfalls*

- Some are fragmented during excision, and the pathologist receives only pieces of the fibrous pseudocyst wall that lack the characteristic mucin.

■ *Pearls*

- The most common mesenchymal tumors of the hand and wrist
- Ganglion cysts, digital myxoid pseudocysts and cutaneous myxoid cysts are likely related lesions or may represent various stages of the same process
- The most important distinction is from superficial angiomyxomas since the latter tend to recur and may be associated with Carney's complex
- Vast majority occur on the hands and wrists (especially of young to middle-aged females)
- Location helps distinguish them from cutaneous focal mucinosis
- If the clinical presentation is characteristic, fragments of a fibrous "wall" containing even small deposits of basophilic mucin are usually adequate for diagnosis in most situations (Fig. 14.33B).

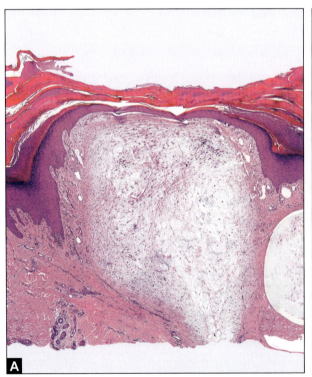
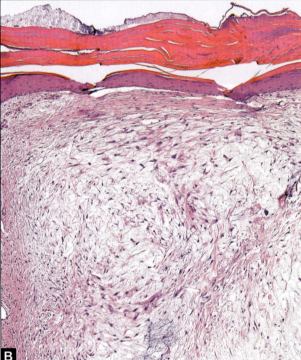

Figs 14.33A and B: Digital myxoid pseudocyst. (A) The features resemble cutaneous focal mucinosis but, as seen here, the lesions occur on acral skin. At the far right of the field, a well-formed cystic space is evident; (B) Spindled and stellate fibroblasts are present, usually in greater numbers than those seen in cutaneous focal mucinosis.

Superficial Angiomyxoma/Cutaneous Myxoma

■ Criteria for diagnosis

- Polypoid or nodular tumors
- Intradermal multilobulated neoplasm composed of cytologically banal spindled cells within a myxoid stroma that almost always contains neutrophils and surrounds adnexal structures (Figs 14.34A and B).

■ Differential diagnosis

- Cutaneous focal mucinosis
- Ganglion cyst/digital myxoid pseudocyst/cutaneous myxoid cyst
- Nerve sheath myxoma
- Acral fibromyxoma.

■ Pitfalls

- Unlike many of its simulators, cutaneous angiomyxomas have a tendency for recurrence

- Superficial angiomyxoma should not be confused with the "aggressive angiomyxoma" that typical occurs within the deep tissues of the genital region or perineum.

■ Pearls

- Local recurrence in 20–30%
- Typically polypoid or nodular
- Stromal neutrophils are a clue to superficial angiomyxoma (though they may vary markedly in number) (Fig. 14.34B)
- Predilection for males; occurs in almost any age
- Trunk is the most common site, followed by the head, neck and limbs
- Multiple angiomyxomas are associated with Carney's complex.
- Tendency for recurrence.

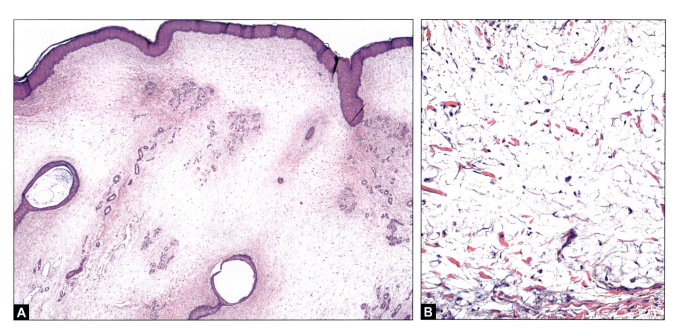

Figs 14.34A and B: Superficial angiomyxoma. (A) Entrapped adnexal structures are often present; (B) The lesional cells are stellate and spindled as they are in most myxoid neoplasms. Although not seen in this field, neutrophils are often present and can be a helpful clue to diagnosis.

Myxoid Spindle Cell Lipoma

■ Criteria for diagnosis

- Mature adipocytes, banal spindled cells and cord-like collagen bundles within a myxoid stroma (Fig. 14.35).

■ Differential diagnosis

- Myxoid/round cell liposarcoma (very uncommon in skin)
- Other myxoid tumors.

■ Pitfalls

- Some cases are almost entirely myxoid with only a few adipocytes to suggest its true nature.

■ Pearls

- Usually contains many more spindled cells than ordinary lipomas
- Contain 13q chromosomal aberrations, as do other spindle cell lipomas, and are the best considered part of the spindle cell lipoma spectrum (see below).

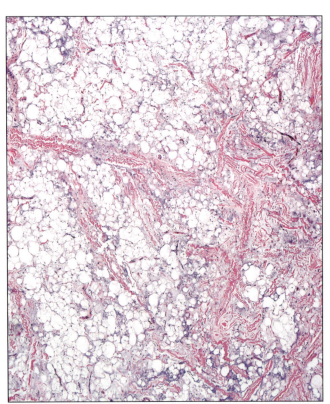

Fig. 14.35: Spindle cell lipoma. Mature adipocytes are surrounded by a fibromyxoid stroma. In some, however, myxoid material predominates.

Acral Fibromyxoma (Figs 14.36A and B)

■ *Criteria for diagnosis*

- Dermal based tumor with a myxoid to fibrous stroma populated by cytologically banal CD34+ spindled cells (Fig. 14.36A).

■ *Differential diagnosis*

- Superficial angiomyxoma
- Neurofibroma
- Dermatofibroma.

■ *Pitfalls*

- Some cases are predominantly myxoid while others are mostly fibrous, making the differential diagnosis broad on initial examination.

■ *Pearls*

- Sometimes referred to as "digital acral fibromyxoma" since there is a predilection for the nails, fingers and toes; some occur on the palm as well (see Table 14.2).
- CD34 and often CD99 are expressed, but S100 is negative, aiding in the exclusion of neural tumors and dermatofibromas.
- Superficial angiomyxoma is predominantly myxoid and usually contains neutrophils.

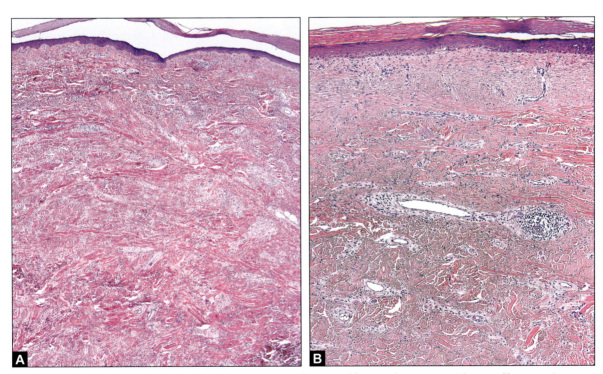

Figs 14.36A and B: Acral fibromyxoma. (A) The tumor has myxoid areas that merge with more fibrous regions; (B) Vascular elements are often prominent, a clue to the diagnosis.

Nerve Sheath Myxoma (Figs 14.37A to D)

■ *Criteria for diagnosis*

- Slow growing, solitary masses
- Myxoid lobules centered within the dermis "compartmentalized" by fibrous bands
- S100+ cells that vary in morphology from spindled or stellate to plump and epithelioid and are arranged singly or in cords and small nests (Fig. 14.37A).

■ *Differential diagnosis*

- Myxoid schwannoma
- Myxoid neurofibroma
- Myxofibrosarcoma (low grade)
- Neurothekeoma.

■ *Pitfalls*

- Moderate pleomorphism of the neoplastic cells in some cases (including cells that are plump, multinucleated or epithelioid) may be overinterpreted as evidence of malignancy (Fig. 14.37B)
- Rare cases overlap with neurothekeomas morphologically (but most nerve sheath myxomas are S100+, while neurothekeomas are not).

■ *Pearls*

- Predilection for young to middle-aged adults with peak incidence in fourth decade
- Females more commonly than males
- Distal extremities, especially the fingers and hand, and head and neck are favored sites (see Table 14.2)
- At low power, the compartmentalized architecture—myxoid lobules surrounded by fibrous septa is characteristic
- Formerly referred to as "myxoid neurothekeomas" but recent studies have demonstrated that these tumors are true peripheral nerve sheath neoplasms derived from schwann cells and should be separated from "neurothekeomas" (which are not of nerve sheath origin) (see Table 14.3)
- In addition to S100, neoplastic cells often express GFAP, CD57 and neuron specific enolase; EMA often highlights a small population of perineurial cells at the periphery of the myxoid lobules
- Myxoid schwannomas may appear similar but usually have a more conspicuous fibrous capsule
- Myxoid neurofibromas usually have a more diffuse growth pattern.

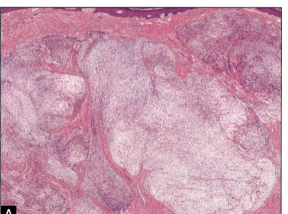
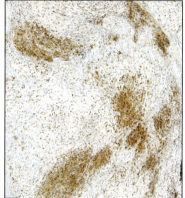
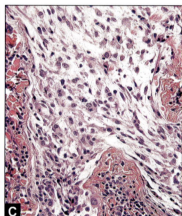
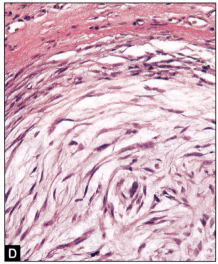

Figs 14.37A to D: Nerve sheath myxoma. (A) Nodules of round, spindled and ovoid cells compose nodules surrounded by fibrous trabecular; (B) Unlike a neurothekeoma, there is a predilection for acral skin and the tumor cells express S100; (C) Moderate pleomorphism of the neoplastic cells occurs in some cases; (D) A loose myxoid stroma is characteristic (but not specific).

Myxoid Neurofibroma

■ Criteria for diagnosis

- A predominantly myxoid stroma containing spindled to ovoid cells (Fig. 14.38)
- Immunohistochemistry:
- S100   + in approximately 50% of lesional cells
- CD34   + in variable number of cells
- EMA   + in scattered cells.

■ Differential diagnosis

- Focal cutaneous mucinosis
- Nerve sheath myxoma
- Digital fibromyxoma
- Myxoid lipoma
- "Neurofibroma-like" low-grade variant of MPNST.

■ Pitfalls

- As in conventional neurofibromas, only approximately 50% of lesional cells express S100
- Neurofibroma-like myxoid MPNSTs are more likely to retain S100 expression.

■ Pearls

- Myxoid neurofibromas are uncommon and have a predilection for the extremities.

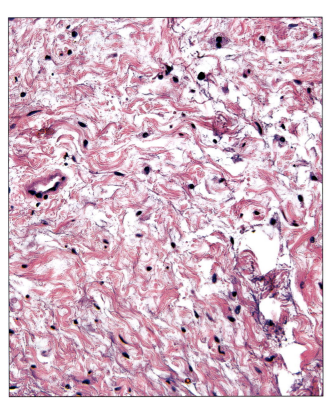

Fig. 14.38: Myxoid neurofibroma. In some neurofibromas, the stroma can be myxoid and more abundant than that of an "ordinary" neurofibroma.

Myxoid Dermatofibrosarcoma Protuberans

▪ *Criteria for diagnosis*

- Clinical, cytologic and immunophenotypic features of a DFSP but with an extracellular matrix that is predominantly myxoid rather than fibrous (Fig. 14.39A).

▪ *Differential diagnosis*

- Deep "aggressive" angiomyxoma
- Low-grade myxofibrosarcoma
- Myxoid neurofibroma
- Myxofibrosarcoma
- Other myxoid sarcomas (e.g. myxoid liposarcoma) (Fig. 14.39B).

▪ *Pitfalls*

- May be easily mistaken for benign myxoid lesions in superficial biopsies
- Some cases closely simulate myxoid liposarcoma on H&E stained material.

- Rare cases exhibit "sarcomatous" areas, which in myxoid variants is likely to resemble myxofibrosarcoma; these regions have diminished or absent CD34 expression.

▪ *Pearls*

- Superficial portions may be mistaken for a benign myxoid tumor
- Unlike myxoid liposarcoma, DFSPs are usually restricted to the dermis and subcutis, express CD34, and do not contain lipoblasts
- Only rare cases are purely myxoid; usually there are at least some foci that resemble conventional type DFSP
- The prognosis of myxofibrosarcomatous differentiation is unclear, but with wide local excision and clear margins, the risk of recurrence and metastasis appears similar to that of conventional DFSPs.

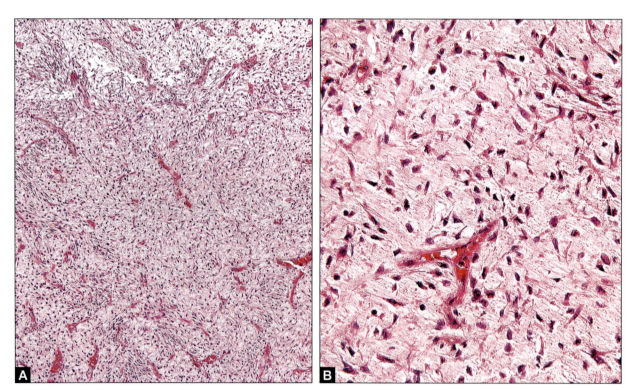

Figs 14.39A and B: Myxoid dermatofibrosarcoma protuberans. (A) The myxoid variant often appears less cellular than ordinary dermatofibrosarcoma protuberans; (B) Thin branching capillaries are more obvious with the decreased cellularity, and may closely resemble myxoid liposarcomas and other myxoid tumors.

Myxofibrosarcoma

■ *Criteria for diagnosis*

- Mutlilobular myxoid tumor composed of spindled and stellate cells, at least some of which exhibit cytological atypia (Fig. 14.40A)
- The cellular density and pleomorphism varies dramatically, and tumors may be classified as low, intermediate or high grade; often, however, a large excision is needed for definitive classification (Figs 14.40B and C)
- High-grade tumors often have marked pleomorphism and are admixed with variable numbers of cells with vacuolated cytoplasm (pseudlipoblasts) (Fig. 14.40C).

■ *Differential diagnosis*

- Myxoid DFSPs
- Myxoid leiomyosarcomas
- Myxoid MPNST
- Myxoid "round cell" liposarcoma.

■ *Pitfalls*

- Superficial areas are often relatively paucicellular and cytologically banal
- Tumor may progress to higher grade with recurrence(s).

- Since myxofibrosarcomas are often highly infiltrative tumors with ill-defined borders that are commonly deceptively hypocellular at their periphery, margins are often underestimated at the time of initial resection.

■ *Pearls*

- Most common soft tissue sarcoma of older adults
- Myxofibrosarcoma-like areas may occur in myxoid DFSP (see myxoid DFSPs)
- Low-grade lesions do not metastasize, but with recurrence, the tumors often become higher grade (and acquire metastatic potential)
- High-grade lesions contain solid areas with pleomorphic cells of the type seen in pleomorphic undifferentiated sarcoma (malignant fibrous histiocytoma)
- Predilection for the lower limbs of older adults and the elderly
- Peak incidence age 50–70
- Up to 70% occur within the deep dermis or subcutis
- Margins must be assessed very carefully, since the periphery of myxofibrosarcomas may be predominantly composed of low-grade areas that are easily overlooked.

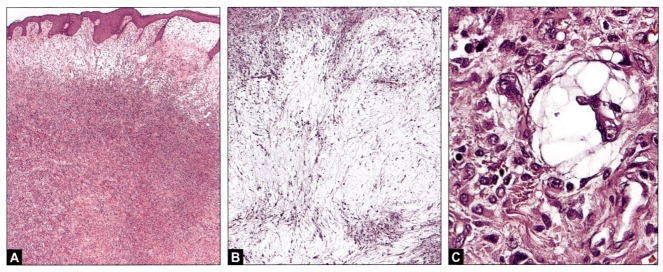

Figs 14.40A to C: Myxofibrosarcoma. (A) The superficial portions of a myxofibrosarcoma may be only sparsely cellular, despite the fact that a densely cellular tumor with moderate or high-grade atypia lies just beneath; (B) The cellularity may vary greatly from region to region. Areas of low cellularity, such as this, can be mistaken for less aggressive (or benign) myxoid tumors; (C) There is a spectrum of histopathologic grade. In intermediate to high-grade tumors, pseudolipoblasts are often seen, large vacuolated cells that very closely resemble lipoblasts but contain acid polysaccharides rather than lipid.

Myxoid Liposarcomas
(Round Cell Liposarcoma)

■ Criteria for diagnosis

- Usually deep seated tumors; rarely arise within the subcutis but may extend upward into it or occasionally metastasize to it
- Round to oval shaped mesenchymal cells within a myxoid matrix that contains conspicuous thin branching capillaries (Fig. 14.41).

■ Differential diagnosis

- Other myxoid tumors, especially myxoid neurofibroma, myxoid dermatofibrosarcoma protubers and low to intermediate grande myxofibrosarcomas.

■ Pitfalls

- Cases with low cellularity and minimal atypia may be mistaken for various benign myxoid tumors
- Immunohistochemically, there may be expression of S100 protein causing confusion with myxoid neural tumors.

■ Pearls

- Predilection for young to middle-aged adults
- Second most common form of liposarcoma
- Vast majority arise within the soft tissue of the thigh
- Very rarely arise primarily within the retroperitoneum; if one is encountered within the retroperitoneum, a metastasis from another soft tissue site must be excluded
- Prominent mucin pooling creates a "pulmonary edema"-like pattern in some areas
- Typically lipoblasts are small and less conspicuous than in other types of liposarcomas
- Have a marked tendency to metastasize to other soft tissues (before lung or other visceral metastases)
- Continuum of low to high cellularity; grading is based on cellularity, and not all high-grade lesions contain cells that are actually "round" (round cells are not necessary for designating a tumor as high-grade).

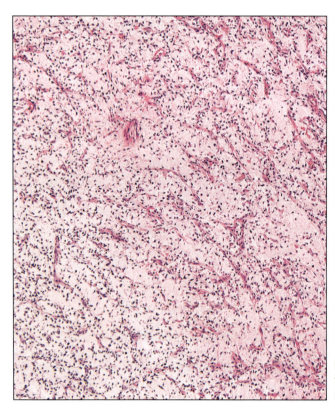

Fig. 14.41: Myxoid liposarcoma. The characteristic appearance is atypical cells scattered within a myxoid stroma that contains numerous thin, branching capillaries.

Acral Myxoinflammatory Fibroblastic Sarcoma (Inflammatory Myxohyaline Tumor)

■ *Criteria for diagnosis*

- Distal extremities, slolwly growing hands and feet subcutis and tenosynovial locations (see Table 14.2)
- Myxoid areas, fibrous areas and areas dominated by inflammation (Figs 14.42A and B)
- Bizarre cells, some with large nucleoli (sometimes resembling Reed-Sternberg cells) (Fig. 14.42C)
- Lage multivacuolated mucin-containing lipoblast-like cells (pseudolipoblasts) similar to those of myxofibrosarcoma.

■ *Differential diagnosis*

- Acral fibromyxoma
- Myxofibrosarcoma
- Other acral tumors.

■ *Pitfalls*

- In cases with extremely dense inflammatory infiltrates, an infectious or inflammatory process may be suspected instead of a neoplasm
- The biological potential is not fully characterized but multiple recurrences are common and metastasis has been documented in several cases.

■ *Pearls*

- High propensity for recurrence; metastases can develop
- Marked predilection for distal extremities, especially the hands
- Most cases occur in fourth and fifth decades but age range is broad.

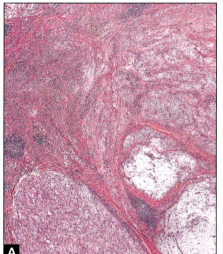
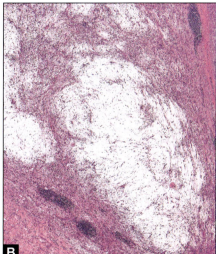
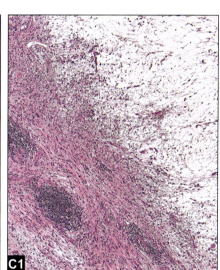
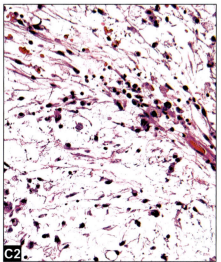

Figs 14.42A to C: Acral myxoinflammatory fibroblastic sarcoma. (A) Dense inflammatory aggregates within a fibrous and myxoid neoplasm are characteristic at low power; (B) There is often an abrupt transition from myxoid to fibrous regions. The aggregates of lymphocytes are frequently found at the periphery of the tumor; (C) Cellularity may be low in some areas, but large cells with bizarre nuclei are apparent. Lymphocytes and plasma cells predominate within the inflammatory infiltrate.

Myopericytoma/Myofibroma

■ *Criteria for diagnosis*

- Slowly growing dermal or subcutaneous nodules
- Multilobulated tumor composed of cytologically banal epithelioid or ovoid cells that encircle small blood vessels in concentric bands (Fig. 14.43).

■ *Differential diagnosis*

- Hidradenomas and other adnexal tumors
- Glomus tumor
- Malignant pericytoma.

■ *Pitfalls*

- Although the perivascular concentric whorls are characteristic, they occur in other tumors as well.

■ *Pearls*

- Vessels often have a "staghorn" (hemangiopericytoma-like) appearance
- Malignant variant is characterized by conspicuous mitotic figures.

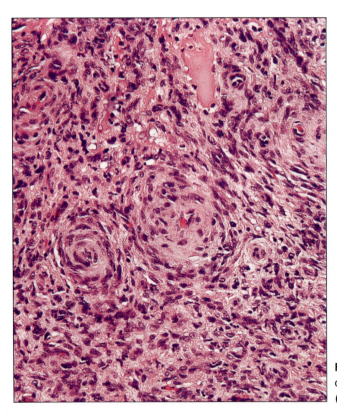

Fig. 14.43: Myopericytoma. The classic feature is epithelioid or ovoid cells that encircle small blood vessels in concentric whorls (the "onion skin" pattern).

Mixed Tumor (Myoepithelioma; Parachordoma)

Criteria for diagnosis

- Myoepitheliomas, mixed tumors and parachordomas likely represent a continuum of closely related tumors composed of cells that express S100 protein and cytokeratins and/or EMA.
- Clinical presentation is usually a firm nodule with a wide spectrum of microscopic features including one or more of the following:
  - Sheets or lobules of neoplastic cells that may be well demarcated or ill-defined (Fig. 14.44A)
  - Cells of varying size that may be spindled, ovoid and histiocytoid with "bubbly" cytoplasm, epithelioid or plasmacytoid, or any combination thereof
  - Variable amounts of stroma that may be myxoid, cartilaginous, fibrous or hyalinized (Figs 14.44B and C
  - No marked cytologic atypia or necrosis; mitotic index fewer than 1–2 per mm^2
- Those with conspicuous ducts and stroma are usually categorized as mixed tumors
- Those with solid or syncytial growth may be classified as myoepitheliomas
- Those in which cells with abundant finely vacuolated "bubbly" cytoplasm (physalliferous cells) are often considered parachordomas (Figs 14.44D and E).

Differential diagnosis

- Epithelioid fibrous histiocytoma (a dermatofibroma variant)
- Glomus tumor, solid pattern
- Neurothekeoma
- Nerve sheath myxoma
- Perivascular epithelioid cell tumor
- Melanoma and Spitz tumors
- Extraskeletal myxoid chondrosarcoma
- Ossifying fibromyxoid tumor
- Chordoma
- Hidradenoma and other adnexal epithelial tumors
- Metastatic carcinoma.

Pitfalls

- The vast array of potential microscopic features often makes for a broad differential diagnosis
- Overlapping features have made terminology confusing and the significance of some parameters (e.g. mitotic index) is not fully characterized; as a result, criteria for malignancy are not well-defined.

Pearls

- Mixed tumors are relatively common and their features are usually straightforward (i.e. a mixture of epithelial cells, some forming ducts within a variably myxoid or chondroid stroma).
- Tumors that more closely resemble myoepithelioma or parachordoma are rare and their histopathologic variability may raise a broad differential diagnosis; for these, the combined expression of S100 and cytokeratins and/or EMA is often very helpful in narrowing it.

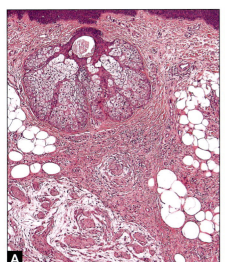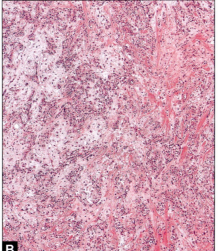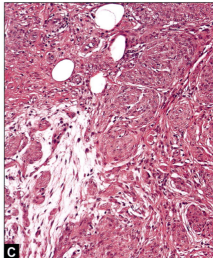

Figs 14.44A to C

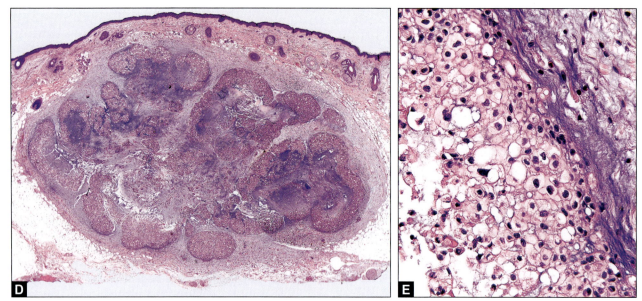

Figs 14.44A to E: (A) Myoepithelioma. The features overlap with mixed tumor, but myoepitheliomas lack ducts and glands. Instead, they are composed of sheets or lobules of cells that are often round, ovoid or somewhat spindled. Admixed within these cells may be mature adipocytes; (B) Mixed tumor. Mixed tumors of the skin (chondroid syringomas) are characterized by epithelioid cells that form small ducts or glands with discernible lumens distributed within a myxoid, chondroid or hyalinized stroma; (C) Myoepithelioma. Like the other tumors within this spectrum, myoepitheliomas usually contain myxoid stroma, at least focally; (D) Parachordoma. Similar to many myoepitheliomas, parachordomas are typically composed of sheets of epithelioid cells within a distinctive myxochondroid matrix; (E) Parachordoma. Physaliferous cells—cells with bubbly-appearing vacuolated cytoplasm—are considered characteristic and have been part of the rationale for considering these tumors distinct. Again, they are more similar to mixed tumors and myoepitheliomas than they are different.

Perivascular Epithelioid Cell Tumor

■ *Criteria for diagnosis*

- Cells with clear to lightly eosinophilic cytoplasm, usually with a radial arrangement around vessels (Fig. 14.45A)
- Epithelioid and/or spindled cells (often both types are present) (Fig. 14.45B)
- Multinucleated cells, cells with a central zone of eosinophilic cytoplasm surrounded by a zone of clear cytoplasm (resembling "spider cells" of adult rhabdomyoma) (Fig. 14.45C)
- Evidence of melanocytic and smooth muscle differentiation.

■ *Differential diagnosis*

- The differential is broad and depends on which morphologic features predominate (spindled vs epithelioid), but the most common considerations are:
- Clear cell variants of many adnexal tumors
- Melanoma
- Metastatic carcinoma (particularly renal cell carcinoma, since these may contain cells with clear cytoplasm)
- Clear cell sarcoma
- Gastrointestinal stromal tumor.

■ *Pitfalls*

- Up to one third of cases express S100 protein, which may cause confusion with melanoma or clear cell sarcoma.

■ *Pearls*

- HMB-45 is positive in over 90% of the cases, Melan-A in over 70%, MiTF in 50%, and SMA in 80%
- Rarely, there is expression of cytokeratins and CD117
- Ultrastructurally, there are features of both smooth muscle differentiation and melanocytic differentiation (in the form of melanosomes)
- Few large case series exist due to the rarity of the tumors but current evidence suggests classification into one of the three categories including: (1) benign; (2) uncertain malignant potential and; (3) malignant
- Local recurrence in approximately 20%; metastases in 13%
- Liver, lung and bone are the most common sites of metastasis.

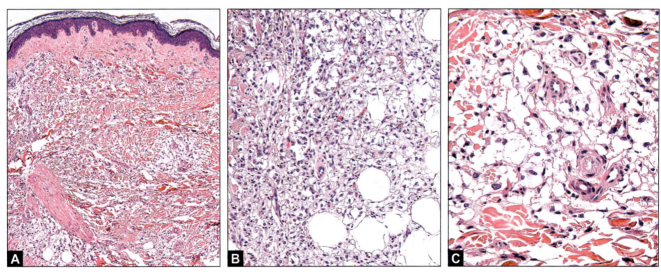

Figs 14.45A to C: Perivascular epithelioid cell tumor. (A) In this example, cells with clear cytoplasm are arranged in clusters throughout the dermis around the vasculature; (B) Clear cytoplasm is usually a distinctive feature. The cells are epithelioid and may closely resemble clear cell variants of adnexal, melanocytic, or metastatic tumors; (C) Nuclear size and shape may vary, and multinucleated cells may be present. Some cells have eosinophilic cytoplasm centrally. Thin eosinophilic strands may extend through the surrounding a rim of clear cytoplasm, simulating the so-called "spider cells" of an adult rhabdomyoma.

Glomus Tumor, Solid Pattern

▪ *Criteria for diagnosis*

- Small, red to blue papule or nodule, most often on the distal extremities (especially the digits)
- Circumscribed lobules of monomorphic round cells that express SMA but are negative for desmin, endothelial cell markers (e.g. CD31) and cytokeratins (Fig. 14.46A).

▪ *Differential diagnosis*

- Mixed tumor
- Adnexal tumors (particularly hidradenoma)
- Myoepithelioma

▪ *Pitfalls*

- By definition, solid pattern glomus tumors have inconspicuous vascular spaces and may be mistaken for epithelioid tumors, especially hidradenomas (Fig. 14.46B).

▪ *Pearls*

- Marked predilection for fingers, particularly subungual, followed by palm, wrist, forearm and foot
- Subungual glomus tumors are three times more common in females than in males
- By definition, solid pattern glomus tumors have inconspicuous vascular spaces and may be mistaken for epithelioid tumors, particularly adnexal neoplasms, such as spiradenoma and hidradenoma (Fig. 14.46C)
- Frequently painful (as opposed to glomangiomas, which are larger, usually painless, present at a younger age, and tend to occur on the trunk and upper extremities)
- Derived from modified, smooth muscle cells of the glomus apparatus, a structure involved in thermoregulation.

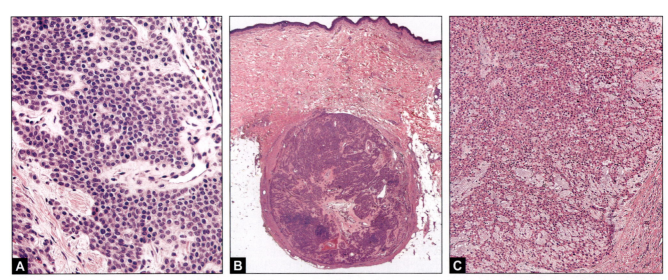

Figs 14.46A to C: Glomus tumor, solid pattern. (A) The glomus cells are monomorphic with regular round nuclei, a feature constant to all patterns. In the solid pattern, however, they often seem to be arranged haphazardly in clusters rather than around vessels; (B) Since vessels are inconspicuous in this type of glomus tumor, they can be mistaken for an adnexal tumor such as a hidradenoma or mixed tumor; (C) The stroma is commonly myxoid or hyalinized, further complicating distinction from mixed tumors and adnexal neoplasms.

Epithelioid Sarcoma

Criteria for diagnosis

- A malignant neoplasm composed of nodules of round, ovoid or polygonal cells that have a distinctly "epithelioid" quality, occasionally with spindled cells as well (Fig. 14.47A)
- Tumor extends into skin from deep soft tissue or very rarely, may be centered within the subcutis or dermis.
- Expression of vimentin along with focal expression of cytokeratins (especially cytokeratin 8) and expression of CD34 in at least 50%.

Differential diagnosis

- Central necrosis within tumor lobules simulates granuloma annulare, rheumatoid nodule and other palisading granulomatous conditions, such as fungal or mycobacterial infection (Fig. 14.47B)
- Giant cell tumor of the tendon sheath (see Table 14.2)
- Fibromatosis, fibrous histiocytoma and other fibrous lesions
- Other epithelioid sarcomas.

Pitfalls

- Mistaking epitheliod sarcoma for a benign process, particularly a palisading granulomatous is one of the most well-known catastrophic mistakes in dermatopathology
- The more superficial portions of the tumor may have fewer mitotic figures and less obvious atypia than the deep regions; (Fig. 14.47C) superficial biopsies may prevent accurate diagnosis.

Pearls

- Epithelioid sarcoma is rare but can have disasterous consequences if it is missed
- Since it can closely simulate palisading granulomatous conditions, it should be considered in the differential diagnosis of palisading lesions on the distal extremities (Fig. 14.47D).

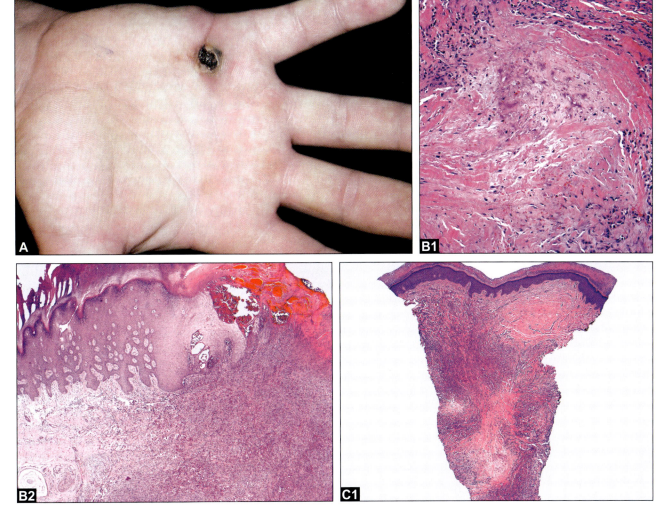

Figs 14.47A to C1

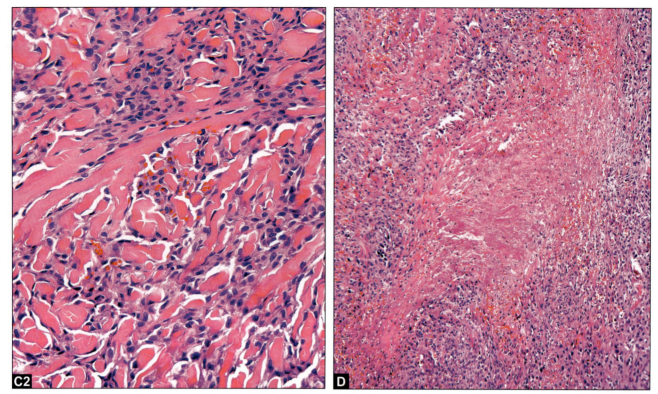

Figs 14.47A to D: Epithelioid sarcoma. (A) This young man presented with an eroded necrotic nodule on the palm; (B) There is marked epidermal hyperplasia, ulceration, and necrosis overlying the tumor; (C) In their superficial and peripheral portions, the neoplastic cells may have a very banal appearance; (D) These tumors are notorious for their tendency to resemble palisading granulomatous lesions. Close inspection demonstrates that the central regions are necrotic tumor rather than degenerating collagen.

Epithelioid Hemangioendothelioma

■ *Criteria for diagnosis*

- A tumor composed of round, ovoid or plump spindled endothelial cells arranged in cords or small nests within a hyalinized or chondromyxoid stroma occupying the dermis and/or subcutis (Fig. 14.48A)
- The neoplastic cells may surround a pre-existing vessel but the neoplasm itself by definition does not form vascular lumens (Fig. 14.48B)
- Tumor cells express at least one vascular marker (FLI-1, factor VIII-related antigen, CD31) and usually are focally positive for cytokeratins (especially keratins 7 and 18) (see Table 14.4)
- The clinical features favor markedly.

■ *Differential diagnosis*

- Epithelioid sarcoma
- Epithelioid angiosarcomas
- Hobnail hemangioendothelioma variants
- Metastatic carcinoma
- Adnexal tumors.

■ *Pitfalls*

- Clinical features are usually nonspecific and a neoplasm is often not suspected
- The lack of vascular channels may prevent consideration of a tumor of endothelial origin.

■ *Pearls*

- Formation of vascular lumens by definition is absent in epithelioid hemangioendothelioma; while this is a potential pitfall in recognizing it as an endothelial cell tumor, it also helps to exclude many other vascular neoplasms (Fig. 14.48C).

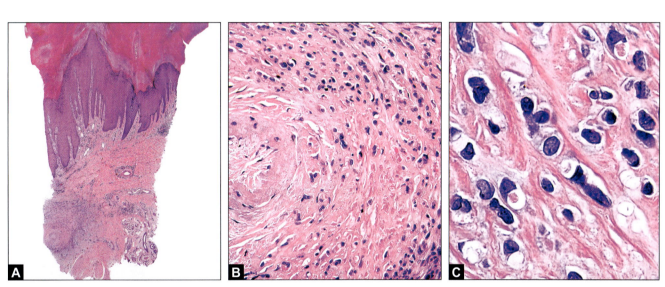

Figs 14.48A to C: Epithelioid hemangioendothelioma. (A) The most striking feature at low power is marked verrucous epidermal hyperplasia, but within the reticular dermis at the lower left is a tumor lobule; (B) Commonly, the tumor cells are distributed concentrically around a central vessel, as in this case; (C) The neoplastic cells are distributed as small clusters of two or three cells or singly. Characteristically, some of the tumor cells contain intracytoplasmic vacuoles that house red blood cells (two of which are evident in this field).

Epithelioid Angiosarcoma

■ *Criteria for diagnosis*

- A malignant neoplasm composed of epithelioid cells that demonstrate evidence of an endothelial origin (e.g. expression of vascular markers, such as FLI-1, CD31, etc.) but tend to express cytokeratins, at least focally (Fig. 14.49).

■ *Differential diagnosis*

- Melanoma
- Carcinomas (primary or metastatic)
- Other epithelioid sarcomas.

■ *Pitfalls*

- When they occur on the breast, they may be mistaken for invasive breast cancer

- Formation of vascular lumens may be inconspicuous with nodular or sheet-like growth of the epithelioid cells dominating the histopathologic picture (Fig. 14.49).

■ *Pearls*

- Even epithelioid variants retain expression of vascular markers.
- Most epithelioid sarcomas have a clinical presentation similar to their non-epithelioid counterparts.

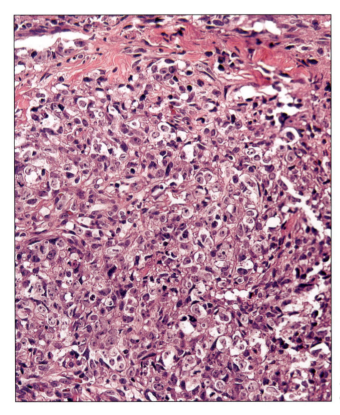

Fig. 14.49: Epithelioid angiosarcoma. It is not uncommon for angiosarcomas to grow as solid sheets of epithelioid endothelial cells with inconspicuous or absent vascular lumens.

Malignant Peripheral Nerve Sheath Tumor, Epithelioid and Myxoid Pattern (Figs 14.50A and B)

■ *Criteria for diagnosis*

- A tumor composed of atypical epithelioid cells arranged in diffuse sheets

■ *Differential diagnosis*

- Nerve sheath myxoma
- Neurothekeoma, myxoid pattern
- Mixed tumor/myoepithelioma
- Melanoma
- Synovial sarcoma (see Tables 14.4 and 14.5)
- Other epithelioid sarcomas.

■ *Pitfalls*

- Unlike spindle cell MPNSTs, the epithelioid variant is more likely to retain S100 expression; this can complicate distinction from nerve sheath myxomas and melanocytic tumors.

■ *Pearls*

- Careful search at the periphery of the tumor for an adjacent neurofibroma essentially confirms the diagnosis but is not present in those that arise de nove, i.e. without a pre-existing neurofibroma
- Heterologous differentiation (rhabdoid areas, angiosarcoma, osteosarcomatous and chondrosarcomatous areas) is seen in approximately 10% and is a clue to diagnosis
- If melanoma is a consideration, careful scrutiny of the epidermis may identify melanoma in situ and exclude MPNST
- Synovial sarcoma is a notorious mimic of malignant peripheral nerve sheath tumor, but almost never involves the skin.

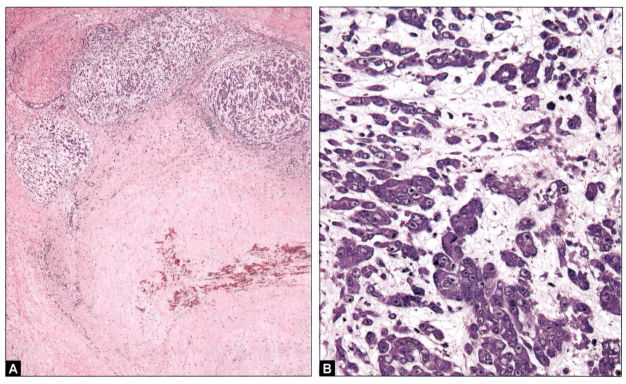

Figs 14.50A and B: Malignant peripheral nerve sheath tumor (epithelioid and myxoid pattern). (A) The discrete lobules of neoplastic cells within a myxoid stroma may resemble nerve sheath myxoma or myxoid pattern neurothekeomas. Even at low power, however, a broad region of necrosis is evident, suggesting malignancy; (B) The cells contain large, vesicular nuclei with prominent nucleoli. A mitotic figure is evident near the center of the field. The combination of marked cytologic atypia and necrosis essentially excludes a benign tumor.

Nevus Lipomatosus Superficialis

■ *Criteria for diagnosis*

- Plaques, polypoid papules or nodules, usually flesh-colored (Fig. 14.51A)
- Mature, cytologically banal adipocytes distributed throughout the entire dermis, particularly around vessels (Fig. 14.51B).

■ *Differential diagnosis*

- Focal dermal hypoplasia
- Ordinary lipoma

■ *Pitfalls*

- Occasionally, closely resembles focal dermal hypoplasia (either sporadic or in the setting of Goltz syndrome).

■ *Pearls*

- Considered as a connective tissue nevus rather than a lipoma variant
- The presence of adipocytes within the dermis is the most obvious feature, but there are often areas of loose dermal collagen, decreased elastic fibers and sometimes a reduction in adnexal structures (supporting classification as a hamartoma/connective tissue nevus)
- Buttocks, thighs and back are favored sites
- Occasionally, closely resembles focal dermal hypoplasia (either sporadic or in the setting of Goltz syndrome).

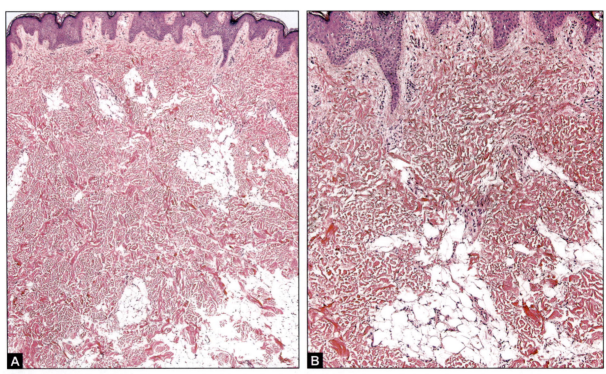

Figs 14.51A and B: Nevus lipomatosus superficialis. (A) This lesion was one of several flesh-colored plaques on the lower back of a young adult male. Discrete lobules of mature adipose tissue are present throughout the dermis; (B) The adipocyte lobules are located predominantly around the blood vessels. Unlike an ordinary lipoma, the lobules are multiple, small and unencapsulated.

Lipomas

■ *Criteria for diagnosis*

- Subcutaneous nodules composed of lobules of mature adipocytes without cytologic atypia (Fig. 14.52A).

■ *Differential diagnosis*

- Well-differentiated liposarcoma/atypical lipomatous tumor
- Adipose differentiation within other tumors (e.g. fibrous hamartoma of infancy, myoepithelioma, lipomatous hemangiopericytoma).

■ *Pitfalls*

- Intranuclear vacuoles are common and must not be mistaken for the vacuolated cytoplasm of a lipoblast
- Several variants of lipoma exist and may be mistaken for various other tumor types (see below) since mature adipocytes may be a small component
- Occasionally, trauma or atrophy can cause variability in adipocyte size causing confusion with well-differentiated liposarcoma/atypical lipomatous tumor (Fig. 14.52B)
- Atypical cells may be inconspicuous in well-differentiated liposarcoma/atypical lipomatous tumor and in some cases only careful examination allows their distinction from ordinary lipomas.

■ *Pearls*

- Lipomas are benign and only seldom recur, even after incomplete excision.

Angiolipoma

- Angiolipomas are a morphologic variant of lipoma in which aggregates of capillary sized blood vessels are present
- Unlike ordinary lipomas, angiolipomas may be painful
- Fibrin thrombi are almost always seen within small vessels, especially at the periphery of the tumor
- Rare examples are very cellular (cellular angiolipoma), and contain numerous spindled cells causing confusion with other spindle cell tumors (Fig. 14.52C).

Chondroid Lipoma

- A variant of lipoma containing mature adipocytes admixed with small lipoblasts, embryonal chondrocyte-like cells, and a myxoid, hyalinized or chondroid matrix (Figs 14.52D and E)
- May be confused with myxoid liposarcoma and extraskeletal myxoid chondrosarcoma
- Like conventional lipoma, it is benign and does not recur locally or metastasize.

Myolipoma

- A variant of lipoma containing mature adipocytes admixed with smooth muscle bundles.

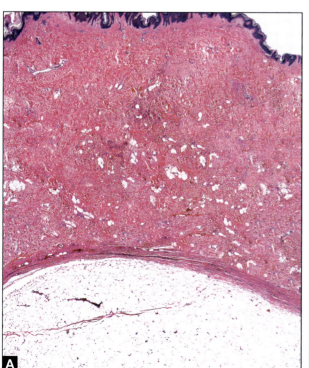

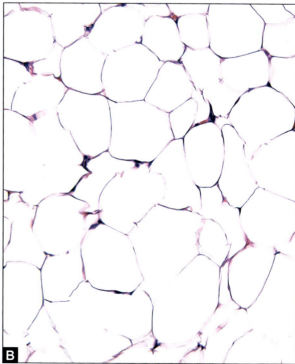

Figs 14.52A and B

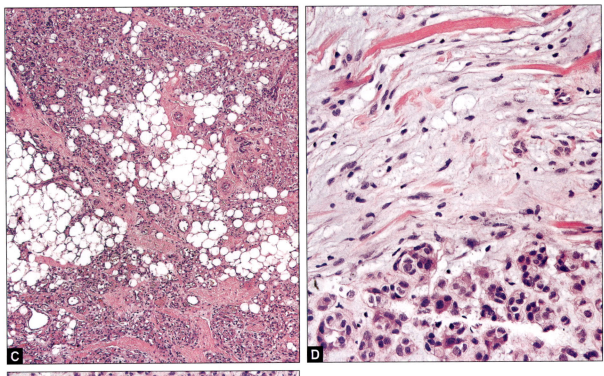

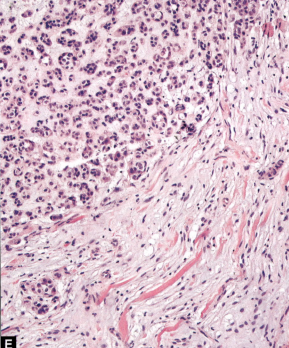

Figs 14.52A to E: Lipoma. (A) In the subcutis, a lobule of mature adipocytes surrounded by a rim of compressed fibrous tissue (capsule); (B) Mature adipocytes with small, peripherally located nuclei make up the entire tumor. The adipocytes should be approximately uniform in size although variability in size may occur as a result of trauma; (C) Angiolipoma. Although many ordinary lipomas contain areas of increased vascular density, the term angiolipoma is often used when this feature predominates. This is a particularly cellular example that could easily be confused with other tumors that have adipose differentiation; (D) Chondroid lipoma. Small chondrocytes accompany mature adipocytes in this lipoma variant; (E) A myxoid or myxohyaline stroma is typical. The adipocytes may be few in number and inconspicuous relative to the chondrocytes.

Spindle Cell Lipoma/Pleomorphic Lipoma/ Myxoid Lipoma

▪ Criteria for diagnosis

- Solitary tumor on the upper back, neck or shoulder of a middle-aged or older adult (Fig. 14.53A)
- Mature adipocytes admixed with cytologically banal spindled cells (spindle cell lipoma), pleomorphic multinucleated cells with a "floret" configuration (pleomorphic lipoma), or a combination of both (Fig. 14.53B)
- Thick collagen bundles within a myxoid stroma, or a myxoid stroma with little collagen (Fig. 14.53C).

▪ Differential diagnosis

- Other variants of lipoma
- Atypical lipomatous tumor/well differentiated liposarcoma.
- Cellular angiolipoma.

▪ Pitfalls

- Occasionally, spindle cells predominate and adipocytes are so few that the differential includes numerous other spindle cell tumors.
- Histopathologically similar tumors may occur in other sites and in younger patients, but are more likely to be atypical lipomas (well differentiated liposarcomas)

- Occasionally, it may be difficult to determine whether the pleomorphic cells represent the benign cells of a pleomorphic lipoma or the bizarre malignant cells of a liposarcoma (Fig. 14.53D).

▪ Pearls

- Spindle cell lipoma, myxoid lipoma and pleomorphic lipoma are closely related lesions or a spectrum of tumors that have overlapping clinical and histopathologic features and have a deletion of 16q or (less commonly) 13q (Figs 14.53E and F)
- Rarely, MDM2 expression may be detected in these tumors (a feature usually encountered in liposarcomas); the significance of this, if any, remains unknown.
- The classic clinical presentation is a subcutaneous nodule on the shoulder girdle of an older male
- The histopathologic features in conjunction with the typical clinical presentation usually cause very little diagnostic difficulty
- Pleomorphic lipomas do not contain genuine lipoblasts (large atypical cells with vacuolated cytoplasm that compress the nucleus, giving it "scalloped" contours).

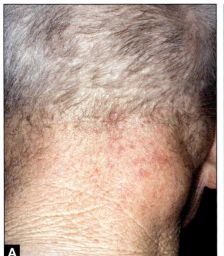
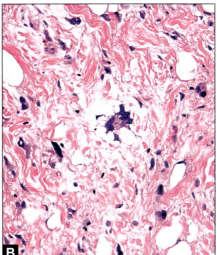
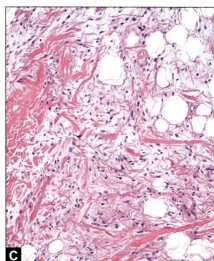

Figs 14.53A to C

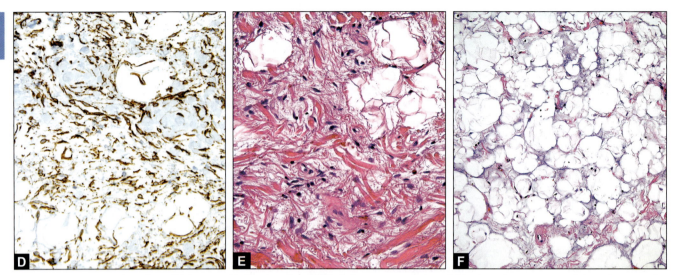

Figs 14.53A to F: (A) Spindle cell/pleomorphic lipoma. Over 85% of these tumors arise within the subcutaneous adipose tissue on the upper back, neck or shoulders of older males; (B) Pleomorphic lipoma. The diagnostic feature of a pleomorphic lipoma is the presence of multinucleated giant cells, particularly those in which the nuclei are arranged at the periphery of the cell (Floret-type giant cells). Unlike malignant lipoblasts, the intracytoplasmic vacuoles do not indent or "scallop" the nucleus; (C) Spindle cell lipoma. Spindle cell lipomas usually are well circumscribed and often have a loose collagenous stroma with thick wavy collagen bundles admixed with collagen strands; (D) The neoplastic cells of spindle cell lipomas and pleomorphic lipomas typically express CD34; (E) Cellularity may vary significantly, but the cells are spindled or slightly ovoid and have banal nuclei; (F) Myxoid lipoma. Recent evidence suggests that myxoid lipomas are related to pleomorphic and spindle cell lipomas. In these tumors, a myxoid matrix is conspicuous. Some spindled cells are present, but they are less prominent than in spindle cell lipomas. Like pleomorphic lipomas and spindle cell lipomas, some have been shown to have 16q or 13q deletions.

Source: Dahlén A, Debiec-Rychter M, Pedeutour F, Domanski HA, Höglund M, Bauer HC, Rydholm A, Sciot R, Mandahl N, Mertens F. Clustering of deletions on chromosome 13 in benign and low-malignant lipomatous tumors. Int J Cancer. 2003;103(5):616-23. Review. PubMed PMID: 12494468.

Hibernoma

■ *Criteria for diagnosis*

- Subcutaneous nodules composed of cells with granular or multivacuolated cytoplasm admixed with a variable number of mature adipocytes and banal spindle cells (Figs 14.54A and B).

■ *Differential diagnosis*

- Granular cell tumor
- Rhabdomyoma
- Spindle cell lipoma
- Histiocytoid neoplasms.

■ *Pitfalls*

- The vacuolated cytoplasm may cause confusion with the lipoblasts of liposarcoma.
- The granular cytoplasm may make distinction from granular cell tumor difficult, and both may express S100

- Rhabdomyomas often have similar cytomorphology and granular cytoplasm
- If spindle cells are numerous, hibernoma may be difficult to differentiate from spindle cell lipoma (and the spindle cells in both express CD34).

■ *Pearls*

- Benign tumors derived from brown fat
- Do not recur if completely excised
- Mallory's phosphotungstic acid-hematoxylin (PTAH) stains may allow identification of cytoplasmic striations, indicating a diagnosis of rhabdomyoma rather than hibernoma
- Lipomas are benign and only seldom recur, even after incomplete excision.

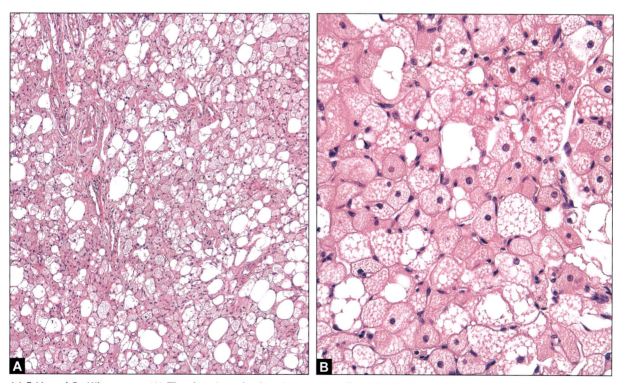

Figs 14.54A and B: Hibernoma. (A) The dermis and subcutis contain cells with abundant clear or eosinophilic cytoplasm admixed with mature adipocytes; (B) The cytoplasm ranges from coarsely granular to vacuolated. The size of the vacuoles varies, but many are relatively small, round and uniform.

Atypical Lipoma/Well-Differentiated Liposarcoma

■ *Criteria for diagnosis*

- A subcutaneous nodule composed of mature adipocytes but also a variable number of multivacuolated lipoblasts and fibroblast-like cells with large hyperchromatic nuclei (Fig. 14.55A).

■ *Differential diagnosis*

- Traumatized/inflamed lipoma
- Fat necrosis
- Fat atrophy
- Reaction to injected silicone
- Pleomorphic lipoma/spindle cell lipoma
- Cellular angiolipoma

■ *Pitfalls*

- In some examples, the atypical cells may be widely scattered and few in number and can be easily be missed without extensive sampling and careful microscopic inspection (Fig. 14.55B)

- Fat necrosis within an ordinary lipoma may lead to variability in adipocyte size and infiltrating macrophages that can simulate an atypical lipoma.

■ *Pearls*

- Rare in the skin
- Locally aggressive tumor that commonly recurs if not completely excised but does not metastasize unlesss "dedifferentiation" occurs
- Exclude fat atrophy and fat necrosis before making the diagnosis of atypical lipoma; these are commonly misinterpreted mimics.

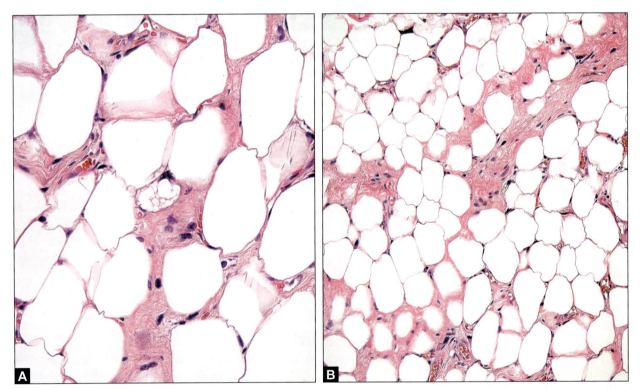

Figs 14.55A and B: Atypical lipoma. (A) In the center of the field is a lipoblast, characterized by multiple cytoplasmic vacuoles that indent the large hyperchromatic nucleus; (B) Most examples resemble ordinary lipomas except they contain scattered atypical cells, such as the one at the top left of the field.

THE VASCULAR TUMORS

Hemangiomas

■ *Criteria for diagnosis*

- Erythematous or violaceous macules or papules; usually solitary but occasionally multiple
- A collection of vessels lined by cytologically banal endothelial cells (Fig. 14.56A)
- No distinctive clinicopathologic features that would warrant classification as one of the specific hemangioma subtypes described below.

■ *Differential diagnosis*

- Other hemangiomas (see below)
- Reactive vascular proliferations (reactive cutaneous angiomatoses, granulation tissue, etc.)

■ *Pitfalls*

- Some of the distinct clinicopathologic hemangioma subtypes contain areas that resemble these nonspecific hemangiomas
- Rarely, angiosarcomas have cytologically banal regions at their periphery that resemble benign hemangiomas.

■ *Pearls*

- Some designate hemangiomas by the architectural configuration that predominates ("cavernous" type, "capillary" type, etc.), but many have a mixture of several architectural patterns, and there is little value in subclassifying hemangiomas without distinctive clinicopathologic features (Fig. 14.56B).

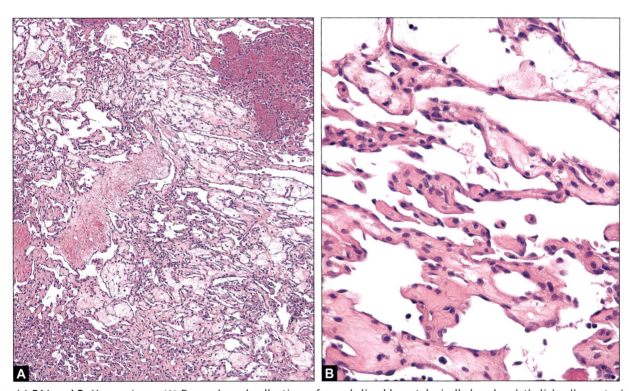

Figs 14.56A and B: Hemangioma. (A) Dense dermal collections of vessels lined by cytologically banal endothelial cells are typical. Although the vessels vary in size and shape, many are the caliber of capillaries; (B) Other hemangiomas have more widely dilated vascular channels and sometimes even broad cyst-like spaces. These have been designated "cavernous hemangioma" by some.

Angioma (Cherry Angioma)

■ *Criteria for diagnosis*

- Red papules composed of a circumscribed collection of congested capillary-sized vessels with hyalinized walls lined by cytologically banal endothelial cells (Fig. 14.57)
- No discrete lobular organization, inflammation/granulation tissue or ulceration that would suggest a pyogenic granuloma/lobular capillary hemangioma.

■ *Differential diagnosis*

- Pyogenic granuloma/lobular capillary hemangioma
- Angiokeratoma
- Hemangiomas.

■ *Pitfalls*

- Rarely, superficial portions of other vascular lesions may resemble cherry angiomas.

■ *Pearls*

- The clinical presentation is usually distinctive; biopsies are usually performed to exclude basal cell carcinoma or for cosmetic reasons.

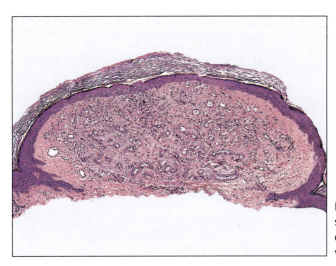

Fig. 14.57: Angioma (Cherry angioma). These small, dome-shaped red papules commonly appear in adults. The dermis is occupied by a well demarcated collection of small capillary sized vessels. An epidermal collarette commonly surrounds the lesion.

Infantile Type Hemangioma

■ *Criteria for diagnosis*

- Densely packed, capillary-sized vessels arranged in lobules, diffusely or both, with involvement of the dermis and often the superficial subcutis (Fig. 14.58A)
- Expression of GLUT-1 within endothelial cells of the lesional vessels (Fig. 14.58B).

■ *Differential diagnosis*

- Pyogenic granuloma/lobular capillary hemangioma
- Vascular malformation
- Other variants of hemangioma.

■ *Pitfalls*

- May have a very high mitotic rate that must not be interpreted as evidence of an aggressive tumor (Fig. 14.58C).

■ *Pearls*

- The clinical presentation (Fig. 14.58D)
- Expression of GLUT-1 aids in differentiating them from other hemangiomas and vascular malformations, an important distinction since juvenile hemangiomas tend to regress spontaneously while vascular malformations do not.

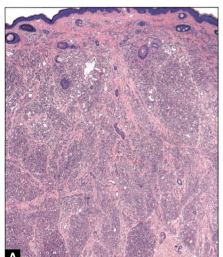
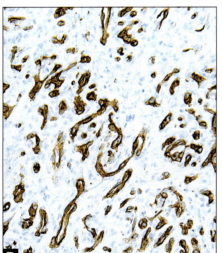
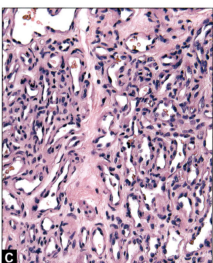

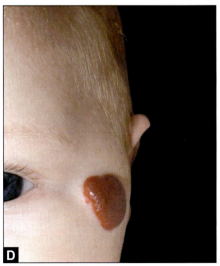

Figs 14.58A to D: Infantile hemangioma. (A) The dermis and superficial subcutis are filled with lobules of small, capillary-sized vessels and closely packed solid-appearing clusters of endothelial cells; (B) The lesional cells almost invariably express glucose transporter 1. The surrounding pericytes and the endothelial cells of intervening normal vessels do not; (C) Mitotic figures are often conspicuous; the endothelial cells are often plump, but they are relatively uniform throughout the entire tumor; (D) Within a few weeks of birth, a red nodule appears and enlarges quickly over a period of 6–12 months. There is a predilection for the head and neck.

Kaposiform Hemangioendothelioma

■ Criteria for diagnosis

- Violaceous papules in an infant or child
- Densely cellular nodules of spindled endothelial cells surrounding small slit-like vascular spaces (resembling Kaposi's sarcoma) (Fig. 14.59A)
- A varying proportion of well-formed vessels that may be capillary-like, angular and branch, or sometimes cavernous.

■ Differential diagnosis

- Juvenile/congenital hemangioma
- Vascular malformations
- Other types of hemangioma.

■ Pitfalls

- The characteristic "kaposiform" areas vary in proportion among lesions and are usually accompanied by regions resembling other types of hemangioma, and incomplete sampling may exclude the characteristic areas (Fig. 14.59B).

- The exact proportion of the tumor that must have kaposiform features is a matter of controversy and appears somewhat arbitrary.

■ Pearls

- Histopathologically, the lesions resemble Kaposi's sarcoma, as the name implies, but clinical features exclude Kaposi's sarcoma
- A consumptive coagulopathy (caused in part by sequestration of blood within the tumor vessels) known as the Kasabach-Merritt syndrome is often cited as a potential complication, but is usually associated with tumors in the deep soft tissue and retroperitoneum and is actually very rare in cutaneous tumors
- The lesional endothelial cells express vascular markers, such as CD31, CD34 and D2-40, but not human herpes virus-8 (HHV-8) or Glut-1.

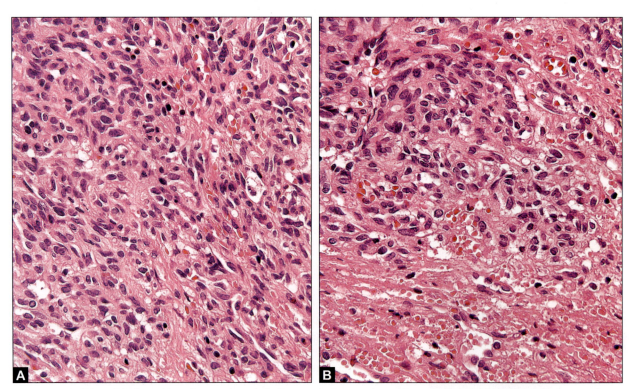

Figs 14.59A and B: Kaposiform hemangioendothelioma. (A) Dense, sheet-like growth of endothelial cells surround inconspicuous slit like vessels; (B) The cells may be elongated or plump and ovoid, as in this focus.

Vascular Malformations

Criteria for diagnosis

- Stable (nongrowing) blue or purple plaques, papules or nodules that are present at birth and do not involute
- A poorly marginated collection of vessels within the dermis and subcutis that vary in caliber and are often separated by intervening areas of normal appearing tissue (Fig. 14.60A)
- Absence of GLUT-1 expression.

Differential diagnosis

- Juvenile/infantile/congenital type hemangioma
- Pyogenic granuloma/lobular capillary hemangioma
- Vascular malformation
- Other variants of hemangioma.

Pitfalls

- Vascular malformations are often excised, but determining the status of margins is usually impossible since lesional vessels cannot be differentiated from the normal vasculature (Fig. 14.60B).

Pearls

- Vascular malformations vary in histopathologic appearance, but in general by comparison to juvenile hemangiomas they are poorly circumscribed and more frequently extend deeply into skeletal muscle or other deep soft tissue
- Many recur repeatedly after excisions, in part because "clear" margins are difficult to achieve as a result of the poor circumscription and deep extent.

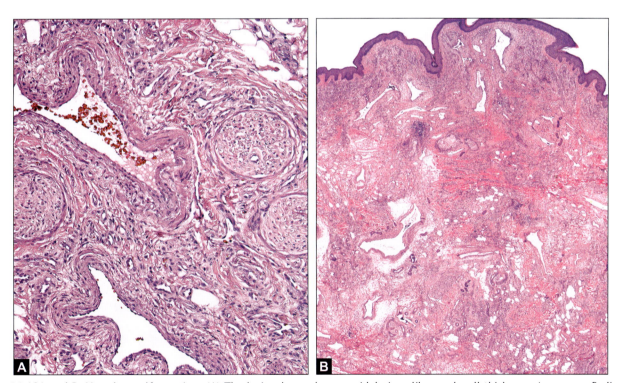

Figs 14.60A and B: Vascular malformation. (A) The lesional vessels vary widely in caliber and wall thickness. A common finding is dilated vessel with thick muscular walls within the superficial dermis; (B) Vascular malformations generally lack the lobular architecture of hemangiomas and have ill-defined borders.

Angiokeratoma

Criteria for diagnosis

- Dilated, thin-walled congested vessels lined by an inconspicuous layer of banal endothelial cells within the papillary dermis that lift the overlying epidermis and cause epidermal hyperplasia that forms a "collarette" around the vessels (Fig. 14.61).

Differential diagnosis

- Pyogenic granuloma/lobulary capillary hemangioma.

Pitfalls

- Rarely, superficial portions of other vascular lesions may resemble cherry angiomas.

Pearls

- The clinical presentation is usually very distinctive.

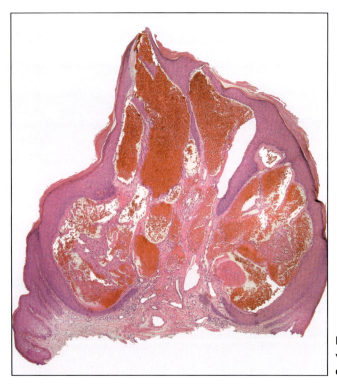

Fig. 14.61: Angiokeratoma. Markedly dilated and congested vessels expand the papillary dermis. An epidermal collarette is often present.

Lymphangiomas and Lymphangioma Circumscriptum

▪ *Criteria for diagnosis*

- Papule(s)
- Irregularly shaped, thin-walled vessels lined by cytologically banal endothelial cells (Fig. 14.62)
- May be filled with pale staining amorphous lymph, erythrocytes or may appear empty.

▪ *Differential diagnosis*

- Angiokeratoma
- Various types of hemangioma
- Vascular malformations.

▪ *Pitfalls*

- Occasionally blood fills the dilated lymphatics, making distinction from hemangiomas and angiokeratomas difficult.

▪ *Pearls*

- Lymphangioma circumscriptum typically presents in infancy but can occur at any age
- Predilection for proximal limbs or limb girdles
- Tend to recur after excision
- Cavernous lymphangioma and cystic hygroma are related lymphatic tumors that often first appear in infancy
- Cavernous lymphangioma usually occurs on the head and neck, the tongue or extremities, and is also prone to recurrence
- Cystic hygroma usually presents as a cystic neoplasm within the soft tissue of the neck, axilla or inguinal region.

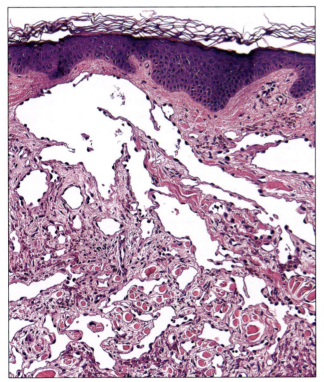

Fig. 14.62: Lymphangioma circumscriptum. The dermis contains dilated, irregularly shaped vascular channels. Often the vessels are clear, as in this case, but the presence of erythrocytes does not exclude the diagnosis. The clinical description may be more helpful in differentiating lymphangiomas from hemangiomas.

Venous Lake

Criteria for diagnosis

- Red or violaceous macules or papules that arise on sun-damaged skin of older adults (Fig. 14.63A)
- Widely dilated, irregularly shaped thin-walled venule with or without red blood cells (Fig. 14.63B).

Differential diagnosis

- Cherry angioma
- AngiokeratomA

Pitfalls

- Superficial biopsy is common and ruptures the vessel, producing nonspecific histopathologic findings, usually diffuse the dermal hemorrhage.

Pearls

- The clinical presentation is usually distinctive
- Unlike angiomas/hemangiomas, venous lakes are solitary vessels
- Most are treated by biopsy performed to exclude other lesions.

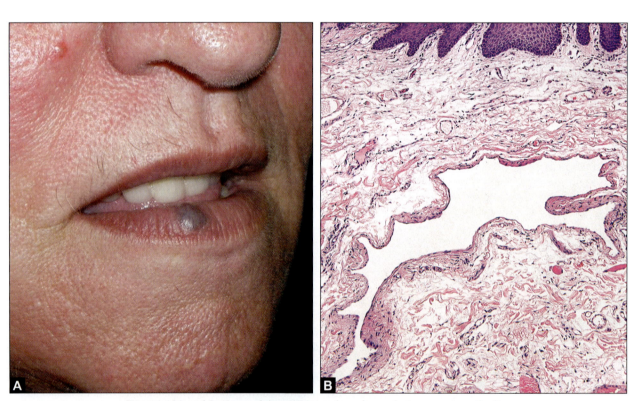

Figs 14.63A and B: Venous lake. (A) A purple red macule is present on the lip; (B) One or more very widely dilated venules occupy the dermis.

Papillary Endothelial Hyperplasia (Masson's Tumor)

■ *Criteria for diagnosis*

- A dermal or subcutaneous nodule that may clinically appear vascular or may be nonspecific
- Irregular papilla and anastomosing cords composed of fibrous or hyalinized stalks or trabeculae covered by cytologically banal endothelial cells that protrude into the lumen of a vessel (Fig. 14.64).

■ *Differential diagnosis*

- Thrombosed blood vessel
- Hobnail hemangioendotheliomas
- Angiosarcoma

■ *Pitfalls*

- When the proliferation is florid, the underlying vessel may be inconspicuous or even obliterated.

■ *Pearls*

- Represents recanalization of a thrombosed vessel in which there is an exaggerated proliferation of the endothelium
- Hyaline cores and fibrin deposits are often seen within the papillae
- Hobnail hemangioendotheliomas have large, rounded endothelial cells that protrude into vascular lumens
- Angiosarcomas have pleomorphic endothelial cells, often with conspicuous mitotic figures, and although they commonly contain papillary structures, they are formed by multilayering or "piling up" of endothelial cells upon one another in angiosarcoma.

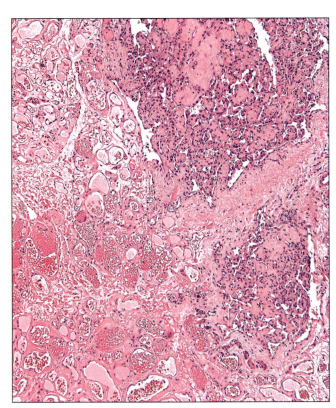

Fig. 14.64: Papillary endothelial hyperplasia (Masson's tumor). Some of the vessels within this benign hemangioma (right-side of image) have developed papillary endothelial hyperplasia characterized by numerous papillae covered by cytologically banal endothelial cells protruding into the lumens.

Pyogenic Granuloma (Lobular Capillary Hemangioma) (Figs 14.65A to C)

Criteria for diagnosis

- Lobules of vessels separated by intervening fibrous tracts
- Most vessels are capillary sized; the vessels are lined by endothelial cells that may plump but are always cytologically banal (Fig. 14.65A).

Differential diagnosis

- Bacillary angiomatosis
- Other types of hemangioma.

Pitfalls

- Rare cases are intravascular and may simulate glomeruloid hemangiomas and other tumors.

Pearls

- Erosion, ulceration, a polypoid shape and surrounding epidermal collarette are characteristic of lobular capillary hemangioma (Fig. 14.65B).

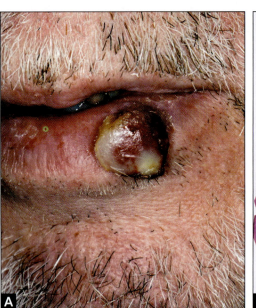

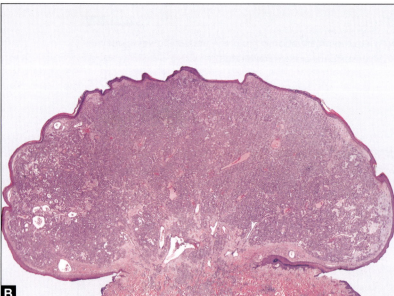

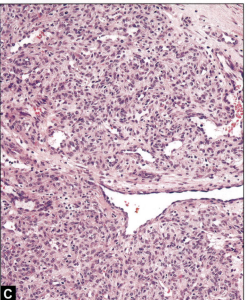

Figs 14.65A to C: Lobular capillary hemangioma (pyogenic granuloma). (A) The lip is a common site but the lesions may arise at almost any site; (B) A polypoid or dome-shaped configuration is typical; (C) Lobules of capillary sized vessels are arranged around larger "feeder" vessels.

Glomeruloid Hemangioma

■ *Criteria for diagnosis*

- Multiple red or violaceous lesions in which a proliferation of small capillary vessels and endothelial cells fill dilated vascular lumens (simulating the appearance of a renal glomerulus) (Fig. 14.66A).

■ *Differential diagnosis*

- Intravascular pyogenic granuloma
- Reactive angiomatoses
- Thrombosed vessels with recanalization
- Kaposiform hemangioendothelioma.

■ *Pitfalls*

- Some cases are easily confused with pyogenic granulomas that are intravascular or composed of widely separated lobules (Fig. 14.66B).

■ *Pearls*

- Strong association of POEMS syndrome (polyneuropathy, organomegaly, endocrinopathy, monoclonal gammopathy, and skin lesions)
- Periodic acid-Schiff-positive globules (representing immunoglobulin collections) are often present (Fig. 14.66C)
- Small collections of red cells which degenerate and become homogenized are common
- Clinical presentation usually allows differentiation from intravascular variant of pyogenic granuloma.

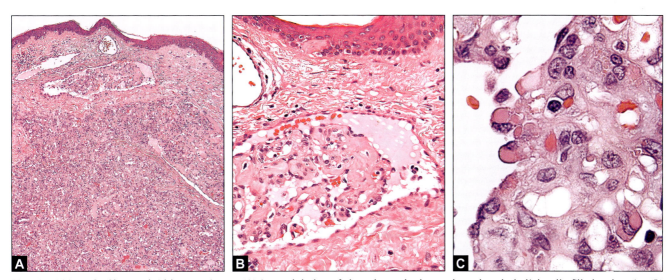

Figs 14.66A to C: Glomeruloid hemangioma. (A) Large lobules of densely packed vessels and endothelial cells fill the dermis; (B) Several of the vascular lobules are surrounded by clear spaces, imparting some resemblance to renal glomeruli; (C) Pale, eosinophilic periodic acid-Schiff positive globules are, such as those at the edge of the lumen in this field, are a characteristic finding. They are believed to be collections of immunoglobulin.

Arteriovenous Hemangioma (Cirsoid Aneurysm)

■ *Criteria for diagnosis*

- A papule or nodule composed of a circumscribed collection of vessels with thick and thin walls (Figs 14.67A and B).

■ *Differential diagnosis*

- Arteriovenous fistula
- Vascular malformation.

■ *Pitfalls*

- Partially sampled lesions can be indistinguishable from vascular malformations.

■ *Pearls*

- Unlike vascular malformations, arteriovenous hemangiomas usually present within adulthood and are well-circumscribed, with little normal appearing tissue between the lesional vessels.

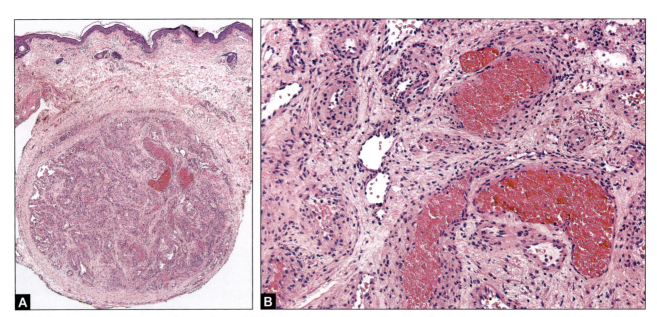

Figs 14.67A and B: Arteriovenous hemangioma. (A)The dermis contains a collection of vessels with varying wall thickness. Unlike a vascular malformation, the lesion is well demarcated; (B) Some of the vessels resemble thin-walled veins while others have the thick, muscular walls of a medium caliber artery.

Hobnail Hemangioma/Targetoid Hemosiderotic Hemangioma

■ Criteria for diagnosis

- A red papule or macule surrounded by an ecchymotic appearing "halo" clinically
- A collection of vessels, some of which are lined by plump but cytologically banal endothelial cells that protrude into the vascular lumen ("hobnail" or "epithelioid" cells) (Fig. 14.68A)
- Hemosiderin deposition within the surrounding dermis.

■ Differential diagnosis

- Hobnail hemangioendotheliomas (Dabska tumor/retiform hemangioendothelioma)
- Early Kaposi's sarcoma
- Ordinary hemangiomas
- Reactive cutaneous angiomatoses.

■ Pitfalls

- Papillary projections, inconspicuous lumens and ill-defined margins occur in some cases, resembling other vascular tumors including Kaposi's sarcoma
- Cases have been reported in which vascular spaces involved the deep dermis and the subcutis (Fig. 14.68B).

■ Pearls

- Some authors now regard these tumors as lymphatic due to their expression of D2-40, a marker of controversial specificity for lymphatics (Fig. 14.68C)
- Features that help in excluding early Kaposi's sarcoma include the presence of fibrin thrombi (rare in Kaposi's sarcoma) and a lack of plasma cells and eosinophilic globules.

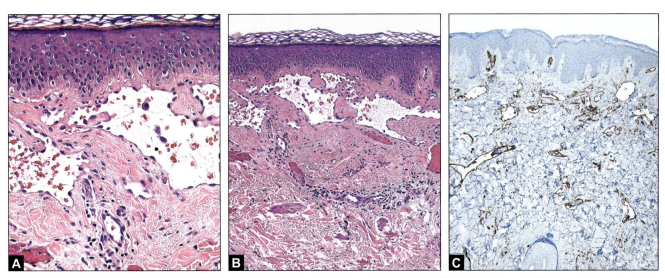

Figs 14.68A to C: Hobnail hemangioma (targetoid hemosiderotic hemangioma). (A) Endothelial cells with large nuclei project into the vascular spaces (hobnail appearance). Intraluminal papillae are often present; (B) The dermis contains dilated vascular spaces; (C) D2-40 expression within the hobnail endothelial cells is a characteristic feature. D2-40 is often considered a marker of lymphatic differentiation, but its specificity remains controversial.

Angiolymphoid Hyperplasia with Eosinophilia/Epithelioid Hemangioma (Figs 14.69A to C)

■ *Criteria for diagnosis*

- Variably sized vessels admixed with aggregates of inflammatory cells, usually lymphocytes and often eosinophils, sometimes with lymphoid follicle formation
- Ectatic, thick-walled vessels lined by prominent endothelial cells with an epithelioid appearance within the central regions.

■ *Differential diagnosis*

- Hemangiomas
- Arteriovenous malformation (see below)
- Lymphomas and pseudolymphomas in cases with particularly dense lymphoid aggregates.

■ *Pitfalls*

- A "histiocytoid" pattern may be present in which the endothelial cells are large and have abundant somewhat granular cytoplasm, resembling histiocytes/macrophages.

■ *Pearls*

- A marked tendency to occur on the head and neck, particularly around the ear
- Considered by some to be a particular type of vascular malformation
- The endothelial cells may have granular cytoplasm and resemble macrophages
- Inflammation may be minimal in some cases, but in others it is dense so as to obscure the vessels and endothelial cells.

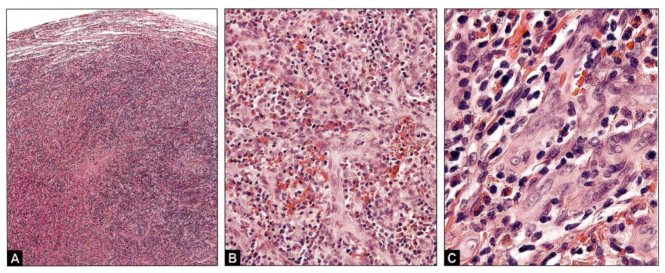

Figs 14.69A to C: Angiolymphoid hyperplasia with eosinophilia/epithelioid hemangioma. (A) These are typically rounded, well circumscribed tumors (although this feature may only be evident if the lesion is removed in toto). They are often mistaken for enlarged lymph nodes on clinical examination; (B) The persistence of both designations for this tumor (angiolymphoid hyperplasia with eosinophilia and epithelioid hemangioma) is illustrated here. Anastomosing vessels formed by large, epithelioid endothelial cells are present, but just as conspicuous is the dense infiltrate of eosinophils and lymphocytes; (C) In some areas vascular lumens cannot be visualized, and the large epithelioid endothelial cells may be mistaken for macrophages.

Postradiation Atypical Vascular Proliferation

■ *Criteria for diagnosis*

- Erythematous patches, papules or plaques that arise within irradiated skin
- An increased complement of ectatic, irregularly shaped vessels some of which have thin anastomosing lumens that extend between dermal collagen bundles (Fig. 14.70)
- Vessels lined by endothelial cells that are plump (sometimes "hobnail"-like) but lack hyperchromasia, pleomorphism and multilayering (Fig. 14.70).

■ *Differential diagnosis*

- Postradiation angiosarcoma
- Reactive cutaneous angiomatosis
- Hemangiomas

■ *Pitfalls*

- Angiosarcomas, especially at their periphery, may contain similar-appearing areas and may be very difficult to exclude without adequate sampling and correlation with clinical features.

■ *Pearls*

- This diagnosis is most often made in breast skin exposed to radiation for the treatment of carcinoma
- Many lesions are more localized and circumscribed than angiosarcomas; these appear to have a low propensity for progression to angiosarcoma
- More extensive lesions may be indistinguishable from low grade angiosarcoma, and warrant excision if possible (Fig. 14.70).

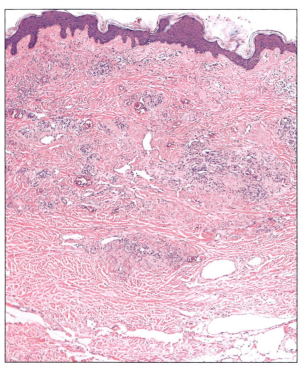

Fig. 14.70: Postradiation atypical vascular proliferation. Anastomosing vessels fill the dermis in this skin that was irradiated years earlier. The vessels vary considerably in size and shape, as do the endothelial cells that line them. The lesion is poorly demarcated and extends into the deep dermis and subcutis. Some areas are difficult to differentiate from low-grade angiosarcoma.

Glomus Tumor, Glomangioma Pattern (Glomulovenous Malformation)

■ *Criteria for diagnosis*

- Conspicuous dilated vascular spaces with monomorphic glomus cells within their walls or the adjacent stroma (Figs 14.71A and B)
- Smooth muscle and hyalinized collagen often prominent.

■ *Differential diagnosis*

- Hemangiomas (especially those with a cavernous or capillary pattern)
- Vascular malformations.

■ *Pitfalls*

- The glomus cells may be inconspicuous in some cases (only one or two layers surround the vessels in some examples) causing the lesion to be mistaken for a hemangioma.

■ *Pearls*

- Less common than solid pattern glomus tumors
- Compared to solid pattern glomus tumors, glomangiomas are usually larger, lack large solid areas, are usually ill-demarcated, occur more often in children, and are often painless
- Common on the hand and forearm, they are more likely to occur on the trunk and proximal extremities than the conventional type.

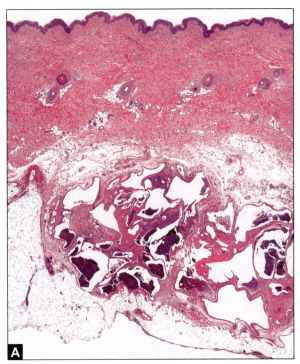
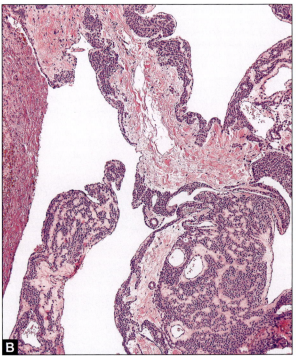

Figs 14.71A and B: Glomus tumor, glomulovenous pattern. (A) A well localized collection of dilated vessels occupies the subcutis. At low power, the glomus cells may be inconspicuous; (B) Close inspection reveals an increased complement of round, monomorphic glomus cells.

Spindle Cell Hemangioma (Figs 14.72A to C)

■ *Criteria for diagnosis*

- Dusky red or purple nodules either single or grouped, that are composed of irregularly shaped, angular vessels surrounded by dense aggregates of spindled to ovoid cells, imparting some resemblance to Kaposi's sarcoma (Figs 14.72A and B)
- Intracytoplasmic vacuoles within a subset of the neoplastic cells.

■ *Differential diagnosis*

- Kaposi's sarcoma
- Other hemangiomas.

■ *Pitfalls*

- On occasion, the intracytoplasmic vacuoles are so large that they may be mistaken for adipocytes

- Some lesions are difficult to differentiate from Kaposi's sarcoma clinically and microscopically (but HHV-8 is invariably negative).

■ *Pearls*

- Predilection for the distal extremities of children and young adults (hand/arm most frequent site)
- Over 50% are multifocal
- Often painful
- Develop slowly and remain indolent (despite the fact that multiple lesions may develop at the site, they do not metastasize)
- Occasionally associated with Maffuci's syndrome and Klippel-Trenaunay-Weber syndrome

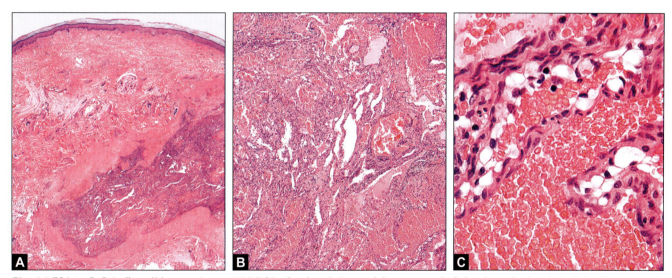

Figs 14.72A to C: Spindle cell hemangioma. (A) Within the dermis is a nodule composed of closely packed endothelial cells surrounding vascular spaces with irregular angled and branched contours; (B) The vascular spaces are slit-like (similar to those of Kaposi's sarcoma) or have irregular angular contours; (C) Some of the neoplastic cells contain intracytoplasmic vacuoles.

Hobnail Hemangioendotheliomas (Figs 14.73A to C)

(Dabska Tumor, Papillary Intralymphatic Angioendothelioma and Retiform Hemangioendothelioma)

■ Criteria for diagnosis

- Ill-defined plaques within the skin or subcutis
- Hobnail endothelial cells that protrude into vascular lumens and intraluminal papillae
- A variably dense lymphocytic infiltrate may be present.

■ Differential diagnosis

- Hobnail hemangioma/targetoid hemosiderotic hemangioma
- Angiolymphoid hyperplasia with eosinophilia/epithelioid hemangioma
- Papillary endothelial hyperplasia
- Angiosarcoma.

■ Pitfalls

- Plump endothelial cells may be overinterpreted as atypical or malignant
- Classification is confusing and controversial
- The terminology is confusing; hobnail hemangioma and hobnail hemangioendothelioma are similar in name but not in prognosis; the former is benign while the latter has low-grade or intermediate malignant potential.

■ Pearls

- Hobnail hemangioendotheliomas have low-grade malignant potential that they tend to recur and may metastasize to regional lymph nodes; however, death from the tumor is rare

- Considered by some to be separate entities, Dabska tumor and retiform hemangioendotheliomas overlap histopathologically and have similar clinical behavior
- Both are thought by many to originate from lymphatics rather than blood vessels, and the name "papillary intralymphatic angioendothelioma" has been used synonymously
- Dabska tumors have a predilection for children and adolescents, while retiform hemangioendotheliomas are more common in adults
- Angiolymphoid hyperplasia with eosinophilia/epithelioid hemangioma usually lacks the intraluminal papillary formations
- Hobnail endotheliomas also exhibit intraluminal papillae and epithelioid cells that protrude in lumens; however, their vessels are usually well-formed and separated by normal dermis rather than diffusely anastomosing, and they do not exhibit the same degree of cellularity (Figs 14.73B and C)
- Angiosarcoma can be very difficult to distinguish, but in hobnail hemangioendotheliomas the endothelial cells do not "pile up" on one another (multilayering) (Fig. 14.73C)
- Angiosarcoma almost never occurs in children and adolescents and therefore, would not be confused with Dabska tumors.
- Angiosarcomas have more cytologic atypia, mitotic activity and endothelial multilayering than hobnail hemangioendotheliomas.

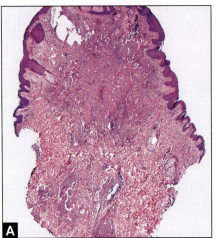 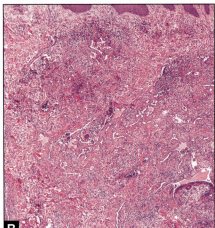 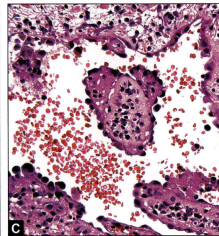

Figs 14.73A to C: (A) Hobnail hemangioendothelioma. (A) At low magnification, the dermis contains variably dilated vessels, as well as solid-appearing growth of endothelial cells; (B) Many of the vascular channels have irregular contours. Anastomosing vessels are obvious, and the appearance may closely simulate angiosarcoma; (C) Papillae lined by endothelial cells are characteristic. Cells lining the vascular channels and the papillae have large nuclei and protrude into the lumens (hobnailing). The same features can be seen in angiosarcomas, but in angiosarcomas the endothelial cells form layers on top of one another.

Kaposi's Sarcoma

◼ *Criteria for diagnosis*

- Erythematous or violaceous papules, plaques or nodules (Fig. 14.74A)
- Clinical history of immunocompromise (HIV infection, immuno-suppressive medicatinos, etc.) or elderly men of Mediterranean ancestry
- Dermal proliferation of blood vessels, at least some of which have narrow, slit-like contours (Fig. 14.74B)
- HHV-8 positivity within endothelial cells.

◼ *Differential diagnosis*

- Kaposiform hemangioendothelioma
- Angiosarcoma
- Spindle cell hemangiomas.

◼ *Pitfalls*

- The histopathologic features of early lesions may be very subtle, and it may not even be recognized as a vascular/endothelial cell lesion
- Narrow, slit-like vessels are nearly always present, but not uncommonly, the periphery contains capillary-sized or cavernous vessels that may be mistaken for a conventional hemangiomas, especially in small biopsies

- Fully evolved lesions may contain dense sheets of spindled or fusiform cells that obscure the vascular spaces and resemble other types of spindle cell tumors.

◼ *Pearls*

- *Early lesions*: Subtle increase in endothelial cells surrounding narrow inconspicuous vascular spaces
- *Established lesions*: Diffusely anastomosing slit-like or angular, branching vascular spaces dissecting between dermal collagen bundles with dense aggregates of spindled and fusiform endothelial cells
- Extravasated erythrocytes, lymphocytes, plasma cells and eosinophilic "globules" are commonly encountered within the lesion (Fig. 14.74C)
- Chronic Kaposi's sarcoma is generally an indolent tumor with mortality of approximately 15% after a course of up to 10 years
- Chemotherapy and radiation therapy are preferred overall surgical management.

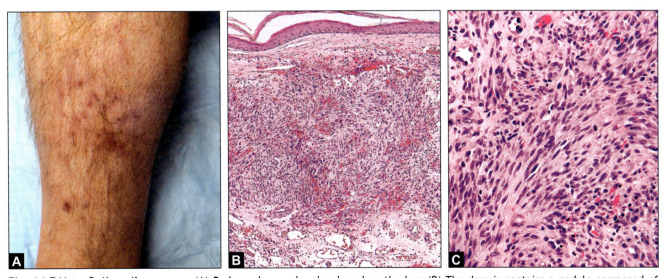

Figs 14.74A to C: Kaposi's sarcoma. (A) Red purple papules developed on the leg; (B) The dermis contains a nodule composed of spindled cells and extravasated erythrocytes surrounding narrow slit like spaces; (C) High magnification reveals mitotic figures and collections of plasma cells.

Cutaneous Angiosarcoma (Figs 14.75A to E)

■ *Criteria for diagnosis*

- Ill-defined ecchymotic macules or plaques
- A dermis occupied by irregular vascular channels lined by atypical endothelial cells that form aggregates or papillary structures at least focally (Fig. 14.75A).

■ *Differential diagnosis*

- Hobnail hemangioendotheliomas
- Atypical fibroxanthoma.

■ *Pitfalls*

- The tumors are deceptive clinically and often involve what were thought to be adequate surgical margins when examined histopathologically
- A significant number appears to be multifocal, further complicating attempts at complete excision
- Low-grade variants may have only subtle endothelial cell atypia, low cellularity and narrow, relatively inconspicuous vascular channels; benign-appearing vascular channels are commonly present at the periphery of the more obviously malignant areas (making sampling error particularly trechearous) (Fig. 14.75B)

- High-grade variants may be epithelioid and pleomorphic making distinction from carcinomas, melanomas and AFXs difficult in some cases.

■ *Pearls*

- The skin is the most common site of angiosarcomas.
- The characteristic presentation is ecchymotic lesion(s) on the scalp or forehead of older adults, particularly elderly men
- Patients often delay medical attention since the lesion resembles a "bruise"
- Prognosis is relatively poor; this may be partly related to the delay in seeking medical attention, and/or the diffusely infiltrative, poorly demarcated tumor borders
- Angiosarcoma is very rare in children and young adults, and a lesion that resembles angiosarcoma should prompt consideration of a hobnail hemangioendothelioma (Dabska tumor) or kaposiform hemangioendothelioma
- Angiosarcomas have more cytologic atypia, mitotic activity and endothelial multilayering than vascular tumors with benign or intermediate malignant potential, including hobnail hemangioendotheliomas (Fig. 14.75C).

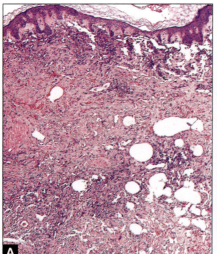 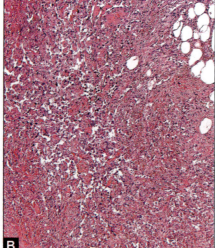 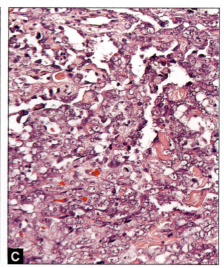

Figs 14.75A to C

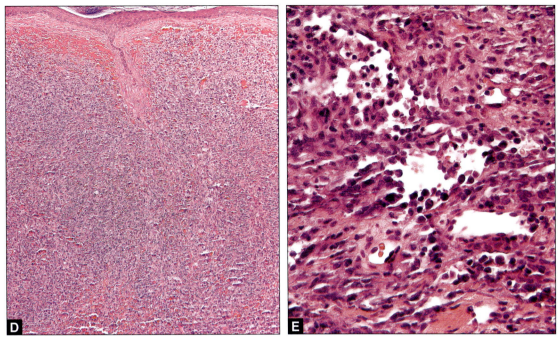

Figs 14.75A to E: Cutaneous angiosarcoma. (A) A dermis containing solid-appearing clusters of cells around vessels with irregularly shaped lumens is a common finding; (B) Some are much more cellular and contain endothelial cells that seem to be "floating" in diffusely anastomosing vascular spaces; (C) Cytologic atypia and mitotic figures may be striking in some examples; (D) Occasionally, the endothelial cells of an angiosarcoma are spindled, arranged in dense sheets and approximately close to the epidermis, resembling an atypical fibroxanthoma; (E) This angiosarcoma has areas that resemble a hobnail hemangioendothelioma. However, notice that the endothelial cells are piled up, one upon another (endothelial multilayering). This is generally not seen in hemangioendotheliomas.

Atypical Fibroxanthoma (Figs 14.76A to E)

■ *Criteria for diagnosis*

- A firm nodule on sun damaged skin (Fig. 14.76A, Table 14.6)
- Confined to the dermis (with at most focal extension into the superficial subcutis) (Fig. 14.76B)
- Pleomorphic population of spindled, ovoid and multinucleated cells that express CD10 but are negative for S100, cytokeratins and desmin (Fig. 14.76C).

■ *Differential diagnosis*

- Atypical fibrous histiocytoma
- Spindle cell or undifferentiated variants of squamous cell carcinoma (Fig. 14.76E)
- Pleomorphic sarcoma
- Pleomorphic leiomyosarcoma
- Pleomorphic angiosarcoma
- Pleomorphic melanoma
- High-grade myofibrosarcoma

■ *Pitfalls*

- In some cases, spindled cells arranged in fascicles predominate and the characteristic pleomorphic cells are rare
- Spindle cell and undifferentiated variants of squamous cell carcinoma may be difficult to exclude since keratin expression in these tumors may be patchy and some cases contain AFX in apparent contiguity with a recognizable squamous cell carcinoma of the skin

- Extension of a deep seated pleomorphic sarcoma superficially into the overlying skin may be identical to AFX, as is a cutaneous pleomorphic sarcoma (see below)
- CD10 expression is frequent in AFX but is by no means specific, as many other sarcomas are CD10-positive (see Table 14.2)
- Like many other neoplasms, scattered dendritic cells/histiocytes, and lymphocytes are often present and may express S100 and CD31, respectively; this must be differentiated from expression of these markers by tumor cells.

■ *Pearls*

- Outside the typical context (i.e. sun-damaged skin of the head and neck of an elderly person), a pleomorphic malignant-appearing tumor in the dermis should be considered as a superficial extension of a deep seated pleomorphic sarcoma until proven otherwise (AFX occurs only exceptionally outside of this clinical scenario)
- Cases occurring in other sites and in younger patients likely represent AFH rather than AFX
- A significant proportion of cases occur in conjunction with a squamous cell carcinoma
- Cells with foamy cytoplasm, osteoclastic-like giant cells and osteoid may be present
- Atypical fibroxanthoma, despite its pleomorphism and high mitotic index, recurs only infrequently; metastases are rare if strict diagnostic criteria are applied
- A helpful immunohistochemical panel includes S100, CD10, pan-cytokeratin, CD31, smooth muscle actin and desmin (see Table 14.2).

Table 14.6: Immunophenotype of cutaneous tumors with spindled and pleomorphic cells					
Tumor	S100	CD10	Cytokeratin	Smooth Muscle Actin	Desmin
AFX	−	+	+/−	− (occasionally +)	−
Melanoma	+	−	−	−	−
Spindle cell squamous carcinoma	−	− (occasionally +)	+	−	−
Angiosarcoma	−	− (occasionally +)	−	−	−
Leiomyosarcoma	−	− (occasionally +)	−	Usually +	Usually +

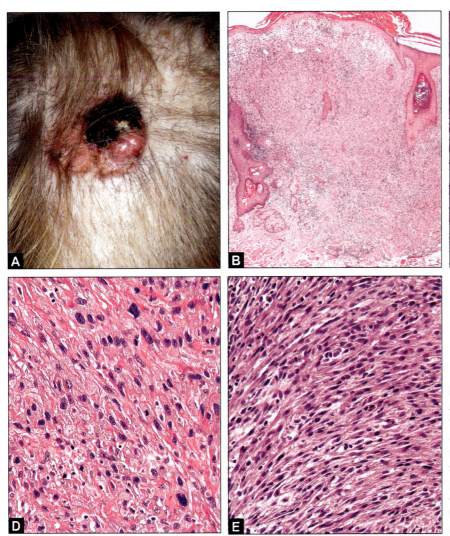

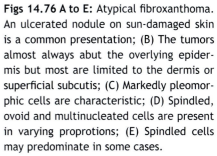

Figs 14.76 A to E: Atypical fibroxanthoma. An ulcerated nodule on sun-damaged skin is a common presentation; (B) The tumors almost always abut the overlying epidermis but most are limited to the dermis or superficial subcutis; (C) Markedly pleomorphic cells are characteristic; (D) Spindled, ovoid and multinucleated cells are present in varying proprotions; (E) Spindled cells may predominate in some cases.

Pleomorphic Sarcoma

■ *Criteria for diagnosis*

- Infiltrative tumor composed of mitotically active atypical pleomorphic and/or spindled cells identical to those of AFX (Fig. 14.77A)
- Extension into the subcutis (and possibly beyond).

■ *Differential diagnosis*

- Atypical fibroxanthomas
- Melanoma
- Myxofibrosarcoma, high-grade
- Spindled squamous cell carcinoma
- Superficial portions of deep seated high-grade sarcomas (Fig. 14.77B).

■ *Pitfalls*

- In biopsies that do not include the subcutis, pleomorphic sarcoma cannot be reliably differentiated from AFX.

■ *Pearls*

- Pleomorphic sarcomas have a significant risk of metastasis, unlike AFX.

- AFX, by definition, does not exhibit more than minimal involvement of the subcutis
- The superficial portions of myxofibrosarcoma are myxoid, contain thin, curvilinear vessels, and usually lack the dense cellularity and marked pleomorphism of pleomorphic sarcoma (Fig. 14.77C)
- Melanoma can often be excluded by identifying an in situ component and by strong and diffuse S100 expression
- Spindle cell squamous cell carcinoma often has regions of conventional squamous cell carcinoma, and the cells often express p63
- Involvement of the skin by a deep seated high-grade sarcoma cannot be excluded without adequate clinical information and imaging studies.

Pleomorphic Variants of Other Sarcomas

- Pleomorphic liposarcoma
- Pleomorphic MPNST
- Pleomorphic leiomyosarcoma
- Pleomorphic rhabdomyosarcoma.

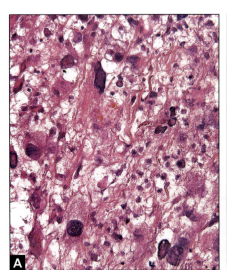 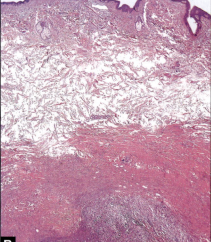 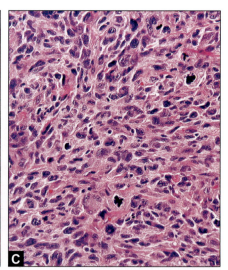

Figs 14.77A to C: Pleomorphic sarcoma. (A) Like atypical fibroxanthoma, the cells may be spindled, epithelioid or a combination of the two; (B) Superficial extension into the skin from a deep-seated sarcoma, as seen here, can simulate an atypical fibroxanthoma histopathologically, although in this example the lack of upper dermal involvement essentially excludes an atypical fibroxanthoma. Cutaneous tumors with morphologic and immunohistochemical features similar to atypical fibroxanthoma but occur outside the typical context of atypical fibroxanthoma should be categorized simply as pleomorphic sarcoma; (C) Marked pleomorphism and a high mitotic index are crucial diagnostic features, as is the absence of any features that suggest melanoma, poorly differentiated squamous cell carcinoma or other cutaneous tumor that may be pleomorphic.

Giant Cell Tumor of the Tendon Sheath (Tenosynovial Giant Cell Tumor)

■ *Criteria for diagnosis*

- A tumor that is attached to (or is within the immediate vicinity of) a tendon sheath
- Nodules with even, rounded contours composed of varying proportions of mononuclear cells, xanthoma cells and multinucleated giant cells surrounded at least partially by a rim of fibrous connective tissue (Figs 14.78A to C).

■ *Differential diagnosis*

- Tendon sheath fibroma
- Palisading granulomatous lesions, especially deep granuloma annulare and rheumatoid nodule
- Tendinous xanthoma
- Foreign body granuloma.

■ *Pitfalls*

- The proportions of the multiple cell types that make up the tumor can vary greatly; some contain very few giant cells.
- A rare but disasterous pitfall is mistaking an epithelioid sarcoma for a giant cell tumor of the tendon sheath (some regions of an epithelioid sarcoma may be cytologically banal, and occasionally they may contain giant cells).

■ *Pearls*

- The most common location is the finger (interphalangeal joint in particular)
- Female predominance (2:1)
- Any age but predilection for fourth to sixth decades
- Most common neoplasm of the hand/fingers
- Less frequent in the toes and larger joints (ankle, knee, wrist and elbow)
- The tumor arises within the synovial space around tendons (flexor and extensor) the but arising from a tendon sheath composed of nodules with even, rounded contours
- The capsule usually does not encompass the entire tumor; small nests are usually found outside of it (Fig. 14.78D)
- Mitotic figures are common; 3–5 per 10 HPFs is average (1–2 per mm2), but some contain up to 20 per 10 HPFs (approximately 12 per mm2).
- Metastasis can occur but is extremely rare.
- Mitotic index may suggest a lesion that is more likely to recur, but neither mitotic index nor the rare finding of tumor cells within a vein has been established as a risk factor for metastasis.

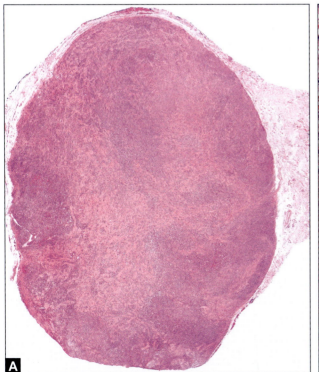

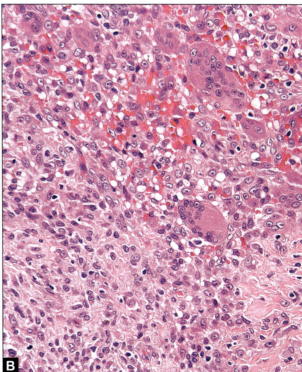

Figs 14.78A and B

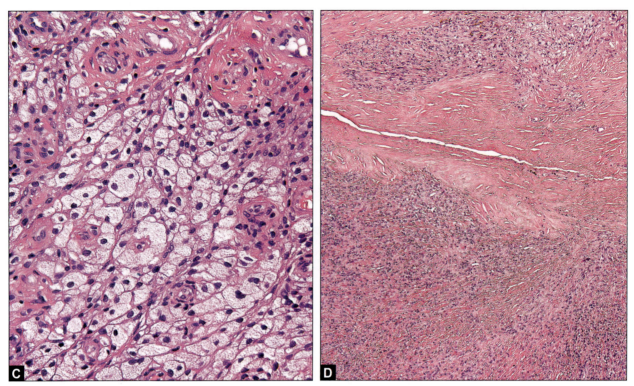

Figs 14.78A to D: Giant cell tumor of the tendon sheath. (A) The tumors are well demarcated and have rounded, smooth contours; (B) Although mononuclear cells usually predominate, multinucleated giant cells are almost always present (although occasionally they may be few in number); (C) Xanthoma cells are often found in clusters, especially at the periphery of the tumor; (D) Nests of tumor cells are often found "outside" of the fibrous capsule, a finding of no significance.

Granular Cell Tumor

▣ Criteria for diagnosis

- Painless nodules (or multiple nodules in 10% of cases)
- Round or polygonal cells with granular cytoplasm arranged in variably sized clusters and nests, or as solitary cells within the dermis and subcutis (Figs 14.79A and B).

▣ Differential diagnosis

- Histiocytic tumors, especially xanthomas and reticulohistiocytomas
- Rhabdomyomas
- Malignant granular cell tumor (see below)
- Granular cell variants of dermatofibroma and leiomyomas.

▣ Pitfalls

- Marked squamous hyperplasia is common, overlying granular cell tumors and may be misinterpreted as squamous cell carcinoma

- The cells of granular cell variant dermatofibroma and leiomyoma may be identical (except for different immunohistochemical properties; see below)
- The differences between malignant and benign granular cell tumors may be subtle (see below).

▣ Pearls

- Round or polygonal cells with granular cytoplasm arranged in variably sized clusters and nests, or as solitary cells within the dermis and subcutis.

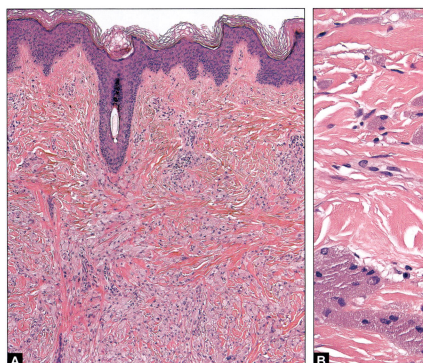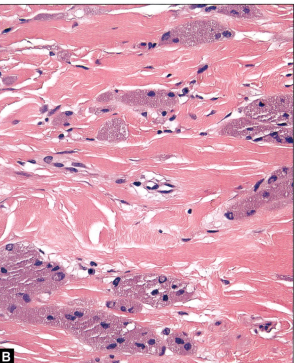

Figs 14.79A and B: Granular cell tumor. (A) Round to polygonal cells with abundant cytoplasm occupy the dermis; (B) The cytoplasm is pale pink or amphophilic and finely granular

Malignant Granular Cell Tumor

■ *Criteria for diagnosis*

- Cells similar to benign granular cell tumor, but the following features suggest malignancy (see Table 14.5):
  - Larger size (greater than 2 centimeters)
  - Infiltrative growth
  - Mitotic index of more than 2 per 10 HPF

- Spindled granular cells arranged in fascicles (Fig. 14.80A)
- Ulceration of epidermis
- Necrosis (usually focal)
- Lymphovascular invasion
- Marked cytologic atypia in some cases (Fig. 14.80B).

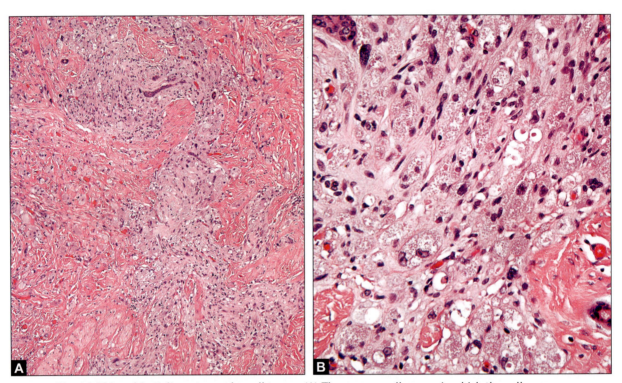

Figs 14.80A and B: Malignant granular cell tumor. (A) There are usually areas in which the cells assume a spindled shape; (B) Cytologic atypia is more severe than benign variants.

Merkel Cell Carcinoma
(Cutaneous Neuroendocrine Carcinoma)

■ *Criteria for diagnosis*

- Collections of cells with scant cytoplasm and large nuclei (high nuclear:cytoplasmic ratio) (Fig. 14.81A)
- Expression of keratins by immunohistochemistry, usually with a perinuclear "dot" in the majority of cells (Fig. 14.81B)
- Absence of features characteristic of neuroendocrine carcinomas from other sites metastatic to the skin (e.g. no expression of TTF-1, no evidence of other primary neuroen_ docrine carcinomas)

■ *Differential diagnosis*

- Lymphomas and other hematolymphoid tumors (especially diffuse large B-cell lymphoma, pre-B-cell and pre-T-cell lymphoblastic leukemia/lymphomas, and other 'blastic'-appearing tumors).
- Metastatic neuroendocrine carcinomas (e.g. small cell carcinoma of lung)
- Ewing's tumors (Fig. 14.81C)
- Other poorly differentiated tumors.

■ *Pitfalls*

- Lack of leukocyte common antigen expression (LCA) does not exclude lymphoma entirely since certain 'blastic' lymphomas do not express LCA (see below).

■ *Pearls*

- Metastatic neuroendocrine tumors are usually the primary differential diagnostic consideration
- When the differential diagnosis includes hematolymphoid tumors/lymphomas, immunohistochemistry for terminal deoxynucleotidyl transferase (TdT) should be performed (in addition to LCA) since "blastic" lymphomas will express TdT but not LCA.

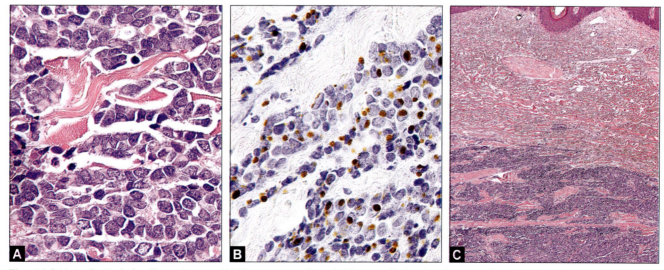

Figs 14.81A to C: Merkel cell carcinoma. (A) The tumor cell nuclei have a distinctive fine granular chromatin pattern; (B) Keratin positivity with a perinuclear "dot" distribution (seen here with cytokeratin 20) is characteristic; (C) Closely packed sheets of neoplastic cells fill the dermis. At low power, the features resemble lymphoma and various undifferentiated tumors (e.g. Ewing sarcoma).

BIBLIOGRAPHY

1. Billings SD, Folpe AL. Cutaneous and subcutaneous fibrohistiocytic tumors of intermediate malignancy: an update. Am J Dermatopathol. 2004;26(2):141-55

2. Billings SD, Folpe AL. Diagnostically challenging spindle cell lipomas: a report of 34 "low-fat" and "fat-free" variants. Am J Dermatopathol. 2007;29(5):437-42.

3. Cheah AL, Billings SD. The role of molecular testing in the diagnosis of cutaneous soft tissue tumors. Semin Cutan Med Surg. 2012;31(4):221-33.

4. Clarke LE, Frauenhoffer E, Fox E, Neves R, Bruggeman RD, Helm KF. CD10-positive myxofibrosarcomas: A pitfall in the differential diagnosis of atypical fibroxanthoma. J Cutan Pathol. 2010;37(7):737-43.

5. Clarke LE, Lee R, Militello G, Elenitsas R, Junkins-Hopkins J. Cutaneous epithelioid hemangioendothelioma. J Cutan Pathol. 2008;35(2):236-40.

6. Clarke LE, Zhang PJ, Crawford GH, Elenitsas R. Myxofibrosarcoma in the skin. J Cutan Pathol. 2008;35(10):935-40.

7. Clarke LE. Fibrous and fibrohistiocytic neoplasms: an update. Dermatol Clin. 2012;30(4):643-56.

8. Dahlén A, Debiec-Rychter M, Pedeutour F, Domanski HA, Höglund M, Bauer HC, Rydholm A, Sciot R, Mandahl N, Mertens F. Clustering of deletions on chromosome 13 in benign and low-malignant lipomatous tumors. Int J Cancer. 2003;103(5):616-23. Review. PubMed PMID: 12494468.

9. Fetsch JF, Laskin WB, Hallman JR, Lupton GP, Miettinen M. Neurothekeoma: an analysis of 178 tumors with detailed immunohistochemical data and long-term patient follow-up information. Am J Surg Pathol. 2007;31(7):1103-14.

10. Fletcher CD, Unni KK, Mertens F. Pathology and Genetics of Tumors of Soft Tissue and Bone. World Health Organization Classification of Tumors. Lyon. IARC Press; 2002.

11. Gardner JM, Dandekar M, Thomas D, Goldblum JR, Weiss SW, Billings SD, Lucas DR, McHugh JB, Patel RM. Cutaneous and subcutaneous pleomorphic liposarcoma: a clinicopathologic study of 29 cases with evaluation of MDM2 gene amplification in 26. Am J Surg Pathol. 2012;36(7):1047-51

12. Goh SG, Calonje E. Cutaneous vascular tumours: an update. Histopathology. 2008;52(6):661-73.

13. Goldblum JR, Weiss S. Enzinger and Weiss's Soft Tissue Tumors. 5th ed. St. Louis: Mosby; 2008.

14. Hunt SJ, Santa Cruz DJ Vascular tumors of the skin: a selective review. Semin Diagn Pathol. 2004;21(3):166-218.

15. Laskin WB, Fetsch JF, Miettinen M. The "neurothekeoma": immunohistochemical analysis distinguishes the true nerve sheath myxoma from its mimics. Hum Pathol. 2000;31(10):1230-41.

16. Lucas DR. Angiosarcoma, radiation-associated angiosarcoma, and atypical vascular lesion. Arch Pathol Lab Med. 2009;133(11):1804-9.

17. Mahajan D, Billings SD, Goldblum JR. Acral soft tissue tumors: a review. Adv Anat Pathol. 2011;18(2):103-19.

18. Mentzel T. Cutaneous lipomatous neoplasms. Semin Diagn Pathol. 2001;18(4):250-7.

19. Patel RM, Downs-Kelly E, Dandekar MN, Fanburg-Smith JC, Billings SD, Tubbs RR, Goldblum JR. FUS (16p11) gene rearrangement as detected by fluorescence in-situ hybridization in cutaneous low-grade fibromyxoid sarcoma: a potential diagnostic tool. Am J Dermatopathol. 2011;33(2):140-3.

20. Thomas C, Somani N, Owen LG, Malone JC, Billings SD. Cutaneous malignant peripheral nerve sheath tumors. J Cutan Pathol. 2009;36(8):896-900.

21. Troiani BM, Welsch MJ, Heilig SJ, Helm KF, Clarke LE. A firm nodule on the arm. Cutaneous myoepithelioma. Arch Dermatol. 2011;147(4):499-504.

22. Wood L, Fountaine TJ, Rosamilia L, Helm KF, Clarke LE. Am Cutaneous CD34+ spindle cell neoplasms: Histopathologic features distinguish spindle cell lipoma, solitary fibrous tumor, and dermatofibrosarcoma protuberans. J Dermatopathol. 2010;32(8):764-8.

CHAPTER 15

The Cutaneous Hematolymphoid Neoplasms

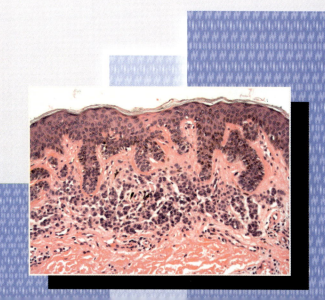

INTRODUCTION

The diagnosis of cutaneous hematolymphoid neoplasms can be hard. A seemingly endless array of lymphomas and leukemias can show up in skin. Complicated immunohistochemical panels and molecular tests may be necessary to differentiate them. Even then, a firm diagnosis usually requires clinical and laboratory data. Moreover, the understanding of hematolymphoid neoplasms is rapidly evolving, resulting in reclassification every few years. Unlike most of their counterparts within blood and lymph nodes, many skin hematolymphoid tumors are composed of just a few neoplastic cells that are easily obscured by the much denser "background" inflammatory cell infiltrate. As a result, simply telling benign from malignant may be difficult or even impossible in some situations. Nevertheless, a few basic principles which can simplify things dramatically are as follows:

- *Use pattern analysis*: Most texts and classification systems group hematolymphoid neoplasms by lineage (e.g. B-cell vs T-cell). Unfortunately, this assumes that you already know the lineage. Few of us can subtype lymphocytes on H&E, of course, and rather than enduring the time-consuming study of the H&E, many pathologists reflexively order a "standard" IHC panel at the mere sight of round blue cells. This is understandable, but often produces a differential diagnosis that is too limited and excludes entire categories of neoplasms. Instead, try assigning infiltrates to one of a few basic patterns as explained in the lecture. This prompts consideration of a broader differential diagnosis and usually a more prudent choice of immunohistochemical stains.
- *Remember the mimics*: The most common cutaneous lymphomas have more benign simulators than any other type of tumor. Early mycosis fungoides, CD30+ lymphomas and others share so many features with benign inflammatory dermatoses that distinction is simply not possible in some cases. Even dense collections of large, atypical-appearing cells can be caused by viral infections or drugs. Thus, never make a diagnosis of lymphoma without carefully excluding a benign simulator. If you cannot, simply state the differential in your report. There is nothing more embarrassing than hearing that the "lymphoma" you diagnosed was cured by permethrin cream—after the entire ICU staff developed scabies.
- *Insist on clinical information*: Mycosis fungoides (MF), for example, cannot be diagnosed without knowledge of the clinical course. In fact, MF is defined in part by its clinical course, and definitive diagnosis requires evidence that lesions are progressing or have progressed in the typical fashion (i.e. from patches to plaques to tumors).

- *Don't overreach*: Even with a thorough clinical history, not every case can be diagnosed on a single biopsy. When this happens, a diagnosis of "atypical lymphocytic infiltrate" or simply "lymphoma" accompanied by a comment that explains the differential is better than pretending to know something with certainty when you don't.

THE EPIDERMOTROPIC/ADNEXOTROPIC PATTERN (TABLE 15.1)

T-Cell Pseudolymphomas (Figs 15.1A to D)

■ *Criteria for diagnosis*

- A cutaneous infiltrate composed predominantly of T-lymphocytes that simulates lymphoma clinically and histopathologically but proves to be reactive rather than neoplastic.

■ *Differential diagnosis*

- T-cell lymphomas
- T-cell dermatoses (e.g. actinic reticuloid, lichen planus, lichen sclerosus, etc.)
- Drug eruptions, insect bite reactions, viral infections.

■ *Pitfalls*

- Some T-cell pseudolymphomas contain clonal T-cell populations
- Cause is not always identifiable; many are due to viruses, drugs or insect bites.

■ *Pearls*

- Features favoring pseudolymphoma over genuine lymphoma are
  - Mixed infiltrate (T-cells, B-cells, eosinophils, neutrophils, macrophages, etc.)
  - B-cell aggregates surrounded by T-cells (recapitulating lymphoid follicles)
  - Onset within days to months of new medication(s)
- Look carefully for viral cytopathic effect as a clue to a viral induced pseudolymphoma
- No clear-cut diagnostic criteria exist for T-cell pseudolymphomas; diagnosis requires clinical correlation
- Occasionally definitive diagnosis is only possible by excluding other entities, which may require months or occasionally even years.

Table 15.1: Common benign mimics of hematolymphoid neoplasms

Pattern	Neoplasm	Benign Mimics
Epidermotropic / adnexotropic	Mycosis fungoides	Lymphomatoid drug eruption
		Lymphomatoid contact dermatitis
		Actinic reticuloid
		Lichen sclerosus
		Pigmented purpuric dermatoses
		Pityriasis lichenoides
		Secondary syphilis
		Lichenoid keratosis
	CD8+ aggressive epidermotropic lymphoma	Actinic reticuloid
		Pityriasis lichenoides
	ATLL	Actinic reticuloid
	LyP Type B	Pityriasis lichenoides/PLEVA
Dermal +/− subcutis	Mycosis fungoides, Plaque/tumor stage	Lymphomatoid drug eruption
		Insect bite reaction
		Secondary syphilis
		Borreliosis/Lyme disease
		Tumid lupus
		Lupus panniculitis
	CD30+ LPDs	Lymphomatoid drug eruption
		Insect bite reaction
		Scabies infestation
		Viral infections
		Orf
		Milker's nodule
		Herpes viruses
		Molluscum contagiosum
	Langerhans cell histiocytosis	Scabies infestation
		Insect bite reaction
		Xanthogranulomas
	B-cell lymphomas	Lymphomatoid tattoo reaction
		Lupus panniculitis
		Lymphomatoid drug eruption, B-Cell Predominant
		Secondary syphilis
		Acral pseudolymphomatous Angiokeratoma
		Other B-Cell pseudolymphomas
	Gamma-delta T-cell lymphoma	Lupus panniculitis
	NK/T-cell lymphoma	Wegener's granulomatosis
		Other 'granulomatous vasculitides'
	Leukemia cutis and blastic plasmacytoid dendritic cell Neoplasm	Extramedullary hematopoiesis
		Leukemia-like drug eruption
		Leukemia-like reaction to topical irritants
	Small-medium T-cell lymphoma	Angiolymphoid hyperplasia with eosinophilia
	Mastocytosis	Urticaria
		Urticaria-like inflammatory processes
Subcutis	Subcutaneous panniculitis-like T-cell lymphoma	Lupus panniculitis

(ATLL: Adult T-cell leukemia/lymphoma; LyP: Lymphomatoid papulosis; PLEVA: Pityriasis lichenoides et varioliformis acuta; LPD: Lymphoproliferative disorder).

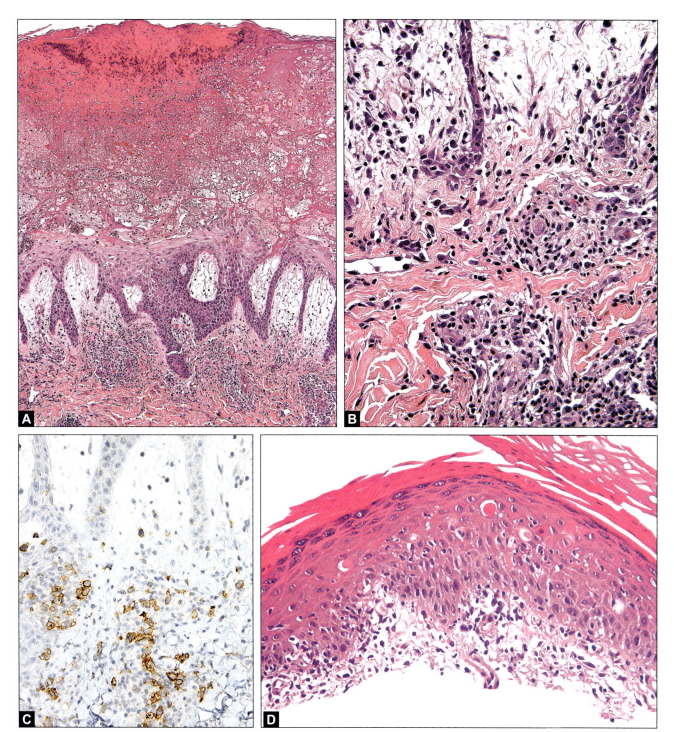

Figs 15.1A to D: T-cell pseudolymphoma. (A) This is but one example of a pseudolymphoma. This patient was originally thought to have lymphomatoid papulosis on clinical examination since there were crops of centrally necrotic papules; (B) Histopathologically there is an infiltrate that contains large lymphocytes within the dermis. However, the degree of spongiosis would be unusual for most lymphomas, including lymphomatoid papulosis; (C) The large cells expres CD30. Large CD30-positive cells are the major constituent of lymphomatoid papulosis, but they are also very common in many other inflammatory processes, particularly insect bite reactions, scabies infestations and viral infections; (D) A well-known simulator of mycosis fungoides is actinic reticuloid, a severe form of chronic photodermatitis. Both may develop erythroderma and exhibit dense lymphocytic infiltrates along the dermoepidermal junction with extension of lymphocytes into the epidermis. Clinical history and correlation with other laboratory data may be necessary to differentiate the two in some instances.

Mycosis Fungoides (Figs 15.2A to G)

■ *Criteria for diagnosis*

- Indolent course; slow progression from patches to plaques to tumors
- Lichenoid infiltrate of benign lymphocytes with scattered neoplastic T-lymphocytes in epidermis, particularly in basal layer
- Skin limited for a protracted period
- Lymph nodes and viscera involved later in course; bone marrow involvement rare
- CD2/CD3/CD4/cutaneous lymphocyte antigen (CLA)   +
- CD7   – often
- CD8   –
- CD30   + (usually large cell transformation)

■ *Differential diagnosis*

- Inflammatory interface dermatoses, such as lichen planus, lichen sclerosus, contact dermatitis, lichenoid drug eruptions and actinic reticuloid
- Sézary syndrome (SS)
- Parapsoriasis
- Lymphomatoid papulosis [LyP (Type B)]
- CD8+ epidermotropic lymphomas (especially CD8+ variant of MF)
- Adult T-cell leukemia/lymphoma (ATLL).

■ *Pitfalls*

- Rare CD8+/CD4– cases of MF exist; they are otherwise typical of conventional MF
- Differentiation of CD8+ MF from CD8+. Aggressive epidermotropic lymphoma is based on clinical course; histopathologic differences cannot reliably differentiate them
- Mycosis fungoides may affect children and adolescents (one of very few primary cutaneous T-cell lymphomas that do so); CD8 positivity is more frequent in these cases
- Rarely, erythroderma develops early in MF and may mimic SS; such cases must be shown to lack the other diagnostic criteria of SS (see below).
- "Loss of CD7" often touted as a clue to MF, but is unreliable by IHC in patch stage MF

- Clonal T-cell receptor (TCR) rearrangement may not be detectable in early lesions
- Benign dermatoses that simulate MF clonal TCR
- Large cell transformation of MF may be CD30+, requiring differentiation from other CD30+ lymphomas.

■ *Pearls*

- By definition, diagnosis requires clinical correlation
- Extent of disease is the most important prognostic factor
- Limited disease has an excellent prognosis (survival similar to that of age-matched persons without MF)
- Extracutaneous dissemination indicates poor prognosis
- Other adverse prognostic factors: Age more than 60 years, elevated lactate dehydrogenase (LDH), large cell transformation
- Large cell transformation is defined as more than 25% large cells
- Evidence-based criteria for diagnosis of early/patch stage MF exist (Table 15.2).

Variants of Mycosis Fungoides

Folliculotropic/adnexotropic variant
- Neoplastic infiltrate centered on follicular epithelium or (less commonly) other adnexal epithelium with relative sparing of epidermis
- Follicular mucinosis common but not invariably present
- Other features similar to conventional MF
- Less responsive to most therapies than conventional MF
- Benign forms of follicular mucinosis occur, and must be excluded.

Pagetoid reticulosis variant
- Histopathologic features similar to conventional MF but only one or several lesions are present and there is no progression.
- Predilection for breast skin.

Granulomatous slack skin variant
- Patients develop folds of lax skin in axilla or groin that contain numerous macrophages and multinucleated giant cells in addition to neoplastic T-cells with the immunophenotype of conventional MF.

Table 15.2: Criteria useful for the distinction of early patch stage mycosis fungoides from inflammatory dermatoses	
More Specific	*Less Specific*
Microabscess formation (Pautrier/Darier)	Pagetoid distribution of intraepidermal lymphs
Lymphocytes in epidermis larger than those in dermis	Exocytosis of lymphocytes with paucity of spongiosis
Halo lymphocytes	Basilar lymphocytes
Four or more contiguous lymphocytes in basal layer	Small or "normal sized" convoluted lymphocytes
Convoluted lymphocytes equal in size to basilar keratinocytes	Papillary dermal fibrosis (wiry collagen)

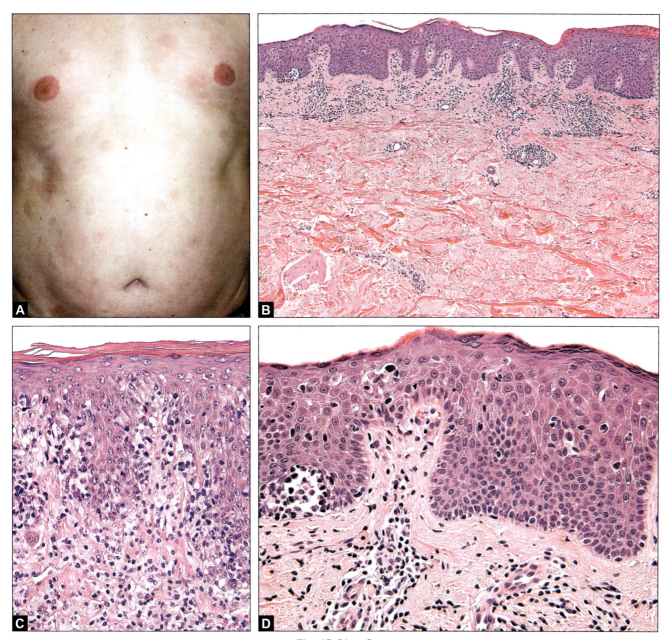

Figs 15.2A to D

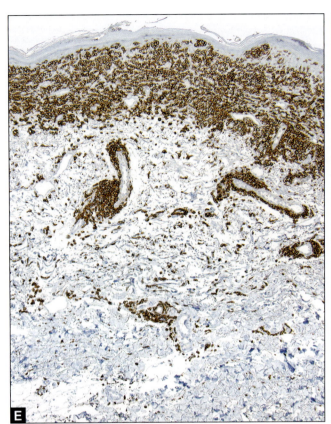

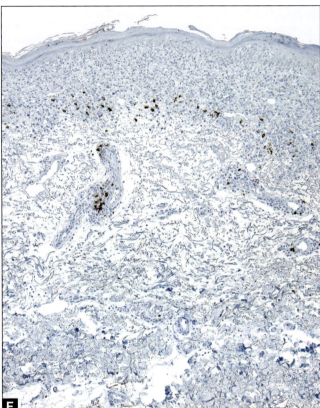

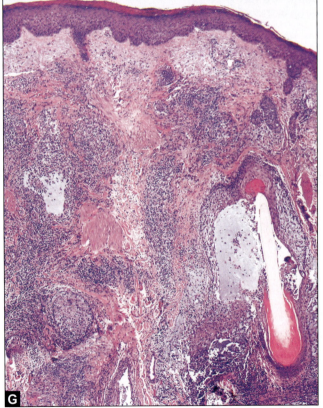

Figs 15.2A to G: Mycosis fungoides. This patient with early stage disease has scattered erythematous patches; (B) At low power, patch stage mycosis fungoides shows a superficial lymphocytic infiltrate with extension of lymphocytes into the epidermis; (C) In classic examples, close inspection will reveal lymphocytes within the epidermis that are larger and more atypical than those within the underlying dermis; (D) When present, sharply marginated clusters of lymphocytes within the epidermis (Pautrier microabscesses) are a very specific feature of early mycosis fungoides. Also note the large lymphocyte in the upper stratum spinosum that is surrounded by a clear 'halo'; (E) In most cases, the neoplastic cells are CD4+; (F) When advanced, as in this case, CD8+ cells make up less than 5% of the infiltrate; (G) Folliculotropic variant. Folliculotropic mycosis fungoided is a variant in which the neoplastic infiltrate preferentially involves the follicular or adnexal epithelium. The infiltrate is often accompanied by "follicular mucinosis"—collections of mucinous material around the follicles as is shown here.

Sézary Syndrome

■ *Criteria for diagnosis*

- Classic triad
  - Erythroderma (Fig. 15.3A)
  - Generalized lymphadenopathy
  - Clonal T-cell population with cerebriform nuclei

One or more of the following secondary criteria

- 1000/mm³ absolute Sézary cell count
- CD4:CD8 ratio more than 10 (by Flow cytometry)
- Abnormal phenotype (loss of one or more T-cell antigens CD2, CD3, CD4, CD5, CD7 and CD26)

■ *Differential diagnosis*

- Mycosis fungoides (although SS tends to be less epidermotropic)
- Other causes of erythroderma (correlation with clinical data, peripheral blood findings and other criteria necessary)

■ *Pitfalls*

- Histopathologic features are nonspecific in more than 30% of skin biopsies (Fig. 15.3B)
- Cannot be differentiated from MF without clinical data and peripheral blood criteria.

■ *Pearls*

- Adults exclusively, usually age 60+
- Onychodystrophy, pruritus, ectropion, alopecia, palmoplantar hyperkeratosis common
- Loss of CD7 and CD26 characteristic of SS
- Aggressive; 5 year survival = 10–20%
- Opportunistic infections are the most common cause of death.

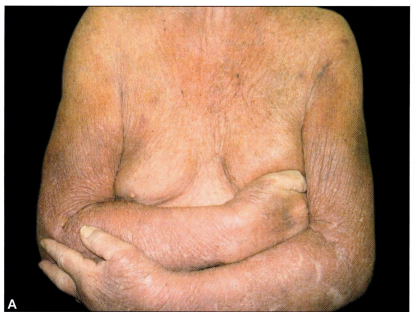
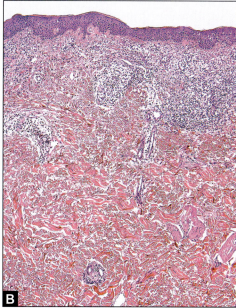

Figs 15.3A and B: Sézary syndrome. (A) Erythroderma is a classic presentation; (B) The histopathologic features may be similar to mycosis fungoides, but often, as in this case, they are nonspecific in skin biopsies without epidermotropism or microabscess formation. Therefore, definitive diagnosis must be based on correlation with laboratory data and clinical features.

Adult T-Cell Leukemia/Lymphoma

■ Criteria for diagnosis

- A clonal T-cell population with monoclonal integration of human T-cell lymphotropic virus-1
- CD25/CD2/CD3/CD5   +
- CD7   –
- CD30   –/+
- Commonly CD4+/CD8–
- Rarely CD4–/CD8+
- Rarely CD4+/CD8+

■ Variants

- *Acute*: Leukemia with markedly elevated WBC count, generalized lymphadenopathy, generalized erythema, papules or nodules, hypercalcemia, constitutional symptoms, elevated LDH, eosinophilia; opportunistic infections common (Fig. 15.4A)
- *Chronic*: Exfoliative rash; mildly elevated WBC count; no hypercalcemia
- *Smoldering*: Rash or papules, lung involvement, normal WBC count, no hypercalcemia.

■ Differential diagnosis

- Broad differential diagnosis since three variants exist, each with different clinical and histopathologic features
- Various other types of T-cell lymphoma and inflammatory processes should be considered in the differential.

■ Pitfalls

- Skin lesions can vary so much in clinical appearance that lymphoma may not be in the clinical differential
- Histopathologic variability among variants; for example, the cells are usually medium to large (Fig. 15.4B) and pleomorphic in the acute type, but small cells predominate occasionally, even in acute type
- Epidermotropism with microabscess formation can be identical to MF (Fig. 15.4B)
- Atypical Epstein-Barr virus (EBV) positive B-cell proliferations (some mimicking Hodgkin lymphoma) may occur (secondary to immunodeficiency resulting from T-cell dysfunction)
- Histopathologic features often nonspecific in "smoldering" type.

■ Pearls

- Most patients from endemic regions: Southwest Japan, Caribbean Islands, South America, Central Africa
- CD25 positivity is a key feature (Fig. 15.4C)
- Skin lesions are the most common site of extranodal involvement and are present in more than 50% of cases
- Widely disseminated nature of disease allows differentiation from indolent primary cutaneous lymphomas
- But a smoldering variant limited to skin may exist.

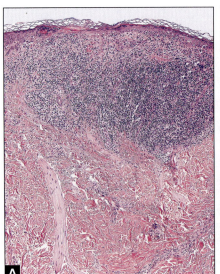 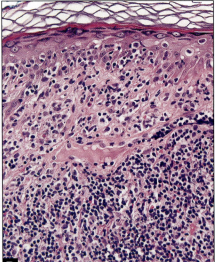 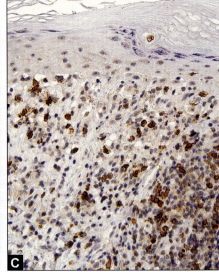

Figs 15.4A to C: Adult T-cell leukemia/lymphoma. (A) This patient presented with erythematous papules and plaques. The infiltrate involves both the dermis and the epidermis; (B) The cells are usually medium to large in size, and the overall appearance may simulate mycosis fungoides, with epidermotropism and microabscess formation; (C) The neoplastic cells are usually CD25 positive. While not specific, CD25 expression certainly supports the diagnosis.

Aggressive CD8+ Epidermotropic Lymphoma

■ *Criteria for diagnosis*

- Aggressive course
- Ulcerated plaques and tumors at onset
- No history of MF or CD8+ LyP
- CD8+ cytotoxic T-cells, usually epidermotropic but also nodular and diffuse dermal aggregates (Fig. 15.5)
- βF1/CD3/CD7/CD8/TIA1   +
- CD4   −

■ *Differential diagnosis*

- γ/δ T-cell lymphoma (see below)
- CD8+ variant of MF
- CD8+ variant of LyP
- Actinic reticuloid
- Subcutaneous panniculitis like T-cell lymphoma (SPTL).

■ *Pitfalls*

- May be difficult or impossible to differentiate from T-cell lymphoma, and the two may represent variants of the same disease
- βF1 is occasionally negative (neoplastic cells may lose expression).

■ *Pearls*

- Diagnosis requires clinical correlation (to exclude MF and LyP).
- Mucosal involvement is common.

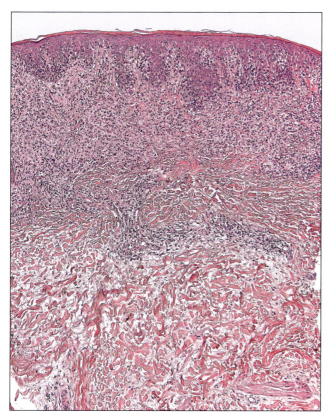

Fig. 15.5: Aggressive CD8+ epidermotropic lymphoma. Many of the features resemble mycosis fungoides, including epidermotropism. The tumor cells are CD8+, but since there is a CD8+ variant of mycosis fungoides, confusion is still possible. The course of this disease, however, is extremely aggressive compared to mycosis fungoides.

Color Atlas of Differential Diagnosis of Dermatopathology

CD30+ Lymphomas/Lymphoproliferative Disorders

■ *Criteria for diagnosis*

- Infiltrate of CD30+ lymphocytes that are large and pleomorphic or immunoblastic-like (Figs 15.6A and B)
- Indolent course
- CD4   +
- CD3, CD5   –/+
- CLA   + [unlike systemic anaplastic large cell lymphoma (ALCL)]
- Anaplastic lymphoma kinase (ALK)   – (unlike many systemic ALCL)
- CD15   – (unlike Hodgkin's lymphoma)
- CD56   –/+
- Interferon regulatory factor 4 translocation   –/+
- Clinical features that differentiate lymphomatoid papulosis from ALCL:

LyP
- Crops of numerous centrally necrotic, crusted papules that regress spontaneous and then recur at another site

ALCL
- One or several grouped plaques or tumors that persist (occasionally regress).

■ *Differential diagnosis*

LyP
- Pityriasis lichenoides

- Insect bite reactions/scabies
- Viral infections

ALCL
- CD30+ pseudolymphomas (same as LyP)
- Melanoma, sarcoma, carcinoma, metastatic tumors
- Secondary skin involvement by systemic variant of ALCL
- Post-transplant lymphoproliferative disorders.

■ *Pitfalls*

- CD30+ lymphocytes common in many non-neoplastic conditions
- Large cell transformation of MF often CD30+; MF must be excluded
- Large atypical cells may simulate sarcoma, melanoma and carcinoma if CD30 not performed (Fig. 15.6C).

■ *Pearls*

- By definition, clinical features (i.e. number and behavior of lesions) determine type
- Extracutaneous dissemination of primary cutaneous ALCL is rare (10%), usually limited to regional nodes, and prognosis remains similar to those with skin-limited disease
- Primary cutaneous ALCL is almost always ALK- [i.e. it lacks the t(2;5) translocation]
- Post-transplant lymphoproliferative disorders are often EBV+.

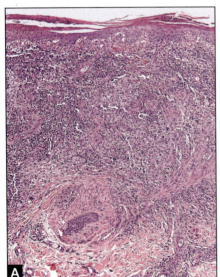
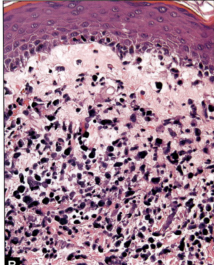
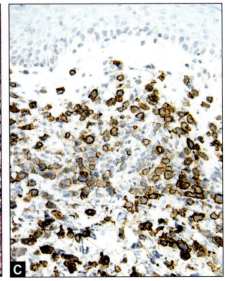

Figs 15.6A to C: Lymphomatoid papulosis. The infiltrates are usually mostly dermal but often result in necrosis of the overlying epidermis; (B) Classic cases are composed of large, markedly pleomorphic lymphocytes; (C) The atypical neoplastic cells exhibit strong diffuse CD30 expression.

B-Cell Pseudolymphomas (Figs 15.7A to C)

■ *Criteria for diagnosis*

- A cutaneous infiltrate that contains numerous B-lymphocytes that simulates lymphoma clinically and histopathologically but proves to be reactive rather than neoplastic.

■ *Differential diagnosis*

- Genuine B-cell lymphomas
- Tumid lupus
- Borrelioisis/Lyme disease
- Post-transplant lymphoproliferative disorders and other immunocompromise related lymphoproliferative disorders
- Nodular scabies
- Drug eruptions (B-cell type), vaccine injection site reactions, secondary syphilis, persistent insect bite reactions, viral infections, tattoo reactions, angiolymphoid hyperplasia with eosinophilia (ALHE).

■ *Pitfalls*

- Some B-cell pseudolymphomas may contain B-cell and T-cell clones or "pseudoclones"
- Some B-cell pseudolymphomas probably do evolve into genuine low-grade B-cell lymphomas (particularly marginal zone and follicle center cell type) due to persistent antigenic stimulation
- Cause is not always identifiable.

■ *Pearls*

- Features favoring pseudolymphoma over genuine lymphoma include a mixed infiltrate and recapitulation of "normal" lymph node architecture.
- Dense B-cell infiltrates on the ear, around the nipple and on the scrotum are far more likely to be Borrelia burgdorferi reactions than genuine lymphomas.

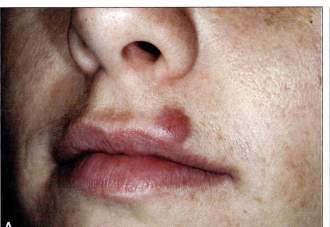
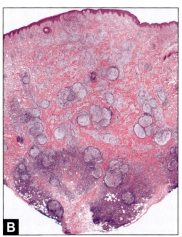
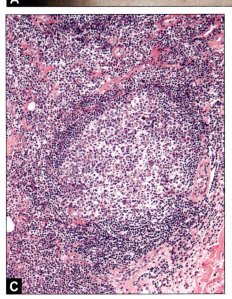

Figs 15.7A to C: B-cell Pseudolymphoma. (A) This solitary lesion on the lip was simply a herpes virus lesion accompanied by an exuberant lymphocytic infiltrate; (B) This is but one example of a reactive B-cell proliferation in the skin that can be confused with a lymphoma. In this case, the numerous lymphoid follicles could potentially be mistaken for a follicular lymphoma (especially since lymphoma was the clinical impression); (C) Close inspection of the lymphocyte aggregates themselves, however, will demonstrate the features of a normal germinal center, including polarization (light and dark areas), as well as numerous tingible body macrophages.

Primary Cutaneous Marginal Zone Lymphoma

▌ *Criteria for diagnosis*

- Indolent behavior
- Solitary or grouped red or violet papules or plaques on trunk or extremities (especially back and upper arms)
- Dermis and upper subcutis containing:
  - B-cells including lymphoplasmatoid cells, plasma cells and marginal zone cells (cells with abundant pale cytoplasm and small indented nuclei, sometimes referred to as centrocyte-like or monocytoid-like B-cells) (Figs 15.8A and B)
  - Evidence of clonality (see below)
  - Scattered centroblast and immunoblast like B-cells but no confluent growth of large cells
  - Reactive T-cells +/– other inflammatory cell types
- Evidence of clonality:
  - Monotypic expression of light chains detected by IHC or ISH
  - Clonal rearrangement of immunoglobulin heavy-chain gene detected by molecular methods
- CD20/CD79a/ B-cell lymphoma 2 (BCL2)   +
- CD5/CD10/BCL6   –

▌ *Differential diagnosis*

- B-cell pseudolymphoma
- Primary cutaneous follicle center cell lymphoma (PCFCCL)
- Plasmacytoma

▌ *Pitfalls*

- Cases with nodules/follicles may simulate PCFCCL
- Myeloma and other plasma cell neoplasms may simulate primary cutaneous marginal zone lymphoma (PCMZL) with extensive plasmacytoid differentiation
- "Blastic transformation" may occur with multiple recurrences and suggests more aggressive behavior (but is very rare)
- Other types of B-cell lymphoma may exhibit extensive plasmacytoid differentiation and light chain restriction
- Light chain restriction is not evident in all biopsies.

▌ *Pearls*

- Monotypic light chain expression by plasma cells at periphery of nodules is particularly helpful
- In situ hybridization is usually more sensitive than IHC for demonstrating light chain restriction
- Increased number of Ki-67 (MIB-1) + cells at periphery of nodules is characteristic
- Immunocytoma and plasmacytoma likely represent variants of PCMZL
- Rare association with Borrelia infection in Europe but not in United States
- Association with autoimmune diseases is uncommon (coexisting autoimmune disorder suggests secondary cutaneous involvement by underlying systemic marginal zone lymphoma rather than primary cutaneous variant)
- Five year survival, approximately 100%.

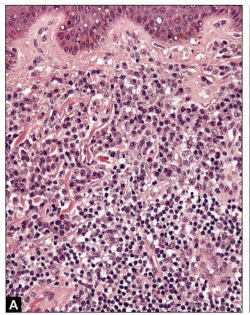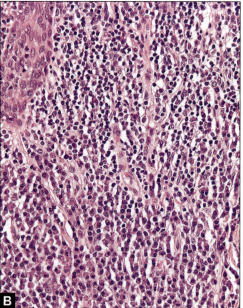

Figs 15.8A and B: Primary cutaneous marginal zone lymphoma. (A) The dermis contains an infiltrate of B-cells that spares the epidermis. The top of the field contains numerous plasma cells, which are commonly numerous at the periphery. The marginal zone cells predominate within the lower half of the field; (B) The marginal zone cells occupy the upper half of the field within this image. They are characterized by with abundant pale cytoplasm and small indented nuclei (sometimes referred to as centrocyte-like or monocytoid-like B-cells). Plasma cells fill the bottom of the field.

Primary Cutaneous Follicle Center Cell Lymphoma (Figs 15.9A to D)

■ *Criteria for diagnosis*

- Relatively indolent
- Solitary or grouped papules, plaques, tumors
- Centrocytes admixed with variable number of centroblasts
- No confluent sheets of centroblasts
- Nodular, diffuse or mixed growth patterns
- CD79a/CD20/PAX5   +
- BCL6   +
- CD10   –/+
- MUM-1   –
- BCL2   – (in neoplastic B-cells)

■ *Differential diagnosis*

- Reactive B-cell pseudolymphomas
- Primary cutaneous marginal zone lymphoma
- Diffuse large B-cell lymphoma
- Secondary involvement of skin by systemic B-cell lymphoma.

■ *Pitfalls*

- Reactive germinal centers may be present, simulating a benign pseudolymphoma
- T-cell rich and macrophage-rich variants exist and these cells may outnumber and obscure the large neoplastic B-cells.

■ *Pearls*

- Lesions often have erythematous border.
- Predilection for head and trunk, especially scalp and back
- Middle aged adults (rather than elderly adults, as in leg-type diffuse large B-cell lymphoma)
- Clues to differentiate PCFCCL from reactive cutaneous lymphoid hyperplasia (B-cell pseudolymphomas with germinal center formation) include:
    - Ill-defined follicles without "polarization" ("light and dark" zones)
    - A monomorphic proliferation of BCL6+ follicle center cells
    - Absence of tingible body macrophages
    - Decreased Ki-67 (MIB-1) index in comparison to reactive germinal centers
    - Absent or attenuated mantle zones
- Secondary involvement of skin by systemic follicular lymphoma must be excluded by staging work-up
- CD10 may be expressed in nodular pattern but is rare in diffuse pattern
- Neither grading nor growth pattern has clinical significance (as it does in systemic follicular lymphoma)
- "Reticulohistiocytoma of the dorsum" and "Crosti's lymphoma" are older terms used for what is now called PCFCCL.

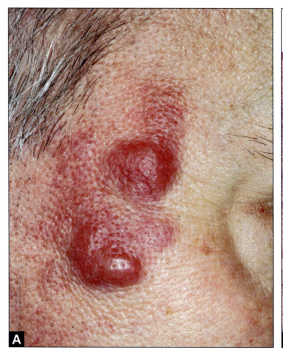

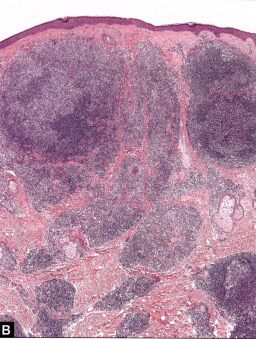

Figs 15.9A and B

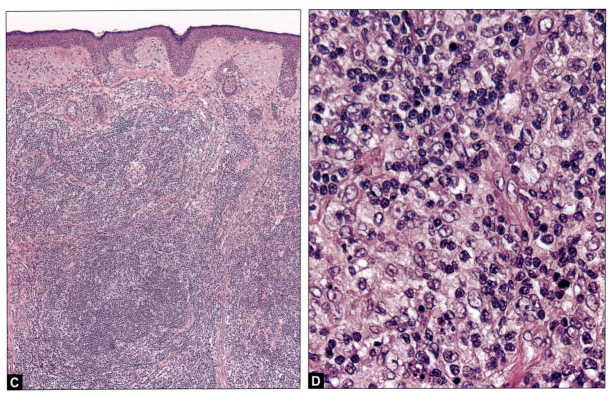

Figs 15.9A to D: Primary cutaneous follicle center cell lymphoma. (A) Erythematous papules and nodules on the head and scalp are a common presentation; (B) Primary cutaneous follicle center cell lymphoma has a follicular or nodular architecture in some instances; (C) In other cases, the infiltrate may be diffuse, with no discernible follicle-like structures; (D) The infiltrate consists of variable proportions of lymphocytes that are small (centrocyte-like) and large (centroblast or immunoblast-like). In this image, the smaller centrocyte-like cells occupy the upper left portion of the field, while larger cells are more numerous near the bottom of the image.

Primary Cutaneous Diffuse Large B-Cell Lymphoma, Leg Type (Figs 5.10A to E)

■ *Criteria for diagnosis*

- Rapidly growing red or violaceous tumors
- Confluent sheets of medium to large B-cell with round nuclei, prominent nucleoli and coarse chromatin (resembling centroblasts and immunoblasts) (Fig. 15.10B)
- Diffuse growth pattern
- BCL2   +++
- BCL6   ±
- CD10   –
- MUM-1   +

■ *Differential diagnosis*

- Primary cutaneous follicle center cell lymphoma with large cells

■ *Pitfalls*

- T-cell rich and macrophage-rich variants exist and these cells may outnumber and obscure the large neoplastic B-cells

- As in other B-cell lymphomas, reactive germinal centers may be present, simulating a benign pseudolymphoma/reactive follicular lymphoid hyperplasia.

■ *Pearls*

- Predilection for legs (less than 10% occur at other sites) of elderly females
- Tend to extend into subcutis (Fig. 15.10C)
- Fewer small reactive lymphocytes than other cutaneous B-cell lymphomas
- Relatively aggressive, with approximately 40% developing extracutaneous disease
- Five year survival 55%
- Multiple lesions at presentation confers worse prognosis.

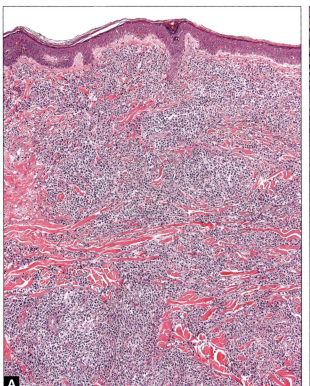 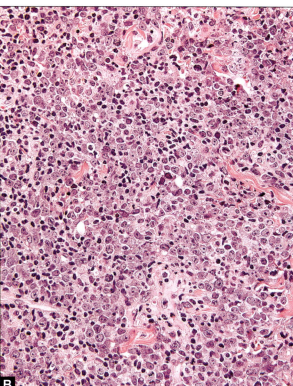

Figs 15.10A and B

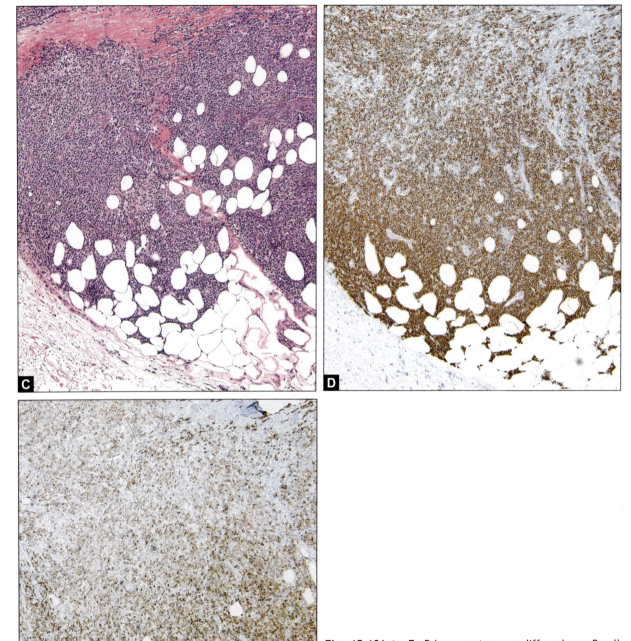

Figs 15.10A to E: Primary cutaneous diffuse large B-cell lymphoma, leg type. (A) The dermis is occupied by a nodular and diffuse infiltrate of large lymphocytes. The epidermis is spared by a thin grenz zone; (B) The tumor cells are arranged in diffuse sheets and have vesicular nuclei, coarse chromatin and prominent nucleoli; (C) Extension into the subcutis is common; (D) The neoplastic cells express CD20; (E) The cells also strongly express B-cell lymphoma-2, providing strong support for the diagnosis when the typical morphologic features are present.

Lymphomatoid Granulomatosis

■ *Criteria for diagnosis*

- An angiocentric and angiodestructive infiltrate of EBV+ B-cells admixed with reactive T-cells (Fig. 15.11A).

■ *Differential diagnosis*

- "Granulomatous vasculitis" (e.g. Wegener's granulomatosis)
- T-cell lymphomas (since T-cells may predominate numerically)
- Epstein-Barr virus + lymphomas and lymphoproliferative disorders (Fig. 15.11B).

■ *Pitfalls*

- Early lesions may contain only a few of the neoplastic B-cells.
- Wegener's and other granulomatous.

■ *Pearls*

- Most cases exhibit at least a few histopathologic findings that the process is reactive rather than neoplastic (infiltrate is mixed, viral cytopathic effect is evident, etc.)
- Progresses to higher grade with time and ultimately may be indistinguishable from diffuse large B-cell lymphoma.

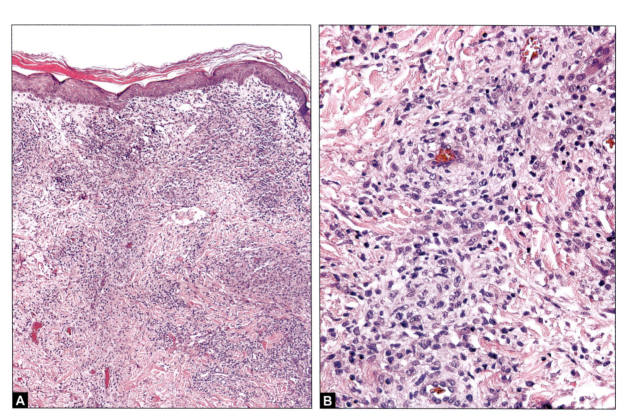

Figs 15.11A and B: Lymphomatoid granulomatosis. (A) The dermis contains a nodular and diffuse infiltrate of inflammatory cells, including small, medium and large lymphocytes; (B) Large cells, many of which resemble macrophages, are centered on blood vessels. The neoplastic large cells are actually B-lymphocytes, and their proliferation seems to be driven by Epstein-Barr virus.

Extranodal Natural Killer (NK) /T-Cell Lymphoma, Nasal Type (Figs 15.12A to C)

■ *Criteria for diagnosis*

- Aggressive course
- Natural killer immunophenotype is most common; a few cases have a cytotoxic T-cell phenotype
- CD3-/CD3 epsilon+/CD2+/CD56+/TIA1+/Granzyme+/EBV+
- Rare CD56- cases must be EBV+ and express cytotoxic markers
- Plaques and tumors on mid-face, trunk and extremities
- Dermis, subcutaneous, occasionally epidermotropic.

■ *Differential diagnosis*

- Lymphomatoid granulomatosis
- Angioimmunoblastic T-cell Lymphoma
- Wegener's granulomatosis (and other granulomatous vasculitides)
- Natural killer cell leukemia involving skin
- Rarely ALCL may express CD56.

■ *Pitfalls*

- Angiocentricity and mixed inflammatory infiltrate common, causing confusion with lymphomatoid granulomatosis, Wegener's, Angioimmunoblastic T-cell lymphoma, etc.
- May be confused with NK-cell leukemia (which involves skins and is also EBV-associated)

- LMP-1 inconsistently expressed; use EBV-encoded RNA for EBV
- T-cell receptor gene usually in germ-line configuration (no T-cell clonality)
- CD56 occasionally expressed in ALCL, so always do CD30 and ALCL
- Hydrovacciniforme-like cutaneous T-cell lymphoma is a rare EBV-associated cytotoxic T-cell lymphoma that affects children in Latin America and Asia and must not be confused with NK/T-Cell lymphoma, nasal type.

■ *Pearls*

- Skin is the second most common site of involvement after nasal cavity/nasopharynx, and treatment is same, so differentiating a "primary cutaneous" form is not necessary
- Median survival 5 months if not limited to skin; 27 months if skin only
- Usually adult men
- Asia, Central American, South America have the highest incidence.

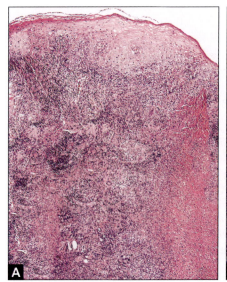 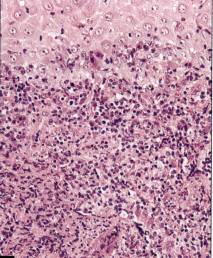 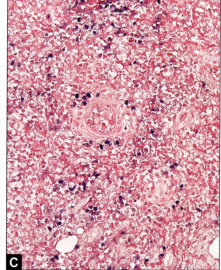

Figs 15.12A to C: Extranodal natural killer/T-cell lymphoma, nasal type. (A) The dermis contains areas of necrosis and a mixed infiltrate that is sometimes not immediately recognizable as lymphoma; (B) Even at high magnification, the infiltrate is polymorphous and includes neutrophils and other reactive cells. Close inspection will reveal large, atypical lymphocytes, however; (C) In situ hybridization for Epstein-Barr virus (EBER-ISH) highlights the neoplastic EBV+ cells arranged around blood vessels.

Blastic Plasmacytoid Dendritic Cell Neoplasm (Figs 15.13A to D)

■ *Criteria for diagnosis*

- Aggressive course
- Dermal and subcutaneous infiltrate of monomorphic but blastic cells (large and undifferentiated cells)
- CD4+/CD56+/CD123+/CD8–/CD7+/CD45RA+/sCD3–/cCD3 epsilon+ (IHC)/TIA–1–/Granzyme B–/Perforin-/TCL1+/EBV–
- T-cell receptor genes in germ line configuration.

■ *Differential diagnosis*

- Leukemia cutis (especially myelomonocytic, lymphoblastic and myeloblastic)
- Natural killer/T-cell lymphoma, nasal type
- γ/δ T-cell lymphoma.

■ *Pitfalls*

- Difficult/impossible to distinguish from acute myeloid leukemia (AML) in some cases
- CD68 may be positive (as in myelomonocytic leukemia)
- Terminal deoxynucleotidyl transferase may be positive (as in lymphoblastic lymphomas).

■ *Pearls*

- Blastic plasmacytoid dendritic cell neoplasm considered a variant of acute myeloid leukemia by most
- Myeloperoxidase and lysozyme negative (differentiates from other types of AML)
- Skin is frequently the site of initial presentation
- Fifty percent have involvement of marrow, nodes, peripheral blood at time of presentation
- Frequent mitoses
- Inflammatory cells, necrosis and aniocentricity/angioinvasion usually absent (differentiates it from NK/T-cell lymphoma)
- CD3 epsilon (detected by IHC) often positive, but surface CD3 (detected by flow cytometry) is absent, differentiating it from T lymphoblastic lymphoma
- Median survival 14 months.

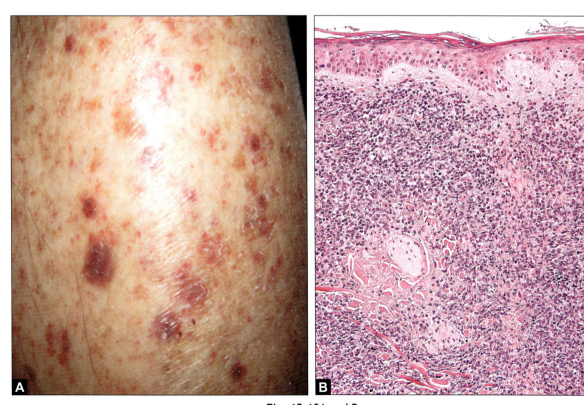

Figs 15.13A and B

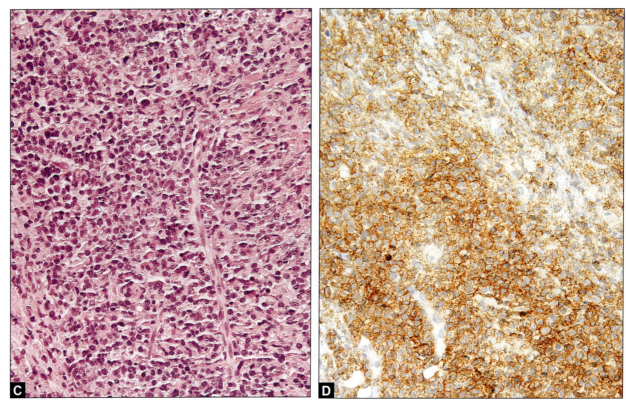

Figs 15.13A to D: Blastic plasmacytoid dendritic cell neoplasm. (A) The clinical presentation is variable, but presentation with skin lesions, as was the case in this patient, is common. Initially, this patient had one red patch on the scalp that was clinically thought to be angiosarcoma. Within days, the patches and plaques became generalized; (B) Even early in their course, the lesions tend to be diffuse sheets of large cells that fill the dermis; (C) The tumor cells are large but are relatively monomorphic; (D) Expression of CD123, a marker of plasmactyoid dendritic cells, is common to these tumors.

Gamma/Delta T-Cell Lymphoma

■ *Criteria for diagnosis*

- Aggressive course
- Disseminated plaques/nodules/tumors, especially on extremities (Fig. 15.14A)
- Involvement of mucosa and other extracutaneous sites
- Apoptosis, necrosis, angioinvasion common
- TCRγ+/βF1–/CD3+/CD5–/CD7CD56+/TIA1+/GranzymeB+Perforin+
- Usually CD4–/CD8+

■ *Differential diagnosis*

- SPTL
- Lupus, especially lupus panniculitis and tumid lupus
- Blastic plasmacytoid dendritic cell neoplasm (BPDCN) (CD56+/CD4+).

■ *Pitfalls*

- Epidermotropic, dermal and subcutaneous involvement may be present simultaneously and may vary among sites biopsied
- "Rimming" common (but not specific)
- βF1 expression may be lost by neoplastic cells, causing an α/β lymphoma to be confused for a γ/δ T-cell lymphoma.

■ *Pearls*

- Current classifications separate γ/δ T-cell lymphoma from SPTL (which is α/β)
- Median survival 15 months (compared to 82% disease specific survival in SPTL)
- Unknown whether a true "cutaneous variant" exists; may be part of a spectrum of "mucocutaneous γ/δ T-cell lymphoma"
- Unlike SPTL, γ/δ T-cell lymphoma tends to involve dermis in addition to subcutis (Fig. 15.14B)
- Spleen, node and marrow involvement rare (unlike most other peripheral T-cell lymphomas)
- T-cell receptor + immunohistochemical staining now available for paraffin embedded sections (Fig. 15.14C).

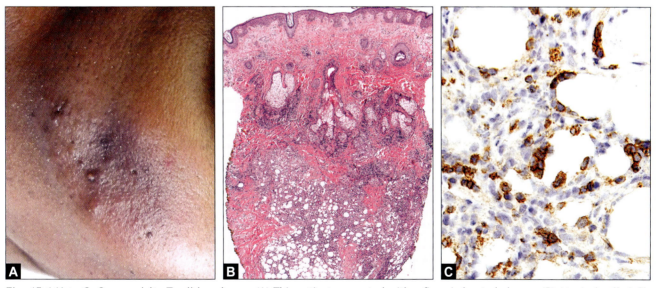

Figs 15.14A to C: Gamma-delta T-cell lymphoma. (A) This patient presented with a firm, indurated plaque; (B) Atypical cells infiltrate the subcutis. Notice that they are also present within the dermis around adnexal structures, a feature that helps to distinguish this entity from subcutaneous panniculitic T-cell lymphoma (see below); (C) The neoplastic cells express the gamma-delta type T-cell receptor, as demonstrated here by immunohistochemistry for T-cell receptor-gamma.

Myelogenous Leukemia

■ *Criteria for diagnosis*

- Papules, plaques or tumors, localized or generalized, composed of dense infiltrates of atypical cells that often infiltrate the dermis diffusely but may also be localized around blood vessels and adnexa (Fig. 15.15).
- Cells commonly are monomorphous but have "blastic" cytologic features including one or more prominent nucleoli and an increased nuclear to cytoplasmic ratio.
- Atypical cells express one or more of the following markers:
  - Myeloperoxidase
  - NASDCL (Leder stain)
  - CD4
  - CD13
  - CD14
  - CD15
  - CD33
  - CD34
  - CD68
  - CD117

■ *Differential diagnosis*

- Cutaneous extramedullary hematopoiesis
- LCH
- Granulomatous dermatitis
- BPDCN (see above)
- Anaplastic large cell lymphoma and other lymphomas.

■ *Pitfalls*

- Leukocyte common antigen often negative
- Expression of CD56 and CD123 may occur in some cases of AML, making distinction from BPDCN difficult
- S100 may be expressed by some forms of AML causing potential confusion with Langerhans cell histiocytosis (LCH) and other dendritic cell neoplasms
- CD34 is a sensitive but very nonspecific marker of leukemic cells
- Phenotype of cutaneous lesions may differ from that in peripheral blood and bone marrow (flow cytometry may provide a more accurate representation of the true phenotype).

■ *Pearls*

- Since classification of AML is now largely based on specific translocations/molecular markers and flow cytometric immunophenotyping, and the phenotype of skin lesions may differ from that of bone and peripheral blood, specific immunophenotyping by IHC on skin biopsies is generally not recommended

- If the biopsy is performed in order to establish the diagnosis of relapsed leukemia, knowledge of the immunophenotype obtained from prior flow cytometry studies may help identify IHC markers more likely to be positive within the skin biopsy
- More "mature" forms of AML are those most likely to involve the skin (e.g. myelomonocytic AML)
- Mucosa is commonly involved in addition to skin
- "Aleukemic leukemia cutis" describes skin lesions of AML in patients without other evidence of leukemia; all of these patients eventually develop leukemia, usually soon after skin lesions appear
- No significant difference in prognosis has been shown between patients with cutaneous involvement and those without it.
- Skin involvement by chronic myelogenous leukemia and myelodysplastic syndromes occurs but is rare
- Look for concomitant infections since patients are immunocompromised secondary to chemotherapeutic drugs, post-transplant immunosupression or the leukemia itself.

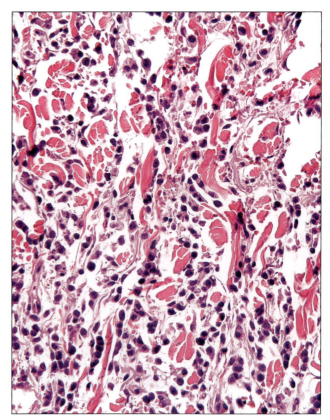

Fig. 15.15: Myelogenous leukemia.

Langerhans Cell Histiocytoses
(Other Histiocytic/Dendritic Cell Tumors)

■ *Criteria for diagnosis*

- Clonal infiltrate of Langerhans cells that are ovoid and devoid of dendritic cell processes (Figs 15.16A and B)
- CD1a (Fig. 15.16C)   +
- S100   +
- CD4   +
- Langerin   +
- Birbeck granules   +
- Vimentin   +
- CD68   +
- HLA-DR   +

■ *Differential diagnosis*

- Rosai-Dorfman disease (benign sinus histiocytosis with massive lymphadenopathy)
- Juvenile xanthogranuloma, reticulohistiocytoma and other forms of xanthogranuloma
- Dendritic cell tumors.

■ *Pitfalls*

- CD4 positivity may lead to confusion with a T-lymphocyte neoplasm if other markers are not used

- Osteoclast-like giant cells, eosinophils, neutrophils and lymphocytes may accompany LCH cells and sometimes the inflammatory milieu predominates, obscuring the underlying Langerhans neoplasm
- Differentiation of congenital self-healing LCH (Hashimoto-Pritzker) from other forms of LCH requires clinical correlation and follow-up to exclude progression/systemic disease
- Association between LCH and T-lymphoblastic lymphoma.

■ *Pearls*

- Clinical course is related to staging at presentation
- Survival 99% or greater with unifocal disease but only 33% for infants or young children with multisystemic disease who do not rapidly respond to therapy
- Involvement of bone marrow, liver and lung are high-risk factors
- Progression from solitary lesion to multisystem involvement occurs, usually in infants
- Extent of disease is a more important prognostic factor than age
- Hemophagocytic syndrome is a rare complication
- Unifocal disease is more common in older children and young adults.

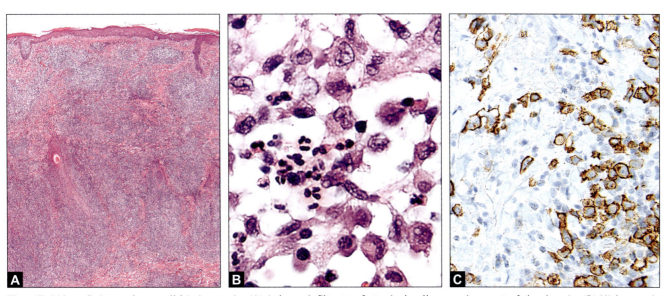

Figs 15.16A to C: Langerhans cell histiocytosis. (A) A dense infiltrate of atypical cells occupies most of the dermis; (B) High magnification reveals the typical Langerhans cell nuclei, which are often described as "C-shaped" or "reniform"; (C) Strong and diffuse expression of CD1a is characteristic of Langerhans cells. The staining is membranous, and occasionally a paranuclear "dot" is evident.

Cutaneous Mastocytosis

- Mastocytosis may be limited to the skin (primary cutaneous mastocytosis) or involve other organs in addition to the skin (systemic mastocytosis with cutaneous involvement). In general, the term "cutaneous mastocytosis" is used when there is no evidence of a systemic component.

Telangiectasia Macularis Eruptiva Perstans

■ Criteria for diagnosis

- Patches, papules and macules (Figs 15.17A and B)
- A variably dense infiltrate of mast cells (usually sparse relative to other types of mastocytosis) that is most prominent around the vasculature (Fig. 15.17C)
- No evidence of systemic involvement.

Urticaria Pigmentosa (Maculopapular Cutaneous Mastocytosis)

■ Criteria for diagnosis

- Papules and macules composed of mast cell aggregates that fill the papillary dermis and usually extend into the dermis as diffuse sheets (Figs 15.17D and E)
- No evidence of systemic involvement.

Diffuse Cutaneous Mastocytosis

■ Criteria for diagnosis

- Diffuse thickening of skin without discrete lesions
- Mast cells arranged in a band like distribution in the papillary dermis or in diffuse sheets that occupy the entire dermis (Fig. 15.17F)
- No evidence of systemic involvement.

Solitary Mastocytoma

■ Criteria for diagnosis

- A solitary lesion composed of aggregates of mast cells within the dermis, with or without extension into the subcutis (Figs 15.17G and H)
- No evidence of systemic involvement.

Mast Cell Immunophenotype

- Tryptase   + (most specific marker)
- CD117 (Fig. 15.17I)   +
- CD68   +
- CD33   +
- CD45   +
- CD14/15/16   – (absence helps exclude myelomonocytic leukemia)
- CD25/CD2   + in neoplastic mast cells (but difficult to use in sparse infiltrates)

■ Differential diagnosis

- Systemic mastocytosis (see "criteria" below)
- Inflammatory infiltrates rich in mast cells (e.g. urticaria).

■ Pitfalls

- In adults, urticaria pigmentosa/maculopapular cutaneous mastocytosis (UP/MPCM) may contain mast cells in numbers that do not exceed those of urticarial and other inflammatory processes
- Mast cell aggregates occasionally resemble melanocytic nevi and other neoplasms at first glance
- Systemic mastocytosis must be excluded for definitive diagnosis to be made, yet many adults who have UP/MPCM are eventually found to have systemic disease (see below).

■ Pearls

- Urticaria pigmentosa/maculopapular cutaneous mastocytosis may affect children and adults
- In children, lesions tend to be larger and papules usually predominate
- In adults, lesions are usually more widely disseminated, have a macular appearance and contain fewer mast cells
- In children, cutaneous mastocytosis has a favorable outcome and lesions may regress spontaneously, especially at puberty; systemic involvement seems to be uncommon
- In adults, lesions usually persist and systemic disease is often detected eventually; however, it is usually the indolent form of systemic mastocytosis
- Indolent systemic mastocytosis has a good prognosis (usually a normal life expectancy)
- Adverse prognostic factors include late onset of symptoms, absence of cutaneous lesions, thrombocytopenia, elevated LDH, elevated alkaline phosphatase, hepatosplenomegaly, anemia, bone marrow hypercellularity and peripheral blood smear abnormalities.

■ Criteria for systemic mastocytosis

Major:

- Involvement of bone marrow and/or other extracutaneous sites by aggregates of mast cells (aggregate > 15 mast cells)

Minor:

- More than 25% of mast cells in marrow or other extracutaneous sites have spindled morphology or are atypical.
- Detection of activating point mutation at codon 816 in KIT in extracutaneous mast cell aggregates
- Mast cells in extracutaneous sites express CD2 and/or CD25.
- Serum total tryptase persistently exceeds 20 ng/mL (in absence of a clonal myeloid disorder).

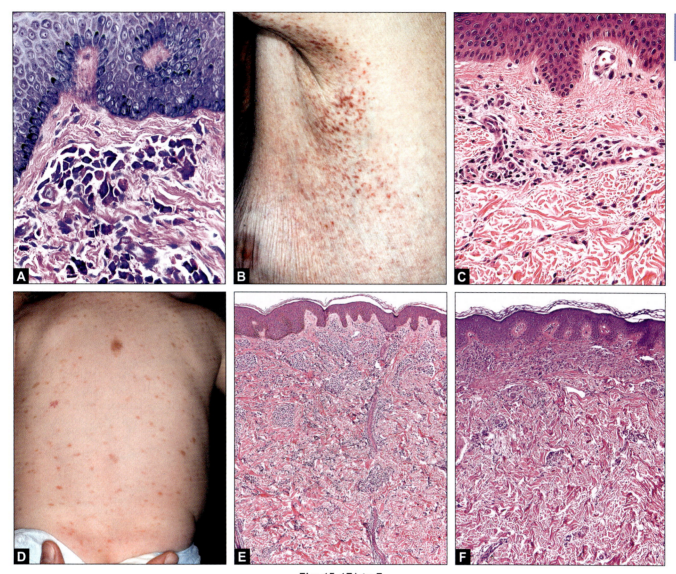

Figs 15.17A to F

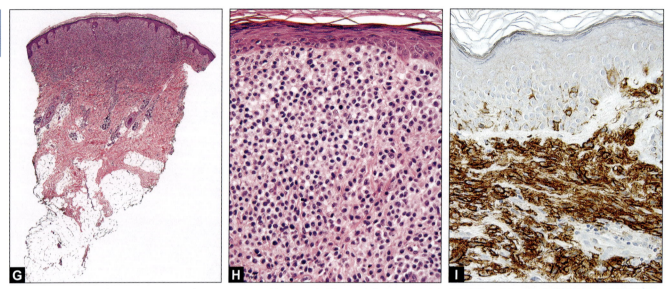

Figs 15.17A to I: Telangiectasia macularis eruptiva perstans. (A) The cytoplasmic granules within mast cells stain purple or dark pink with Giemsa (shown here) and toluidine blue; (B) Small erythematous macules, papules, and patches are common; (C) The mast cells are usually concentrated around vessels, but some are scattered between collagen bundles as well; (D) Urticaria pigmentosa (maculopapular cutaneous mastocytosis). This infant with urticaria pigmentosa has papules and macules with a red-brown "pigmented" appearance; (E) Mast cells form aggregates throughout the dermis; (F) Systemic mastocytosis. A dense infiltrate of mast cells fills the papillary dermis; (G); Solitary mastocytoma. This patient presented with a solitary brown papule. The biopsy demonstrates a dermis occupied by an aggregate of densely packed mast cells; (H) Solitary mastocytoma. At high magnification the mast cells are relatively monomorphic and have round, centrally placed nuclei; (I) Systemic mastocytosis. The mast cell infiltrate is denser than that usually seen in telangiectasia macularis eruptiva perstans, as highlighted here by CD117 (a marker strongly expressed by most mast cells).

Subcutaneous Panniculitis
Like T-Cell Lymphoma (Figs 15.18A to C)

■ *Criteria for diagnosis (Table 15.3)*

- Indolent course
- Pleomorphic infiltrate of small and medium sized α/β cytotoxic CD8+ T-cells confined predominantly to subcutis (Fig. 15.18A)
- βF1+/CD4–/CD8+/CD56–/TCRγ–.

■ *Differential diagnosis*

- Lupus panniculitis/profunda
- γ/δ T-cell lymphoma
- Infectious panniculitis
- Erythema nodosum
- "Atypical lobular panniculitis" (Magro et al.).

■ *Pitfalls*

- ANA may be positive (complicating differentiation from lupus profunda)
- "Rimming" common but not specific to SPTL (Fig. 15.18B).

■ *Pearls*

- Lupus panniculitis is a rare expression of cutaneous lupus, especially if isolated to legs (i.e. lupus panniculitis localized to legs is SPTL until proven otherwise)
- Some reports suggest co-existence of lupus panniculitis and SPTL
- Necrosis, small reactive lymphocytes, macrophages and granuloma formation may occur (rare features in B-cell lymphomas involving subcutis).

Table 15.3: Features of subcutaneous panniculitis like T-cell lymphoma versus γ/δ T-cell lymphoma	
Subcutaneous panniculitis like T-cell lymphoma	γ/δ T-cell lymphoma
5-year survival more than 80%	5-year survival less than 1%
More common	Very rare
Usually limited to subcutis	Usually involves dermis in addition to subcutis
CD8+/CD4– neoplastic cells	CD8–/CD4– neoplastic cells
CD56–	CD56+
Hemophagocytic syndrome rare	Hemophagocytic syndrome more common

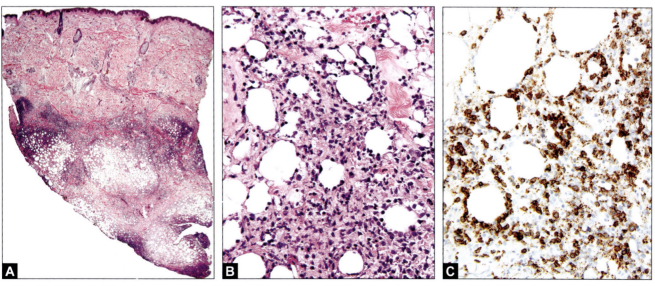

Figs 15.18A to C: Subcutaneous panniculitic T-cell lymphoma. (A) There is a dense lymphocytic infiltrate that is confined to the subcutis; (B) Atypical cells form "rims" around individual adipocytes; (C) The neoplastic cells characteristically express CD8.

1. Burg G, Kempf W, Cozzio A, et al. WHO/EORTC classification of cutaneous lymphomas 2005: histological and molecular aspects. J Cutan Pathol. 2005;32(10):647-74.

2. Cerroni L, Gatter K, Kerl H. Skin Lymphoma: The Illustrated Guide, 3rd edition. Oxford: Wiley-Blackwell; 2009.

3. Criscione VD, Weinstock MA. Incidence of cutaneous T cell lymphoma in the United States, 1973-2002. Arch Dermatol. 2007;143:854-9.

4. De Leval L, Harris NL, Longtine J, et al. Cutaneous B-cell lymphomas of follicular and marginal zone types: use of Bcl-6, CD10, Bcl-2 and CD21 in differential diagnosis and classification. Am J Surg Pathol. 2001;25(6):732-41.

5. El Shabrawi-Caelen L, Kerl H, Cerroni L. Lymphomatoid papulosis: reappraisal of clinicopathologic presentation and classification into subtypes A, B and C. Arch Dermatol. 2004;140:441-7.

6. Feuillard J, Jacob MC, Valnesi F, et al. Clinical and biologic features of CD4 CD56+ malignancies. Blood. 2002;99:1556-63.

7. Glusac EJ. Criterion by criterion, mycosis fungoides. Am J Dermatopathol. 2003;25(3):264-9.

8. Leinweber B, Colli C, Chott A, et al. Differential diagnosis of cutaneous infiltrates of B lymphocytes with follicular growth pattern. Am J Dermatopathol. 2004;26(1):4-13.

9. Magro CM, Crowson AN, Kovatich AJ, et al. Lupus profundus, indeterminate lymphocytic lobular panniculitis and subcutaneous T-cell lymphoma: a spectrum of subcuticular T-cell lymphoid dyscrasia. J Cutan Pathol. 2001;28:235-47.

10. Shapiro PE and Pinto FJ. The histologic spectrum of mycosis fungoides/Sezary syndrome (cutaneous T-cell lymphoma). A review of 222 biopsies, including newly described patterns and the earliest pathologic changes. Am J Surg Pathol. 1994;18(7):645-67.

11. Smoller BR, Bishop K, Glusac EJ, et al. Reassessment of histologic parameters in the diagnosis of mycosis fungoides. Am J Surg Pathol. 1995;19:1423-30.

12. Swerdlow SH, Campo E, Harris NL, et al. World Health Organization Classification of Tumors of Hematopeoiteic and Lymphoid Tissues. Lyon: IARC Press; 2008.

13. Willemze R, Jaffe ES, Burg G, et al. WHO-EORTC classification for cutaneous lymphomas. Blood. 2005;105(10):3768-85.

Index

Page numbers followed by *f* refer to figure and *t* refer to table

Color Atlas of Differential Diagnosis of Dermatopathology

Color Atlas of Differential Diagnosis of Dermatopathology

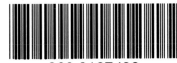

DATE DUE

			PRINTED IN U.S.A.